UCAT Success Toolkit

19

Key skills to boost your scores

Anna Greathead and Masuda Rahman

Foreword by Dr Mahibur Rahman MB BCh MSc FRCGP

self Timed

(1) Abstract = 36/55 = 650

(2) quantitative = 28/36 = 770

(3) verbal = 24/44 = 600

(4) decision = 20/29 = 670

ISBN: 978-1-907902 03-1

First published in 2019 in Great Britain by

Emedica Publications

Birmingham

0121 744 6433

www.emedica.co.uk

Anna Greathead has been a UCAT expert since 2011 – having taken the test every year since then. She also presents UCAT sessions of different lengths at numerous schools around the country. Her highest ever UCAT score was 3350 and she has always made the top decile.

Masuda Rahman is an E-Learning expert with extensive experience in preparing people for on screen testing.

Thank you to:

Hannah Dryden

Susan Farrell

Naomi Greathead

Alan Hodkinson

Harry Naylor

Lydia Poniatowska

Amber Ross

For their contributions to this book

Foreword

Applying to study medicine or dentistry can be a daunting process, with multiple exams, assessments, applications and interviews to prepare for.

Your performance in the UCAT can play an important part in determining whether or not you are offered an interview, and in some medical schools, whether you receive an offer.

Whilst this is an aptitude test, having a thorough understanding of the types of questions, learning techniques to tackle each section, and practising time, can help improve your performance.

The *UCAT Success Toolkit* will help you plan your preparation, learn useful tips and techniques for each section, and through worked examples, develop the skills and confidence that will enable you to achieve your peak performance on the day of the test.

I hope that you will find it informative, enjoyable and a useful guide to your preparation.

You are embarking on a lifelong learning journey towards a challenging and rewarding career, and I wish you every success with this first step and for the years to follow.

Dr Mahibur Rahman MB BCh MSc FRCGP

Medical Director

Emedica

Contents

Introduction

The UCAT is a must for anyone who wants to study medicine or dentistry. There are some universities which don't use it or who hardly consider it but for 2020 entry at least two thirds of medical schools and around half of dental schools do.

You might be tempted to avoid the UCAT altogether by stealthily populating your UCAS form entirely based on avoiding it, but the reality is that this strategy will most likely land you face to face with the BMAT!

The very fact that you are seriously considering the pursuit of such a demanding university course and career means you are likely to be very experienced in taking, and doing well in, examinations, you probably sailed through your GCSEs without much strain and with excellent grades. You might even enjoy exams and find them easy.

However, it is important to remember that the UCAT exists for one reason alone; to differentiate the very bright and very able from the bright and able applicants. In this exam, like no other you're likely to have taken so far, you're genuinely being tested against your intellectual and academic peers rather than the population at large. In short – almost everyone taking it has always found school easy and has always done well so it's going to be harder to be top of this class!

This should not scare you though. If you want to pursue a career in dentistry or medicine then you are going to have to show qualities beyond academic talent and mere cleverness. A demanding career requires other skills such as insight, subtlety, perspective, the ability to cope with uncertainty, resilience and composure and it is these nearly unquantifiable characteristics that aptitude tests such as the UCAT attempt to measure.

This guide will help you prepare for the UCAT. Each question type will be explained and broken down – we'll show you exactly what skills are being tested and how to approach them. Whilst the UCAT is designed to test aptitude rather than learning, potential rather than achievement, it is still a test you can prepare for. You can't revise for it (the potential subject matter would require you to memorise all of Wikipedia just for Verbal Reasoning) but you can fully familiarise yourself with the format, hone your technique, improve your speed and learn to avoid common pitfalls so that you can showcase the very best and fullest range of your capabilities.

The Basics

If you are applying to Medical or Dental School in the UK and are taking the UCAT you will need to register for and take it the summer BEFORE you apply to university. If you are planning to go to university immediately after taking your A-levels this will mean you take UCAT in the summer between years 12 and 13.

Before you take the test, you must register with Pearson Vue who administer the test. Registrations open in May and you can sit the test between July and October. It costs between £65 and £100 and is taken at Pearson Vue testing centres across the UK. A bursary scheme is available for people from low income households to help with this expense. If you have special educational needs then you may be eligible for extra time in each section. Further details and practical advice on registration, booking and special arrangements is provided in the Registration and Booking section.

The UCAT is a five part, two hour, multiple choice exam taken entirely onscreen with strict time controls for each section. If you finish one section with time to spare you're not allowed to have extra time for another. There is no negative marking so it's important to answer every question - you won't lose any marks for getting it wrong so take a guess if you are stuck.

Agonising over one question while the clock ticks away might gain you 1 mark, but lose you 10 marks on questions you leave unanswered for lack of time.

The UCAT Format section gives further details of exam timings and section lengths. There is an introduction to each question type and advice on improving your techniques later in the book.

There are four cognitive sections for which you will receive a numerical score and one non-cognitive (attitude and behavioural) section for which you will receive a banding. Your score from all sections will automatically be forwarded to all UCAT universities that you apply to. Scores vary from year to year, an average section score is around 600 meaning a total raw score average should be 2400. This varies between sections and from year to year. An average score of 700 per section will usually put you in the top 25%.

Universities use the UCAT score in very different ways, some look at your overall score, others at the average section score. Some have a lower limit below which a student who doesn't meet it in any section will not be interviewed.

Strategy and Planning

If you're taking your UCAT halfway through your A-levels – which most people do – then you're already very busy. If you're taking your UCAT because you want to get into medicine via another route such as post-graduate or as a career change you're also likely to be busy! Putting in the hours to do as well as possible may be very hard. You may have lots of good intentions; to prepare and revise thoroughly then find the hours available to you are few. We're all good at finding excuses to avoid the things we don't want to do – see if any of these seem familiar!

> "UCAT is an aptitude test, there's no point in practising much because that's the whole point – you can't revise for it!"
>
> "I am working really hard on my A-levels – there's no point sacrificing my A-level grades to get a good UCAT result."
>
> "I am great at this sort of thing – I passed the 11+, my IQ is off the chart...."
>
> "It's so HARD, and sooo BORING...."

Of course, all these comments are true in their own ways! UCAT is an aptitude test but if you go into the exam room without knowing what to expect you will waste time trying to understand the format of the test, you won't be up to speed with some of the skills you need to do well in it and some of it will almost certainly confuse you. It may test aptitude but preparation will allow you to show off your aptitude to its full potential!

Your A-level grades are vitally important to your university application and it is true that a great UCAT result won't compensate for getting three B grades instead of three A grades. However, even three brilliant A-levels won't compensate for a poor UCAT in some universities. You really need to do both! The UCAT is timed so you can prepare for the test and take it in the summer break. At this time you should be less busy with your academic life – although it's not much fun using your last summer at school to study, it will (I promise!) be worth it!

You may well already be very good at taking tests (you're going to have to be if you're pursuing a successful career in medicine or dentistry!). The difference being that everyone taking this test is very clever and has shown them self to be very good at taking tests. Relying entirely on your (unquestioned!) natural ability without being prepared to put in a bit of effort doesn't bode well for a good UCAT result or a good career.

Almost no-one finds the UCAT easy and still fewer find it fun! However, this guide will give you all you need to gradually break down the UCAT into manageable and doable chunks. As you start to master the different sections, your scores will get better and better and the sense of achievement you feel may even manifest itself as enjoyment!

What we suggest....

Start Early

Depending on exactly when you are reading this, our first tip may be redundant, but we really would recommend that you start your UCAT preparation early. Many years of observation seem to suggest that there is a strong correlation between starting early and doing well.

- Aim to take your UCAT before you return to school for the autumn term so that you're free to concentrate on your A-levels in September.
- Find out exactly when you finish year 12 so you can book your UCAT as soon as possible. Some test centres and dates book up quickly. It's also cheaper if you take it early.
- Start thinking about preparing for the UCAT three months or so before your test date.

Little and often

One of the advantages of starting early is that UCAT doesn't have to become a life-filling, all-encompassing slog. A few hours of UCAT preparation a week for three months is not only infinitely more pleasant than 16 hours a day for a week but likely to be more effective too.

- Aim to spend an hour or so a day looking at the UCAT. You can do a question type per day for a couple of weeks to find out where your strengths and weaknesses lie.
- Be disciplined with the UCAT. Sit at your desk or computer for the allotted time and avoid all distractions. It's only an hour!
- Find a time of day when you feel alert.

Structure your revision

There are as many ways of preparing for a test as there are candidates sitting it. There isn't a hard and fast 'right' or 'wrong' way and you will know what methods work well for you. You may find it worth considering the following when planning your preparation:

- Books and paper materials are portable and easy on the eyes, but the test is on screen and your reading speed may differ between paper and screen. It is a good idea to get some practice on screen.
- Start by working on your technique, study section by section and take some time to make sure you know exactly what is being asked of you for each section and what is not!
- Once you have understood each question type work on your timing. Do as much practice as you can under strictly timed conditions.
- The whole test is over 2 hours long and you need to switch thinking styles quickly. It's worth doing a full mock at least once during your preparation, more if possible.
- Studying with a friend can be very helpful and motivating. It can also help you get a realistic idea of how you are doing.
- There may be one section that you find particularly tricky and it can be tempting to focus all your efforts on improving in that section to the detriment of the others. Try to spread your efforts across all sections, even a section you find easier will benefit from practice and an increase in speed.

Look after yourself

Turning up for your UCAT a broken shell of a person is unlikely to result in a great score! Remember to look after your own health and wellbeing during this busy and stressful period. There are lots of ways to do this, here are some:

- Drink plenty of water – being hydrated will help everything.
- Get enough sleep – you won't do your best at anything if you're fatigued. A good sleep pattern is vital so avoid long lie-ins and lots of late nights.

- Eat well – a balanced diet and regular meals will optimise you and your performance.
- Avoid chemical 'assistance' – coffee, alcohol, tobacco (or other illicit or unwise substances) may help you stay awake during, or relax after study, but the overall effect on your health will be negative. Far better to stay awake because you slept well and relax well because you've achieved your goals for the day.
- Ask for help – if you are really struggling then asking for help is always the best course of action.

Registration and Booking

The UCAT is booked online. The website for the UCAT consortium is UCAT.ac.uk and includes links to the booking pages at Pearson Vue the test administrators.

- Registration opens in May which is couple of months before the first test date.
- Set up an account. You need to set up a Pearson Vue account. This is no different from setting up any other online account, you'll need an email address, and you'll need to devise a password and so on. You will also be asked some questions which may seem a little peculiar – such as the profession of your parents! These are purely for tracking trends in the diversity of applicants and you can opt not to answer if you would really prefer not to.
- Your name. It may be odd to be asked to think about this but the name you book your test in must be exactly the same as it appears on the photographic ID you will use when you check in for your test. If you have ever changed your name, go by a nickname or alias or have more than one version of your name or middle name or initial that you do not use consistently then you must think carefully about entering this information. It is also strongly recommended that you use your name in exactly the same form for UCAT as you will for UCAS – you do not want the UCAT score you worked hard for assigned to someone else!
- ID - This is more difficult than you may think because the ID must be from a prescribed list and also include your signature. If you plan to use your passport make sure this was NOT issued before you turned 16 as this WILL NOT have your signature on it. Other ID options include a driving licence (provisional is fine). If you are a UK candidate you can also ask your school to sign a form, with your photograph, confirming your identity. Instructions on exactly what this form must say are on the UCAT website. Remember that this may be quite difficult to arrange when your school is closed for the summer. For non-EU candidates, the acceptable ID forms are slightly different. Please check the website for details. In short, ID must be original, approved, current and signed.
- The bottom line. You will need a debit or credit card to pay (Visa or Mastercard). The UCAT costs £65 if you take it in the EU before the end of August. After that the price increases to £87. The content of the test does not change, the higher price simply reflects increased demand later in the cycle. People sitting the UCAT outside of the EU pay £115. If you qualify for a bursary your full test cost will be covered and you won't have to pay anything. You need to apply for this via the UCAT website.
- Where? Once on to the 'booking screen' you use your postcode to find a test centre either 5, 10 or 20 miles away. If you live in an urban area you're likely to have a few choices. If you live a rural area or small town then you may only have one. Select the one most convenient to you (bear in mind this may not be the closest – consider public transport links, parking and so on).
- When? Then you get the chance to book your date and time slot. The earlier you do this the more choice you will have. Time slots are in 30 minute intervals usually from 8am to 5pm. Again, consider what is realistic when choosing. An 8am test will get it 'over and done with' but if you arrive stressed out having overslept or missed the bus you won't perform at your best. If you book the test and something unexpected arises you can reschedule it with one clear day's notice but we would recommend you only take this option as a last resort.
- How? This is your opportunity to opt to take the SEN UCAT. Here you are given extra time in each section. If you have a Special Educational Need which ordinarily means you get extra time for exams, then you will probably benefit from taking this option. At this stage you don't need to provide proof

of your SEN but later on the Universities will need to see documentation. Your score will be invalidated if you do not provide the requested documentation – check the EXACT requirements before booking.

The UCAT Format

The sections are always presented in the same order as shown in the table below:

Section	Questions	Arrangement
Verbal Reasoning	44	11 passages of text with 4 questions associated with each
Decision Making	29	Mixed questions
Quantitative Reasoning	36	Sets of data (graphs, tables, charts) with 1 or 4 questions associated with each
Abstract Reasoning	55	11 sets of related shapes / question type groupings with 5 questions associated with each
Situational Judgement Test	69	About 20 scenarios with between 3 and 6 questions associated with each one.

Each section includes one minute for reading the instructions (two minutes for SEN candidates).

Section	Questions	Section time	Time per question
Verbal Reasoning	44	1 min reading, 22 minutes for questions	30 seconds
Decision Making	29	1 min reading, 31 minutes for questions	64 seconds
Quantitative Reasoning	36	1 min reading, 25 minutes for questions	42 seconds
Abstract Reasoning	55	1 min reading, 14 minutes for questions	15 seconds
Situational Judgement Test	69	1 min reading, 27 minutes for questions	24 seconds

Taking your UCAT

- ***The week before***. Make sure you have all your documents ready and that you know EXACTLY where the test centre is, do a little drive by if you can, it is better if the first time you make the journey is not the morning of the exam! By this point you should expect to be familiar with all the questions types and be doing a little timing practice each day, preferably in full section size chunks.
- ***Three days before***. At this point if you feel totally unprepared you should consider postponing your test date, you can change your slot online and without penalty as long as you have one clear day between the change request and your test slot. For example if your test is on a Wednesday, the latest you can change it is Monday (Tuesday is your clear day in between)
- ***The day before***. Do your very best not to start your UCAT with any drama! Plan your day tomorrow, paying attention to what, when and where you will eat before the exam, plan your journey with a view to arrive at least 20 minutes before your test slot. Allow plenty of time for unexpected traffic or delays, check for any travel, weather or special events that may affect your journey. Remember that if you arrive late for your exam you may well be turned away and even if you are allowed in you will certainly feel stressed! Make sure you go to bed early.
- ***Before you leave the house***. Eat something! Breakfast is crucial, especially if you're taking a morning test. We understand that in your youthful vitality you may feel immune to a lack of breakfast, but

humour us, just for today! Try to keep to your plan and leave on time and check you have your documents with you before you leave!

- ***Checking in***. You need to check in before your test time and should allow at least 15 minutes for this. You will need a print out of your email confirmation showing the time of your booked test and your photographic ID which also has your signature on it (remember a passport issued before you turned 16 will not be accepted). You are not allowed to take anything into the test room with you. This includes your phone, your bag, your keys and even a bottle of water. You are given a key to a locker to store your things in whilst the test is in progress.
- ***Before you start your test***. Go to the toilet before you go into the test room - if you need to go during the test the clock will not be paused. Once in the test room you will be directed to a numbered cubicle with a computer station. Other people in the room will be taking other tests. The clock starts when you click the onscreen dialogue box to say you are ready. Before you begin check that you have been given the correct equipment (a spiral bound set of laminated A4 notepaper and a pen – check the pen works!) and take some time to make yourself comfortable – you will be in this seat for 2 hours so adjust your chair, position your keyboard and mouse to suit you, arrange your ID and locker key out of your way and make sure you have space to keep your notepad close enough to write on. If any equipment is missing or if you need anything raise your hand and a test administrator will come to you.
- ***The test itself***. The opening screen for each section is the instructions. You are allowed to look at this for one minute (or you can click past it). This minute is deducted from your time for answering the questions. If you are fully familiar with the format of the UCAT questions you won't really need to read these pages and can use the time to have a quick stretch or close your eyes for a few seconds/look away from the screen so you are ready and alert for each section. If you start to run out of space on your notepad raise your hand to request a replacement – they will take away the old one and replace it with a new one, however this take up some time and you may wish to bear in mind that anything written on the old one will be lost so try to manage your notepaper so that you can request a replacement between sections of at least between question set.
- ***Timing***. The UCAT section timing is strictly enforced. If you finished Verbal Reasoning early you can start the next section, but you won't get any extra time. You get the option to flag a question for review so if you're not sure you can take a guess, move on and use any extra time at the end to review those questions

Most people will run out of time on most sections. Another reason it is not a good idea to agonise and waste time over a single question is that there are always a few 'sample' questions in the mix – ones which won't be marked but are being tested and developed for the following season. Even if you get it right it won't get you a mark. Keep moving.

The table shows the approximate question you should have reached at various points in each section.

Section	10 minutes in	15 minutes in	20 minutes in
Verbal Reasoning	20/44	30/44	40/44
Decision Making	10/29	15/29	19/29
Quantitative Reasoning	14/36	22/36	29/36
Abstract Reasoning	40/55		
Situational Judgement	29/67	37/67	50/57

- ***Marking***. There is no negative marking on the UCAT – if you get 5 questions right and leave 5 questions blank you get 50%. If you get 5 questions right and 5 questions wrong you get 50%. It is always worth taking a guess if you don't know, or if you are running out of time. You have a minimum of a 20% chance of being right and often a couple of the wrong answers can be easily discounted bringing the random chance of getting it right up to 33% or 50%.

- ***Afterwards***. You will be given a print out of your score immediately after the test ends at the reception desk. Keep this safe as you have to pay for copies. The universities you apply to will be notified directly of your score via UCAS.

Example Timeline - Taking the test on August 15th

May	Register with Pearson Vue Check ID and documents for special arrangements End of year exams
June	Exams wrapping up, start preparing for UCAT Book test slot Submit documents for special arrangements Practice technique for all question types
July	Start practicing in timed conditions Make sure all ID in place before school breaks up Plan your journey to the test centre – do a dry run Start practicing full size sections under exam timing Start timed practice every day – try to eat / sleep well
August	Do timed mocks Remember to look after yourself Take the UCAT like a boss Relax!
September	Investigate universities bearing your score in mind Check for any updates in admissions procedures Get advice from school on your personal statement Plan your UCAS application
October	UCAS application Medical / Dental school UCAS deadline

Introduction to Verbal Reasoning

This is the first section of the UCAT you will see, and some people find it tricky because it appears to be so much simpler than it is! It is important to remember that verbal reasoning for the UCAT is NOT the same as comprehension exercises you may have done before.

You are asked to critically assess a passage of text between 200 and 400 words and to assess the validity of a number of statements associated with the text. You are instructed to treat the text as the truth and to answer based solely on the information given – if the passage says the sky is green, you must answer as if the sky is indeed green.

You will be asked to make logical inferences based on the text (sometimes from quite tenuous implications) and but also to identify what you are cannot infer without further information. The passage text is unlikely to be about something you already know a lot about, but if it is, you'll have to be especially careful to not let your existing knowledge derail you!

There are two formats for verbal reasoning questions used in the UCAT, these are sometimes referred to as old and new style or short and long style questions.

Currently the majority of verbal reasoning questions used in the UCAT are in the long style. In this format you are presented with a question and four statements from which you must choose an answer. You may for example be asked which of the four statements is most likely to be true or most likely to be false. These questions sometimes ask feature wording such as LEAST likely to be untrue (i.e. the same as MOST likely to be true) which can be confusing so it is imperative that you read the questions very carefully.

The four question types in Long Verbal Reasoning are:

1. Incomplete statements such as:

   "Government changes to university funding have resulted in:"

   and then four statements – only one of which can definitely, or most reasonably – complete the sentence according to the text.

2. Except questions such as

   All of the following have been funding streams for universities except:

   then a list of three university funding streams and one funding stream which is not mentioned as being a university funding stream in the text.

3. Most likely questions such as

   Which of the following impact on students studying STEM subjects is most likely?

These questions are tricky as none of the options will be definitely true – one will simply be more likely than the others. With these questions you need to carefully distinguish which word denotes likelihood best – is often or usually more likely for example.

4. According to the passage questions such as

   These questions are easier as the information is contained within the passage, rather that you having to make qualified judgements about what is written. However – these questions can easily catch you out by appealing to your external knowledge. It is imperative that you only use the text for information and not your own general education.

The old or short style questions gives a single statement relating to the text and you are asked to decide (using only the information contained in the text) if the statement is true, false or whether you can't tell without further information. This question type currently represents a minority of the questions used in the UCAT but as it was in use for a long time many older resources may focus on this question type. It is important that you find as many long style questions as possible to practice.

Techniques for Verbal Reasoning

The time pressure is very real and you need to focus from the get go. This is the first section and you need to be ready to work at speed. You have around two minutes per set of set of questions. Each passage of text will be the subject of four questions and time spent carefully reading the text can save time on subsequent questions within that set but spending too long reading may leave you with only a few seconds to actually answer the questions. Skimming text and scanning for key words can be very quick but you risk missing crucial data hidden in a separate paragraph or disguised by a subtle change in wording.

Practice reading at speed – read broadsheet newspapers and practice identifying logical inferences. Read things you do not normally read to get used to reading in context and with unfamiliar words and try to improve your vocabulary - if necessary, read with a dictionary handy to look up unfamiliar words.

Your choice of approach should be based on your own knowledge of your personal reading speed and your ability to scan for sense. Be aware that your reading speed on a screen may be significantly slower than on paper and you need to get used to reading without being able to underline important points.

Vary your approach during practice so that you can see what works for you - different approaches work for different questions

- With shorter texts try reading the entire text carefully. With a longer or more complex texts you may prefer to scan
- Try scanning just enough to get the gist of each paragraph so that later you have an idea of where to look for which type of information. Try reading the question before scanning the text
- Look for any extreme statements – anything very definite – always, never, will, will not, first, last, exclusively. Conversely look out for non-definitive terms - occasionally, usually, mostly.
- Try to identify any known unknowns – missing information, opinions, estimates, data ranges, vague dates, percentages without a total population
- Look for any conflicting information or opinions
- Read carefully! Look out for synonyms and antonyms which make scanning for specific words risky, remember these can pop up in the passage and in the question!
- Use context to make sense of passages that use technical or foreign terms – you don't need to know the meaning of every word to understand the key concepts.

There follow two sample questions for you to attempt. In the exam you would expect to spend around four minutes on these two question sets but here you should take as long as you need.

Verbal Reasoning worked sample 1. Explanations are on page 16

The England National Football Team represents England in football and is controlled by The Football Association, the governing body for football in England. England are the joint oldest national football team in the world alongside Scotland, whom they played in the world's first international football match in 1872. England is one of the United Kingdom's home nations, meaning that it is permitted by FIFA to maintain its own national side. England's home ground is Wembley Stadium, London, and the current manager is Fabio Capello

All England matches are broadcast with full commentary on BBC Radio 5 Live. From the 2008–09 season to the 2011–12 season, England's home qualifiers and friendlies both home and away were being shown live on ITV. Away qualifiers are shown on Sky Sports. England's away qualifiers for the 2010 World Cup were shown on Setanta Sports until that company's collapse. As a result of Setanta Sports' demise, England's World Cup qualifier in Ukraine on 10 October 2009 was shown in the UK on a pay-per-view basis via the internet only. This one-off event was the first time an England game had been screened in such a way. The number of subscribers, paying between £4.99 and £11.99 each, was estimated at between 250,000 and 300,000 and the total number of viewers at around 500,000

1. Which of the following statements is true?

A. The England football team was established in 1872

B. England won the world cup in 1966

C. Gareth Southgate is the current manager of the England team

D. The Scotland football team is over 100 years old ✓

2. All the following statements are true except:

A. There aren't many national football teams with as long a history as England

B. Setanta Sport had collapsed by 2010

C. England football team visited Ukraine in 2009

D. FIFA maintain control of the English FA ✓

3. The typical 'per person' fee to watch the first England pay per view event was:

A. £2.50 - £5.99

B. £4.99 - £11.99 ✓

C. £10

D. £5 - £10

4. Which of the following media outlets is the least likely to be used by an England follower?

A. Radio 5 live

B. BBC TV

C. ITV ✓

D. Pay-per-view TV

Verbal Reasoning sample 2: Explanations are on page 17

Tortoises are a family of land-dwelling reptiles in the order Testudines. Like their marine relatives, the sea turtles, tortoises are shielded from predators by a shell. The top part of the shell is the carapace, the underside is the plastron, and the two are connected by the bridge. The tortoise endoskeleton has the adaptation of having an external shell fused to the ribcage. Tortoises can vary in size from a few centimetres to two metres. They are usually diurnal animals with tendencies to be crepuscular depending on the ambient temperatures. They are generally reclusive animals.

Although the word "tortoise" is used by biologists in reference to the family Testudinidaes only, in colloquial usage, it is often used to describe many land-dwelling Testudines. The inclusiveness of the term depends on the variety of English being used.

British English normally describes these reptiles as "tortoises" if they live on land. American English tends to use the word "tortoise" for land-dwelling species, including members of Testudinidae, as well as other species such as box tortoises, though use of "turtle" for all chelonians is as common. Australian English uses "tortoise" for terrestrial species, including semi-aquatic species that live near ponds and streams. Traditionally, a "tortoise" has feet (including webbed feet) while a turtle has flippers.

5. Which of the following statements is most likely to be true?

A. A turtle is a variety of tortoise

B. There are no nocturnal tortoises

C. Tortoises are not usually social creatures

D. The underside of a tortoise shell is a carapace

6. The distinction between tortoise and turtle is:

A. Whether they live on land or in water

B. Almost non-existent from a biological point of view

C. Based on whether the creature has flippers or feet

D. Often linguistic rather than taxonomic

7. All of the statements are true except:

A. A tortoise's shell shields it from predators

B. The ribcage of a tortoise is fused to the shell

C. The shell of tortoises vary in size

D. A tortoise's shell protects from heat

8. According to the text, from a strict biological point of view, which of the following is true?

A. A tortoise is land-dwelling

B. A tortoise has feet whilst a turtle has flippers

C. Turtles are not chelonians

D. A tortoise is in the family Testudines

Answers for Verbal Reasoning sample 1:

1. Which of the following statements is true?

A. The England football team was established in 1872

B. England won the world cup in 1966

C. Gareth Southgate is the current manager of the England team

D. The Scotland football team is over 100 years old

Option A The England football team was established in 1872

A quick scan of the text will reveal the number 1872 which may make you click on 'true'. If you read carefully, the text actually refers to 1872 as being the date for the world's first international football match and not the founding of the national team. However, it is possible that the team was also founded in 1872, it just doesn't say so in the text so you can't tell. The text doesn't explicitly mention when the team was established, nor does it mentioned a date when it wasn't established. Therefore, any questions pertaining to the date the team was established cannot be definitively answered.

Option B England won the world cup in 1966

We all know this is true don't we? But sadly it doesn't say so in the text so England's victory cannot be positively affirmed! Once more this fact cannot be deduced from the text.

Option C Gareth Southgate is the current manager of the England team

Some of the texts may be out of date, or simply incorrect. You may know this for certain. However, there are no points to be gained for spotting factual inaccuracies in the text. Points are scored for answering accurately based on the text. Therefore – though you may know this to be true the text contradicts it and the text must be assumed to be totally true meaning Capello is still the manager. (England manager information correct at the time of going to press!)

Option D The Scotland football team is over 100 years old

A bit of inference must be made here. The facts we know (from the text) is that England football team is the oldest in the world along with Scotland and that the two teams played one another is the first international football match in 1872. Thus – we know that Scotland football team existed in 1872. Whenever you take your UCAT you know that 1872 was more than 100 years old! The correct answer is therefore this option is the correct answer.

2. All the following statements are true except:

A. There aren't many national football teams with as long a history as England

B. Setanta Sport had collapsed by 2010

C. England football team visited Ukraine in 2009

D. FIFA maintain control of the English FA

The correct answer is Option D – this is the only thing in the statement which is 'unknown' and therefore could be untrue. There is little information about the relationship between FIFA and the English FA in the text and certainly not enough to make certain statements about control. Option A is something we can confirm as true – the text says that England and Scotland are the oldest two national football teams in the world so there cannot be 'many' others with as long a history. Option B can be confirmed as true as, although we don't know exactly which the company collapsed, we know that it had already happened by 2009 as the pay per view screening of the 2009 qualifier in Ukraine is described as a result of the collapse. The same event allows us to confirm Option C as verifiable and therefore not the right answer.

3. The typical 'per person' fee to watch the first England pay per view event was:

A. £2.50 - £5.99

B. £4.99 - £11.99

C. £10

D. £5 - £10

This seems blatantly like a question in the wrong place! It's obviously got a numeracy element. However – you do need to read the text carefully to arrive at the right figure. The correct answer is option A and this is also a figure which can be reached by estimating. The range of prices for the event was £4.99 - £11.99 and there were roughly twice as many viewers as subscribers. Therefore – the price per viewer is going to be approximately half the amount of the price per subscriber.

4. Which of the following media outlets is the least likely to be used by an England follower?

A. Radio 5 live

B. BBC TV

C. ITV

D. Pay-per-view TV

Whilst it is impossible to assess numbers for anything but option D all outlets except BBC TV are specified as showing the football matches which makes option B the least likely to be used by an England follower.

Answers for Verbal Reasoning worked sample 2:

5. Which of the following statements is most likely to be true?

A. A turtle is a variety of tortoise

B. There are no nocturnal tortoises

C. Tortoises are not usually social creatures

D. The underside of a tortoise shell is a carapace

A. A turtle is a variety of tortoise

Turtles and tortoises are described at the start of the text as being two different types of reptile within the order of Testudines. Tortoises are differentiated from their "marine relatives, the sea turtles". There is reference the terms being used interchangeably in different versions of English, but these are a matter of opinion and the statement is framed as a definite fact.

Option B. There are no nocturnal tortoises

Tortoises are usually diurnal. This implies that occasionally they may be otherwise. It is therefore possible that some tortoises sometimes may be nocturnal. This is a very definitive statement and while it may be true there are other statements that are more likely to be so.

Option C. Tortoises are not usually social creatures

The passage states "they are generally reclusive creatures". This statement is the most likely to be true making this the correct answer.

Option D. The underside of a tortoise shell is a carapace

The passage actually states the opposite naming the top of the shell as the carapace.

6. The distinction between tortoise and turtle is:

A. Whether they live on land or in water

B. Almost non-existent from a biological point of view

C. Based on whether the creature has flippers or feet

D. Often linguistic rather than taxonomic

The correct answer is Option D.

The passage does not give a clear answer to this question so careful assessment of what is implied and inferred is necessary. The difference between the words is described as colloquial, traditional and based on language. This makes option D seem to most accurately reflect the text given. Option A simply favours the UK usage of the terms, option B may be the case but cannot be shown using the information in the text. Option C is not described in the passage.

7. All of the statements are true except:

A. A tortoise's shell shields it from predators

B. The ribcage of a tortoise is fused to the shell

C. The shell of tortoises vary in size

D. A tortoise's shell protects from heat

The correct answer is D. A tortoise's shell protects from heat

Options A and B are specifically stated within the passage, so we know them to be true. Option C - that a shell would vary in size – can logically be inferred from the fact that tortoises vary enormously in size. We know that the shell must also vary along with the creature because the shell is fused to the creature's ribcage in an adaptation to their endoskeleton. However, there is nothing written about the thermal qualities or uses of a tortoise shell and it just as likely to provide protection from the cold as from the heat, of the options given it is the least likely.

8. According to the text, from a strict biological point of view, which of the following is true?

A. Tortoises are land-dwelling

B. A tortoise has feet whilst a turtle has flippers

C. Turtles are not chelonians

D. A tortoise is in the family Testudines

The correct answer is Option A. Tortoises are land-dwelling

This is a classic example of using scientific language to encourage very careful reading (or careless mistakes!). The fact the opening sentence of the text says that tortoises are land dwelling means all of the other options can be discounted. The difference between a tortoise having feet and a turtle having flippers is mentioned as being 'traditional' (rather than scientific and biological) and the word "tortoise" is in inverted commas referring only to the Australian English use of the word. The word chelonians are only mentioned in the passage where the colloquial use of the word 'tortoise' in American English is discussed and the fact that turtles and tortoises are chelonians is not specified and may or not be true (it is in fact true). Option D is incorrect because the order is defined as the Testudines, the family is the Testudinidae. We know it's only a matter of two letters, but we wanted to remind you to read carefully!

Introduction to Decision Making

This is the newest section of the UCAT and was introduced as a pilot section in the 2016 exam. It replaced Decision Analysis. UCAT is now a scored subtest.

This section features a wide variety of question types – all designed to test your ability to apply logic to reach a conclusion. You will need to be able to evaluate arguments and analyse statistical information.

The question types you'll encounter are:

- Logical puzzles: You will need to use a piece of text, or a data set (such as a map or diagram) along with the information a series of statements to select one of four options which answers the question.

- Syllogism: You will have a statement with information. There will then be five statements which you must assess as being a logical conclusion to draw, or not. The answers options (yes or no) are dragged into position.

- Interpreting information: This is where you have some data from which you can draw conclusions. The answer mechanism is like a syllogism which drag and drop 'yes' or 'no' answers.

- Recognising assumptions: You will be provided with a proposition – the starting part of an argument. You must then select the strongest argument from the four options based on how well they address the original proposition and whether they add useful points.

- Venn diagrams: Here you will be either presented with a complete Venn diagram, an incomplete Venn diagram or information for which you must select the most appropriate Venn diagram from the answer options. The Venn diagrams are often quite complex and don't always follow the strict mathematical rule which suggests no zero sections should exist.

- Probabilistic reasoning: In these questions, you will be given a scenario with a suggested probabilistic conclusion. You then must assess which of the answers – from four options – is right and why.

The proportion of each type of question seems to be about even based on the mock exams on the official website. You should expect to see between 4 and 6 of each question type. They tend to be grouped together but you may see individual questions of any given type at any point as well.

In this section you may need to use the onscreen calculator and you almost certainly will need to use your pen and pad.

Techniques for Decision Making

With so many question types there is no single technique which will be useful to learn for this section. Thankfully – as with the rest of the UCAT – what is being tested is a mode of thinking rather than a technique.

Logic puzzles

It's worth remembering that people do this kind of thing for fun! The text you are given may look something like this:

> Four students (Andrew, Jack, Lucy and Rebecca), took exams on consecutive days from Monday to Thursday. They were studying Art, Biology, English and Maths.

And you will then have a series of statements. One of them will answer the question. The question is likely to be 'Which of the following statements MUST be true?' So, you have to use the information in the bullet points after the text to see if you can deduce the answer. To arrange the information, I recommend you draw a table.

If there is any sequential data, I would fill that in first. Many of the information points could refer to 'before' or 'after'.

Monday	Lucy	Art
Tuesday	Jack	Maths
Wednesday	Rebecca	English
Thursday	Andrew	Biology

You then need to look at the information points you have. They'll need to be read carefully – there may be hidden clues – and repeatedly.

- Lucy took her exam the day before Jack sat his Maths exam
- The art exam happened on Monday, two days before Rebecca sat her exam
- Andrew isn't studying English

Believe it or not – this information is adequate to complete the whole table! It is important to note that sometimes the information will not be enough to complete the whole table but it will always be enough to answer the question. The trick is to select the option which is definitely true, rather than any which could be but might not be also.

Syllogisms

In this question type you are assessing logical conclusions based on (and only on) the data you have been given.

It is important to note words such as all vs some, many vs most, every vs several.

> All the schools in the town required students to wear a school uniform. Most of the uniforms were a traditional tie, blazer and shirt in school colours though a few schools also had a hat! Some schools allowed girls the choice of trousers or a skirt. The most common uniform colour was blue with red and green being less popular.

From here it's important to distinguish between what has been stated and what we might assume. For example:

> All schools wear blue, red or green uniforms

These are the only colours mentioned in the passage but there's nothing to suggest the list of colours is exhaustive. Is this a logical conclusion? No, it isn't.

> Some schools don't require their students to wear a tie

This seems an obvious 'yes' as the word 'most' tells us that not all schools have a tie, blazer and shirt requirement. However – that is a three-part combination. Some schools may require a tie but not a blazer for example. The answer is No again.

> Some schools have a blazer tie, shirt and hat combination in their uniform

As the sentence referring to hats is an 'also' after the traditional combination is detailed the answer here is Yes. It is a logical conclusion.

Interpreting information

The rules of syllogism apply for this question type. Essentially, they are the same except that your initial data comes in the form of a data set rather than a passage of text.

Recognising assumptions

The most important thing in approaching these questions is to disregard your own opinion and don't rely on your existing knowledge.

You will be presented with a statement, or a question, like this:

Schools should ban students from eating junk food on school premises

A. Yes – junk food creates a lot of litter from food packaging

B. Yes – this will contribute to the long-term health of the students

C. No – this is an infringement on the rights of the students to eat what they wish

D. No – Enforcing this could be a lot of additional work for the staff

The best answer is D as it is the only one which doesn't make assumptions. Option A assumes that junk food comes in a lot of food packaging (we may know that to be true, but we are only answering the premise given). Option B assumes any ban would lead to a long-term health gain. Option C assumes that students have the 'right' to eat as they wish – they could be as young as 4. Option D suggests that a ban could lead to extra workload.

Venn Diagrams

This question type is not trying to assess how well you understand Venn diagrams mathematically but how well you can read them as a data source. There are three main types of question in this type

1. Adding up the number of units which fulfil certain qualities by reading a Venn diagram.
2. Placing an example unit into a Venn diagram where sections are labelled
3. Selecting a Venn diagram from options which represent data as given in text form.

Introduction to Quantitative Reasoning

The vast majority of UCAT entrants will be excellent at maths. Almost all will have a grade A*, A or B at GCSE, many will be studying maths at A level. This section should be straightforward… right?

The key here is to comprehend that straight maths skills, whilst useful, won't make 'quantitative reasoning' straightforward. This section of the test has been described as 'maths in the real world' – one thing it certainly isn't is a page full of sums, equations or formulae!

The good news is that the maths is certainly within your grasp – relatively easily! None of the manipulations are above GCSE level and many of them aren't even that hard. The questions aren't to test your raw maths skills but rather your ability to correctly solve problems which have a numerical element. Once again, the importance of reading the question accurately cannot be over emphasised!

The questions will be based around some data – a graph, chart or even a passage of text – around which four to six questions will usually be based. Occasionally you may see a simple data set which only has one question associated with it.

You are provided with some resources to help with this section. There is a simple on-screen calculator (it only has +, -, * and /) laminated note pad and pen – not a wipe clean one though. This enables you to do calculations and keep a record of answers you've already worked out. It is worth keeping a record of the various calculations you do to avoid having to do the same sums over again for the next question.

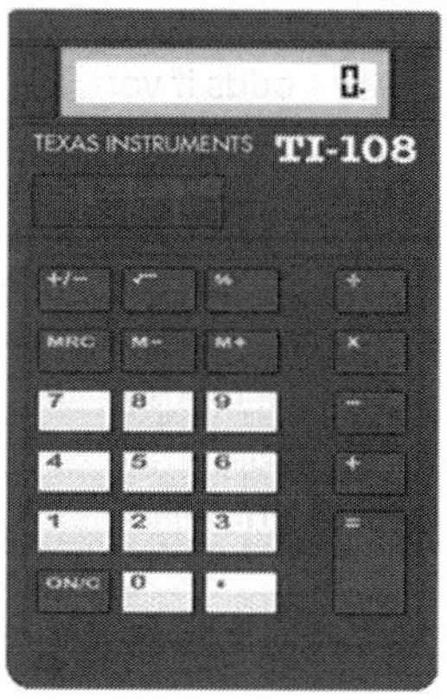

Quantitative reasoning can be the most time pressured of all the UCAT sections. Candidates know they can do the maths but can spend far too long doing endless (and needlessly complex) sums and equations and find their time is up with half the questions unanswered! Being able to quickly identify exactly what the question is asking is key to speeding up - how quickly can you work out what is being asked and what you must do.

Focus your revision for this section on avoiding the most common mistakes and speeding up your calculation methods.

Techniques for Quantitative Reasoning

If you haven't studied maths for a while – or even if you have – a few sessions practising conversions, percentages, area and volume calculations and so on will pay dividends. It's all too easy to do these sums the 'wrong' way around when you are in a hurry and the most common incorrect answers will likely be included as an option to catch you out doing just that! A useful habit to get into is a quick check to see if you answer looks reasonable – does it look bigger or smaller than it should, are you in the right units?

Techniques for improving accuracy

- Look at the data set presented and carefully read any accompanying text. If the data set is very large – the question may be about estimating! No one expects you to do 50 calculations in a single question.
- Note anything unusual in the data – an empty section, a value which is much higher or lower than the others, a different unit
- When making notes remember to label what you have worked out (e.g. Total wages = £360, Tax = £36) you may need the data again.
- Write neatly. Recalculating wastes more time than writing legibly!
- Check your answer is reasonable - think 'is that possible? Some situations need a whole number answer e.g. you can't have 4.5 people.
- Remember average can mean median, mean or mode. Median and mode are usually easier to work out.
- Remember that 1.5 minutes actually means 1 minute 30 seconds – check the units on the answer options.
- If you're really struggling with any data set then take a guess, flag the questions for review, and move on to the next set which may have easier, or at least quicker, maths

Techniques for speeding up!

- The onscreen calculator can be fiddly – Practice using the computer keypad before your test.
- Look at the answer options – are any of them obviously wrong? Any you rule out will improve your odds if you need to guess.
- See if you can estimate the answer using data reading or mental maths; if only one option is close to that then select it!
- Speed calculate using tricks like 560 x 0.9 to find 90% or 560 x 1.2 to increase by 20%, 560 x 0.8 to decrease by 20%.
- Minimise the number of calculations you do on the calculator – every input is a potential mistake and your brain is often faster!
- Round numbers to make mental calculations easier – 72 x 19 is *almost* 70 x 20.

Quantitative Reasoning Worked Samples

Here are two sample questions sets for you to attempt. In the exam you would expect to spend around five minutes on these two question-sets but here you should take as long as you need.

Quantitative Reasoning Worked sample 1. Answers on page 25

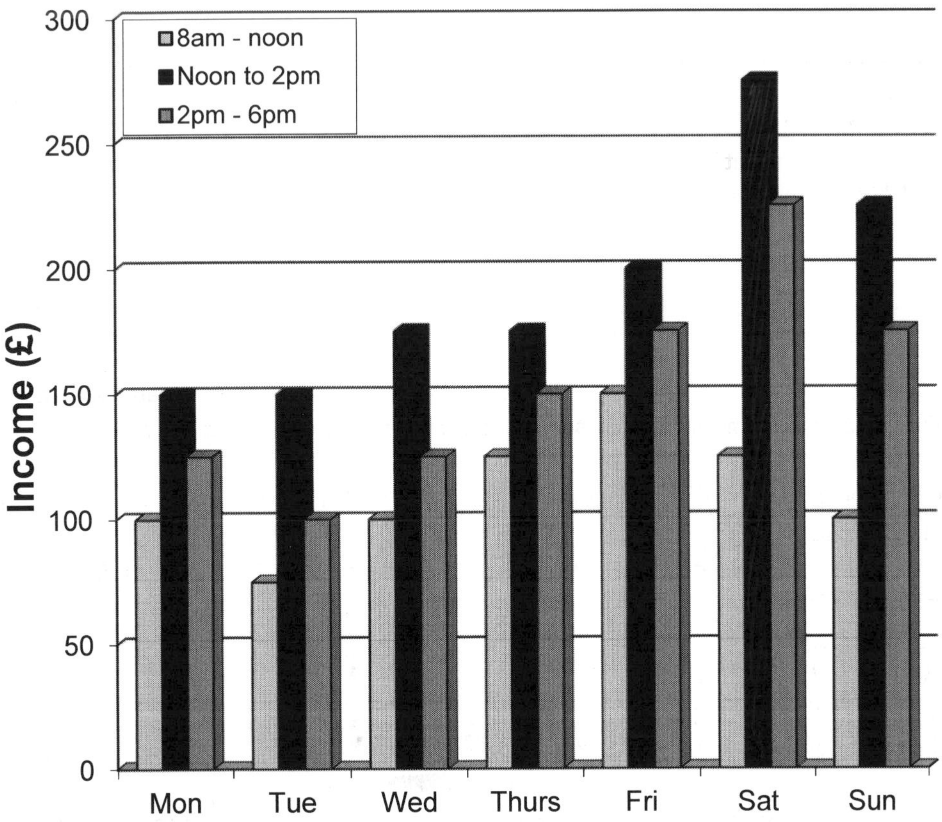

This chart shows average weekly takings for a café at different times of day. The café pays two members of serving staff at a rate of £7.50 per hour. Both of whom work from 8am to 6pm. The café has fixed overheads of £250 per week and makes 50% profit on all sales.

1. How much profit does the café make on breakfast / morning food sales before overheads?

A. £387.50
B. £775
C. £880
D. £1300
E. £1550

2. Some market research suggests that the café would be able to take 40% extra at weekends if they employed a third staff member. How much difference would this make to weekly profits?

A. £75
B. £150
C. £300
D. £225
E. £450

3. How much will the café need to take to make a profit each week?

A. £1050
B. £1300
C. £2100
D. £2600
E. £2601

4. The owner decides to only employ one member of staff for most of the morning on weekdays. She asks one member of staff to come into work at 11.30am instead of 8am. How much more profit will she make in a week?

A. £131.25
B. £150.00
C. £183.75
D. £210.00
E. £262.50

Quantitative Reasoning worked sample 2: answers on page 26

Below is a table detailing global time zones but not allowing for national 'daylight saving' schemes. Please assume all time zones are as detailed in the table unless indicated otherwise.

Place	Time – compared to UTC	Place	Time – compared to UTC
London	0	London	0
Cape Verde	-1	Italy	+1
South Georgia	-2	South Africa	+2
Brazil	-3	Saudi Arabia	+3
Barbados	-4	Dubai	+4
Cuba	-5	Maldives	+5
Mexico	-6	Antarctica - Vostok	+6
Denver - USA	-7	Thailand	+7
Pitcairn Islands	-8	Australia – West Coast	+8
Alaska	-9	Japan	+9
Hawaii	-10	Australia – East Coast	+10
Samoa	-11	Antarctica - Casey	+11
		New Zealand	+12

5. John works in London and wishes to call Maria in Rio de Janeiro, Brazil between 9am and 5pm local time for them both. What time period can John call (London time)?

A. 10am – 3 pm
B. 11am – 4pm
C. 12 noon – 5pm
D. 12 noon – 8pm
E. 1pm – 5pm

6. An aeroplane takes off from the west coast of Australia at 7.30am local time, heading towards South Africa. The flight will take 12 hours. What local time will it be when the plane lands in South Africa?

A. 1.30pm
B. 3.30pm
C. 5.30pm
D. 730pm
E. 9.30pm

7. A ship sailing across the Atlantic Ocean – covering 5 time zones – takes 12 days. The ship changes its clocks an equal amount on each of the 12 days. How much would this be?

A. Forward 25 minutes
B. Backward 25 minutes
C. 25 minutes
D. 42 minutes
E. 2.4 hours

8. Shaun needs to take medication every three hours. He is travelling from the UK to Japan. He plans to take a dose as he takes off at 6pm and will arrive the following day at 11pm local time. How many more tablets will he need for the flight?

A. 4
B. 5
C. 6
D. 7
E. 8

Answers for Quantitative Reasoning worked sample 1.

First impressions regarding this data set.... There might be a lot of adding up as the graph has 21 separate figures. Must remember to read the text beneath.

1. The correct answer is Option A. £387.50.

Total breakfast session takings are £775, 50% of which is profit. £775 divided by 2 = £387.50. The question asks for profit before overheads so there is no need to deduct fixed or variable overhead costs such as staff.

2. The correct answer is Option A. £75

One extra member of staff for weekends = £7.5 x 10 x 2 = £150

Takings at weekends = £1125 of which £562.50 profit. Weekend takings + 40% = £1575 of which £787.5 profit. Additional profit due to extra takings is £225 less the cost of extra staff (£150) = £75.00

Although it looks like you need to do a lot of maths for this actually all you need to do is calculate weekend profits, add 40% and then calculate what one staff member will earn in two days.

3. The correct answer is Option E. £2601

The sums here are easy but the question is easy to misread.

The correct working is 2 x staff members. Staff earn £7.50ph x 10 hours x 7 days (£525 each) + £250 fixed overheads. This adds up to £1300.

We know also that the profit made on food is 50% which means that the café needs to take double the overheads to break even.

Hence the correct answer is option E – as £2600 would be the breakeven figure.

4. The correct answer is Option A £131.25

This question needs to be read very carefully. The graph is a distractor as you don't need to look at it at all. All you need to know is: a) the member of staff will be paid for 3.5 hours less, on weekdays. The easy mistakes to make are misreading that the staff member will start at noon instead of 11.30am or misreading that the staff cut is on all days rather than just weekdays. The wrong answers are in the options.

- So, one less staff member at £7.50 per hour for 3.5 hours less per day (£26.25) for 5 days = £131.25
- However, one less staff member for 4 hours per day for 5 days = £150 (option B)
- One less staff member for 3.5 hours per day for 7 days = £183.75 (option C)
- One less staff member for 4 hours per day for 7 days = £210.00 (option D).

Answers for Quantitative Reasoning worked sample 2.

First impressions regarding this data set… I may need a basic grasp of geography! The table tells me how far ahead (+ numbers) or behind (- numbers) a time zone is from the 0 (UTC).

5. The correct answer is C. 12 noon – 5pm

It is reasonably straightforward to work out that Rio de Janeiro is 3 hours behind London. However, it's important to have read the question and remember that both offices shut at 5pm. John won't want to stay in the office late and more than Maria will want to come in early!

6. The correct answer is A. 1.30pm

The flight will take 12 hours, but the time difference is -6 hours. It takes a bit of mental gymnastics to work it out. One way is to work out the time in the zero zone (i.e. the UK) for the start of the journey: 7.30am – 8 hours = 11.30pm. Add 12 hours and then work out what time that would be in the end of the journey – 11.30am in UK is 1.30pm in South Africa.

7. The correct answer is C. 25 minutes

5 time zones equal 5 hours which equals 300 minutes. 300 divided by 12 is 25. As we don't know if the ship is sailing east or west, we can't know whether the clocks will move forward or backwards.

8. The correct answer is C. 6

The table shows us that Japan is 9 hours ahead of the UK. Therefore 11pm there is 2pm in the UK making Shaun's journey last for 20 hours. If Shaun takes his tablet every three hours after the one he takes at takeoff he will need six.

Introduction to Abstract Reasoning

This section of the UCAT really is.... abstract! A lot of people really struggle with it whilst a lucky few find it obvious and easy! In all likelihood you're in the first group – if you are a member of the second group please feel free to skip forward a section!

This section tests your ability to spot abstract – as opposed to linguistic or numerical – patterns. Whilst tackling it you will need to form hypotheses and test (and possibly discard) them.

Students commonly get frustrated and wonder what this section is testing. It is worth remembering that many aptitude sets – the 11+, IQ tests – all contain questions a lot like this. It might be hard to articulate but abstract reasoning certainly tests an ability that differentiates – even if its relevance is not immediately obvious.

There are 4 different types of question in this section. Most questions presented are the type 1 format.

Type 1 - You will be presented with two sets of shapes labelled "Set A" and "Set B". You will be given 5 test shapes associated with these Sets and asked to decide whether the test shape belongs to Set A, Set B, or Neither.

The rules are independent of each other and may be absolutely different. Sometimes it will be, for example, in Set A there is always a white triangle and in Set B there's always a black square. Other times it will be, for example, in Set A there is always a white triangle and in Set B the number of sides of the black shapes exceeds the number of sides of the white shapes by 3.

Additional questions formats:

Type 2 - You will be presented with a series of shapes and asked to select the next shape in the series.

Type 3 - You will be presented with a statement involving a group of shapes. You will be asked to determine which shape completes the statement. An example of a statement [Shape 1] is to [Shape 2] as [Shape 3] is to ......

Type 4 - You will be presented with two sets of shapes labelled "Set A" and "Set B" and 4 additional shapes. You will be asked to select which of the four additional shapes belongs to Set A or to Set B.

We will work through an example of each question type at the in this chapter but you should concentrate your revision on Type 1 questions as these form the majority of questions.

Techniques for Abstract Reasoning

Trying to spot a pattern in a seemingly random set of pictures can send your eyes, brain and psyche a bit crazy! There are some techniques to help you approach this section with a bit more confidence, but this is the section where the least time is given to answer the most questions. Here, more than anywhere, it is sometimes worth taking a guess if the pattern really does elude detection.

It's worth developing a methodical and structured approach to look at various features in turn. You can develop your own or employ one which is already written. The one below might be worth a try.

- Pattern: Look to see if the patterns are symmetrical, or a rotation, or a mirror image. See what sizes shapes are.
- Count: Look for number of shapes, edges, corners, intersections, right angles, curved lines.
- Place: See if the shapes are positioned specifically – higher or lower, near the edge or touching another shape
- Other: There is often more than one rule and also conditional rules. Check for secondary rules before answering

- Direction: If there are arrows or lines then consider where they are pointing and what they're pointing to.

So – work through PC PLOD! – Pattern, count, place, other and direction!

- Study the simplest square as the rule will apply there and there will be fewest distracting elements.
- Test potential rules in all six boxes in the set, and then all six boxes of the other set – anything that appears in all boxes of a set is significant.
- Remember that the rules are ways of differentiating between Set A and Set B – if something is the same in all Set A and Set B boxes you can only use it to establish that a shape belongs to neither set.
- Not every shape or feature of the pictures is relevant so don't strain to find a pattern which will allow for every detail.
- Sometimes the rule is very simple. If you spot a simple rule then take it as a gift and don't second guess yourself.
- Sometimes a picture just 'looks' more like one set than the other. If you can't see a definite rule then this is as good a way to classify them as any!
- This section is short so don't agonise over any one question - a guess here will work between a 25% and 33% of the time.
- There is an almost infinite selection of possible Abstract Reasoning rules – don't beat yourself up if you don't easily spot every single one

Abstract Reasoning Worked Samples

There follow 18 sample questions for you to try. In the exam you would expect to spend around four and a half minutes on these questions but here you should take as long as you need. Answer start on page 32.

Set A

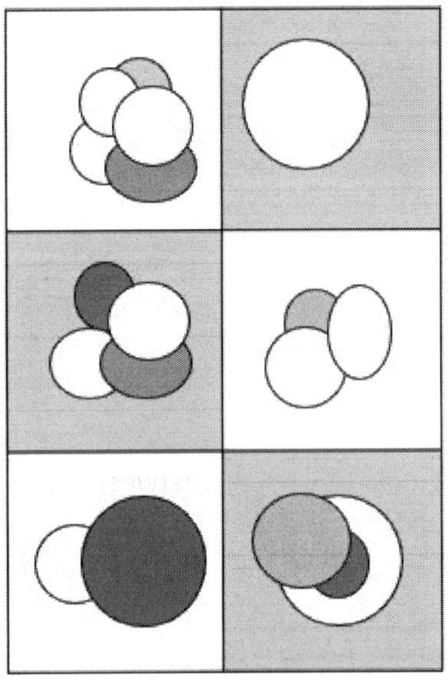

Set B

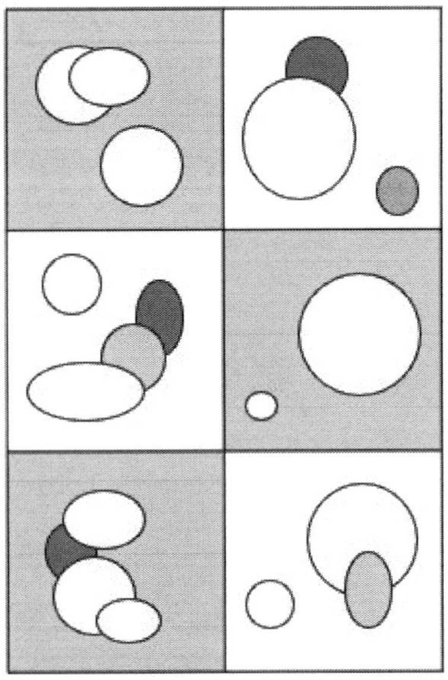

1

Set A
Set B
Neither

2

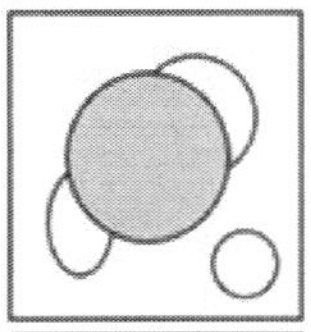

Set A
Set B
Neither

3

Set A
Set B
Neither

4

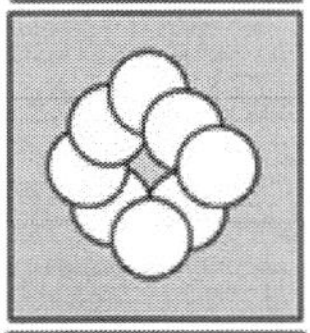

Set A
Set B
Neither

5

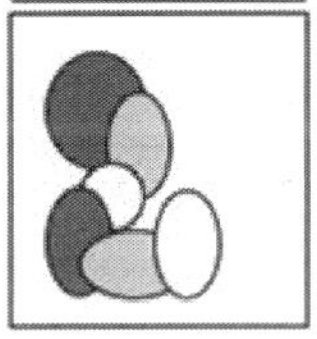

Set A
Set B
Neither

To which of the two sets do the following shapes belong?

Set A

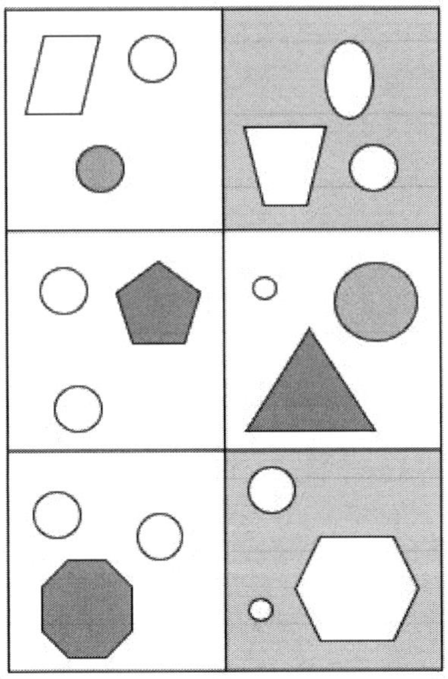

Set B

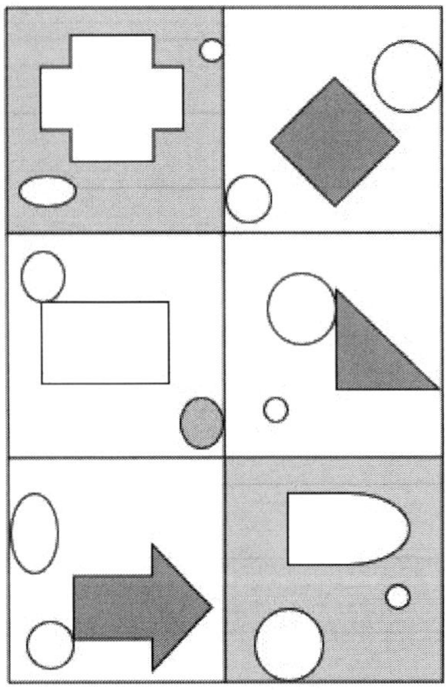

6

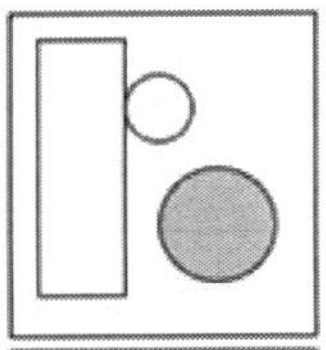

Set A
Set B
Neither

7

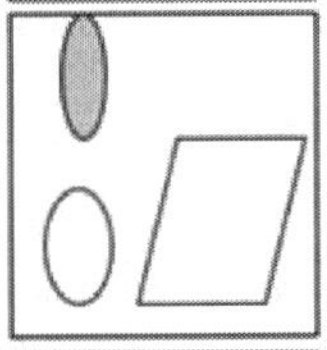

Set A
Set B
Neither

8

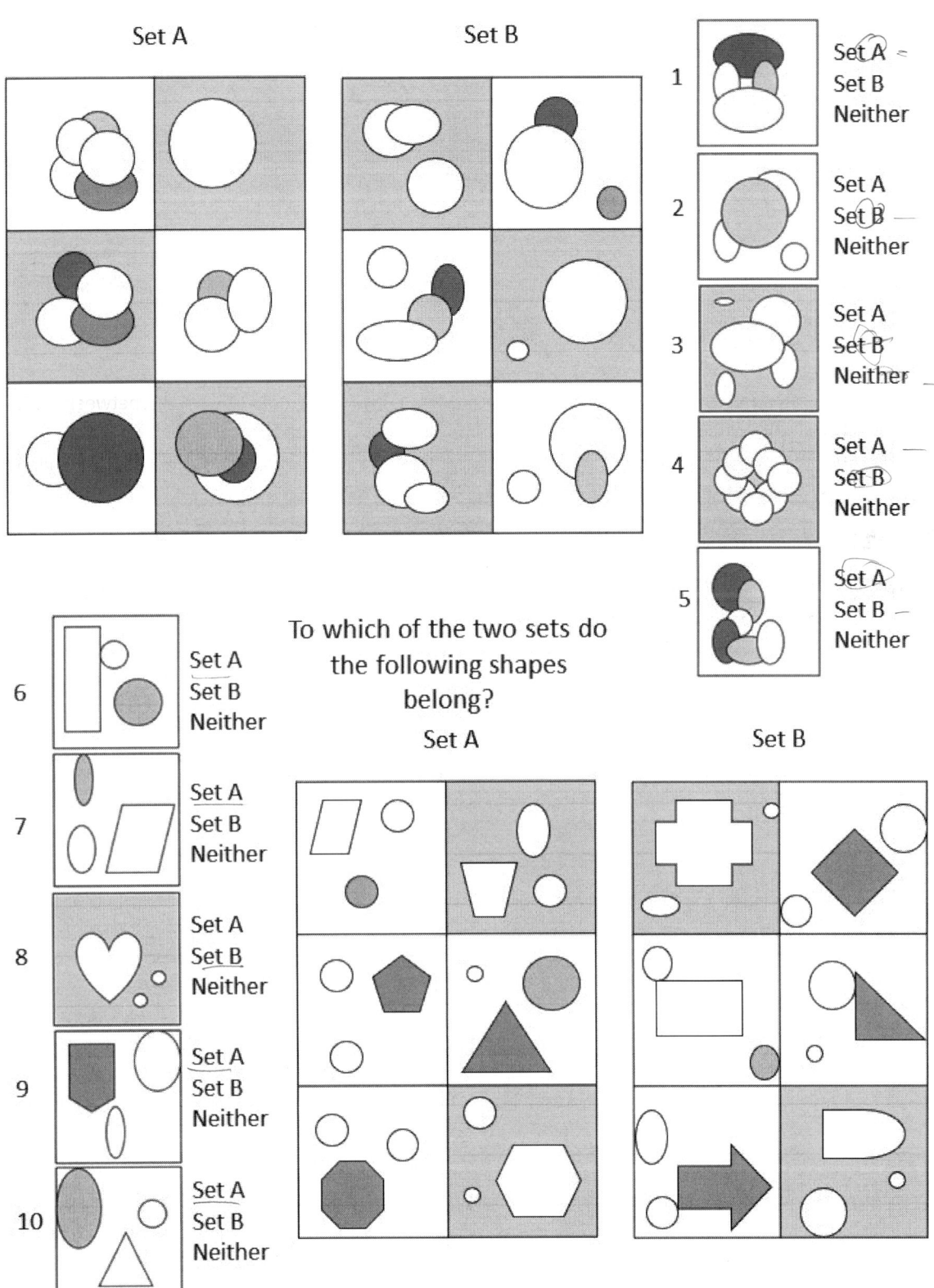

Set A
Set B
Neither

9

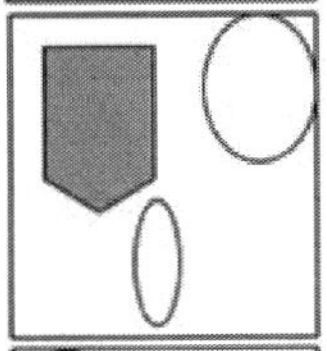

Set A
Set B
Neither

10

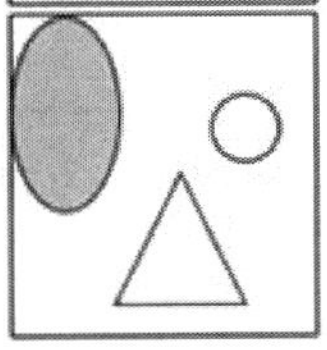

Set A
Set B
Neither

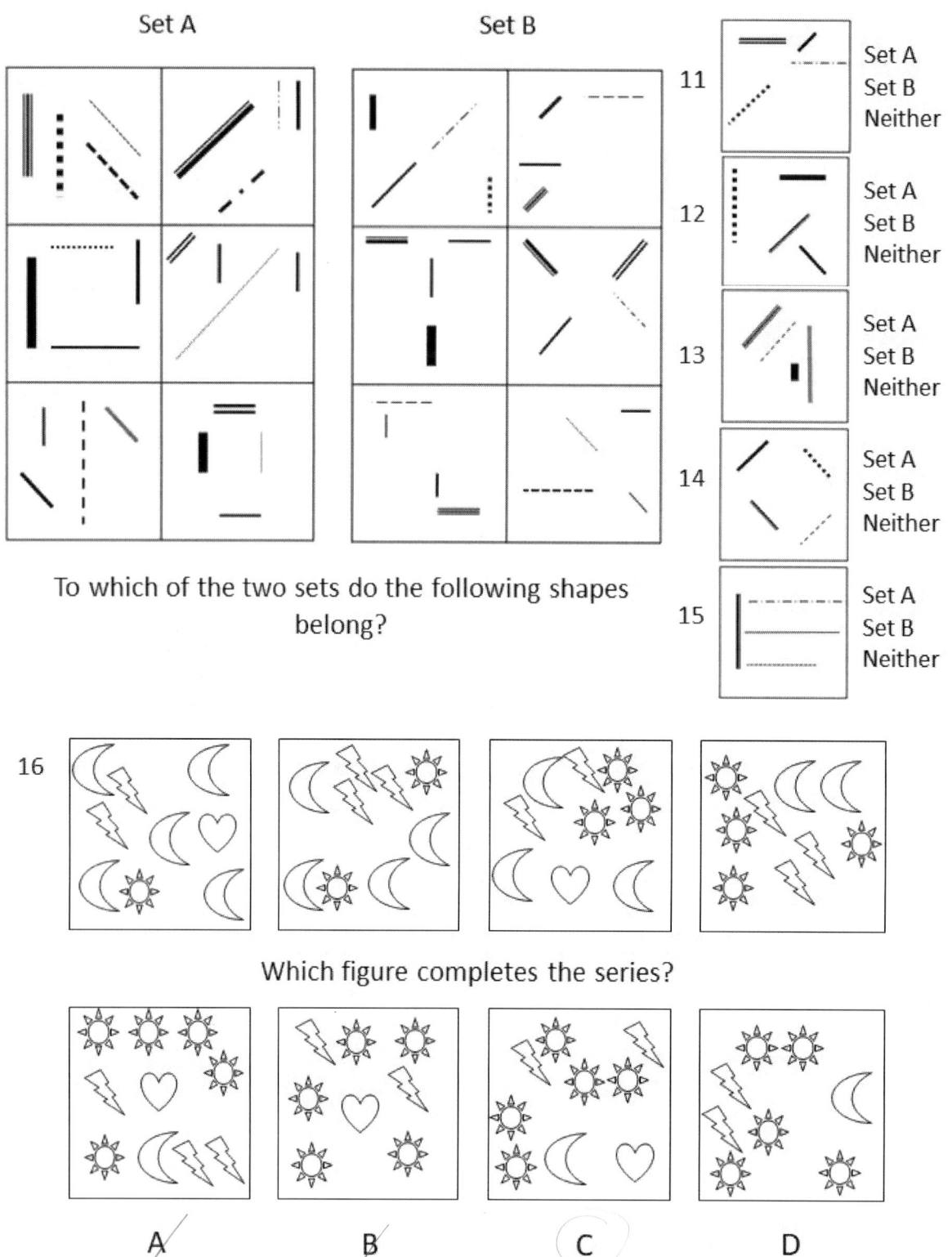

Set A

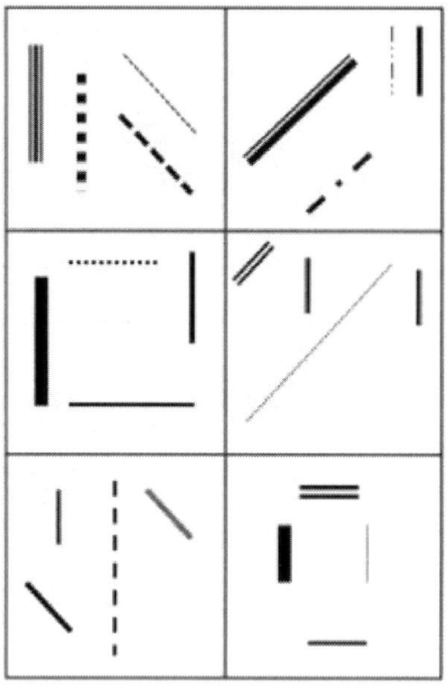

Set B

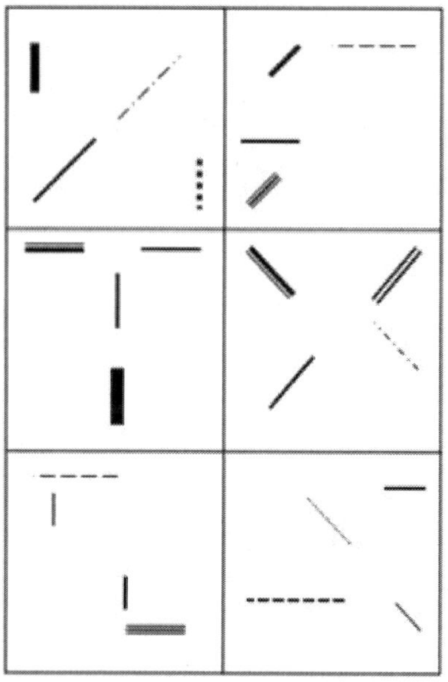

To which of the two sets do the following shapes belong?

11 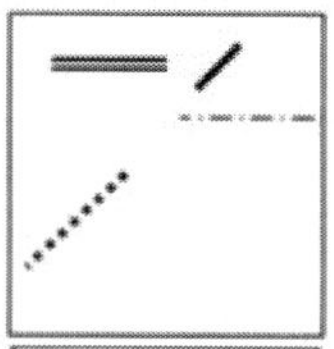
Set A
Set B
Neither

12 
Set A
Set B
Neither

13 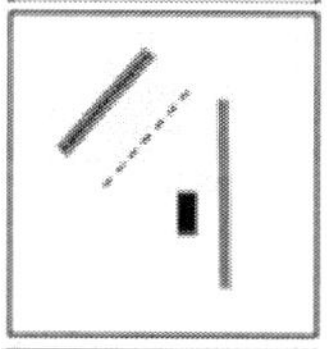
Set A
Set B
Neither

14 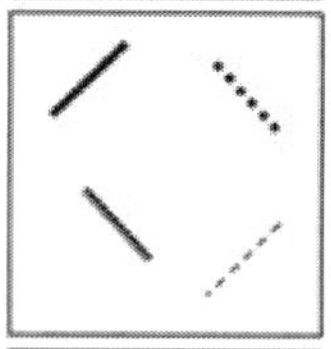
Set A
Set B
Neither

15 
Set A
Set B
Neither

16 

Which figure completes the series?

A B C D

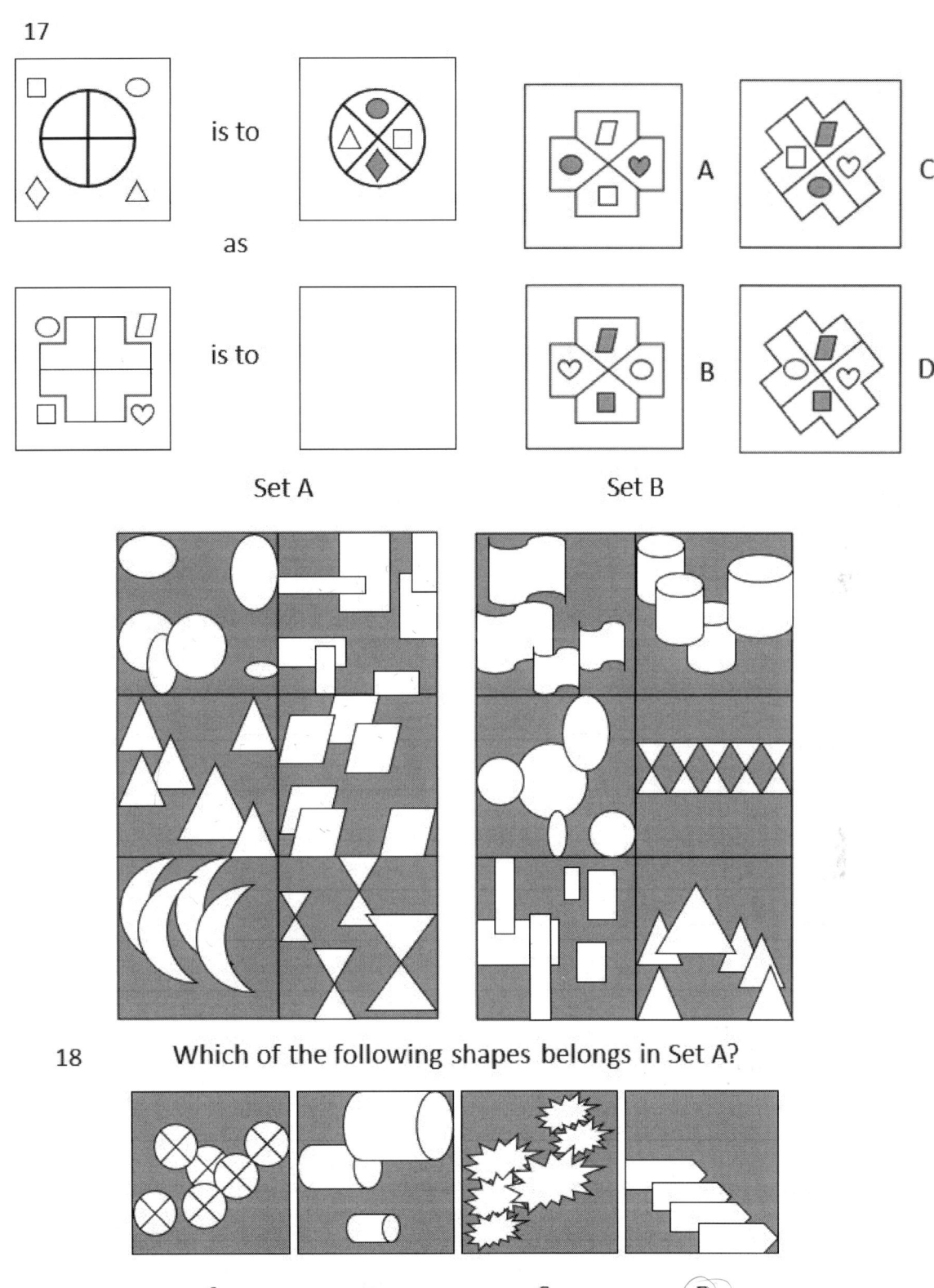

17

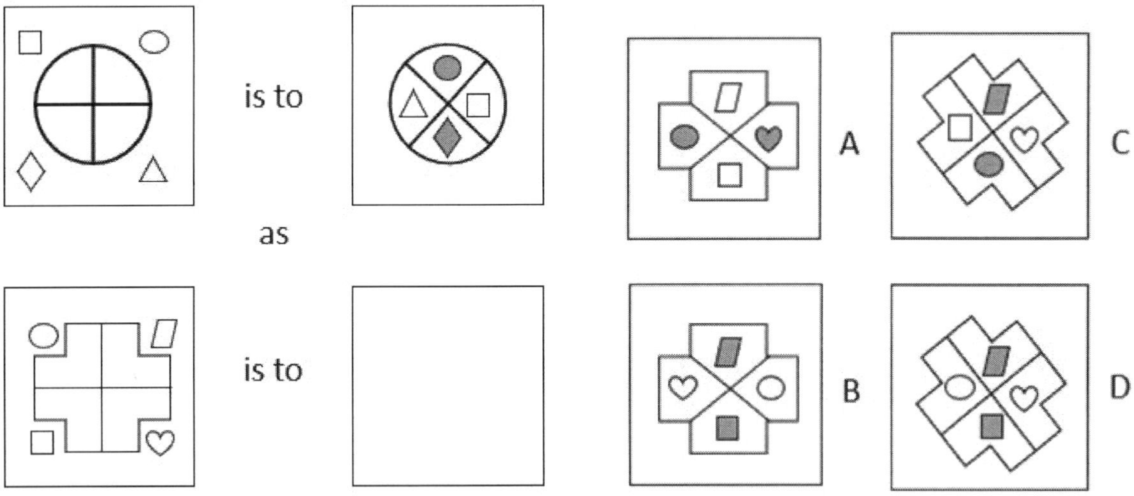

Set A Set B

18 Which of the following shapes belongs in Set A?

A B C D

Worked answer - Abstract Reasoning Type 1 sample 1

First impressions...The collections of circles feature different numbers, and different sizes. There are white, light grey and dark grey circles and white and light grey backgrounds. Most of the circles overlap or are overlapped by other circles.

Pattern: The rule here is to do with whole shapes – we can see lots of shapes but only a few of them are not overlapped by others. **In Set A, we can always see one whole circular shape, in Set B, we can always see two.**

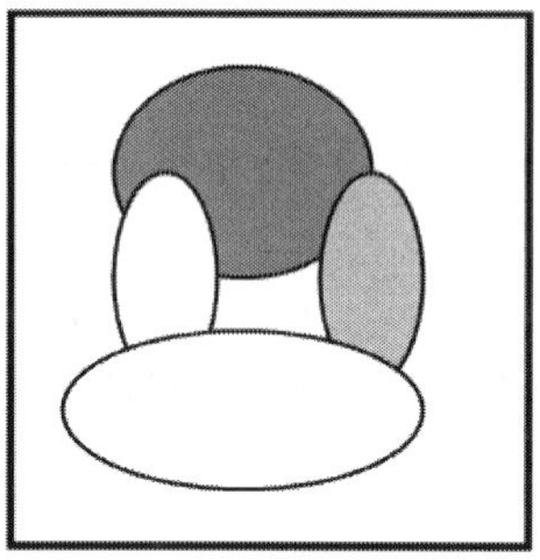

Count: There's no obvious pattern with the number of circles – Set A has pictures with 1, 2, 3, 4 and 5 circles whilst Set B has 2, 3, 4 and 5. Colour seems irrelevant – both sets have a seemingly even split of white, light and dark grey. Size, similarly, seems to be irrelevant.

When you know this rule classifying the new pictures is easy. This picture only has one whole visible circular shape so must fit into set A.

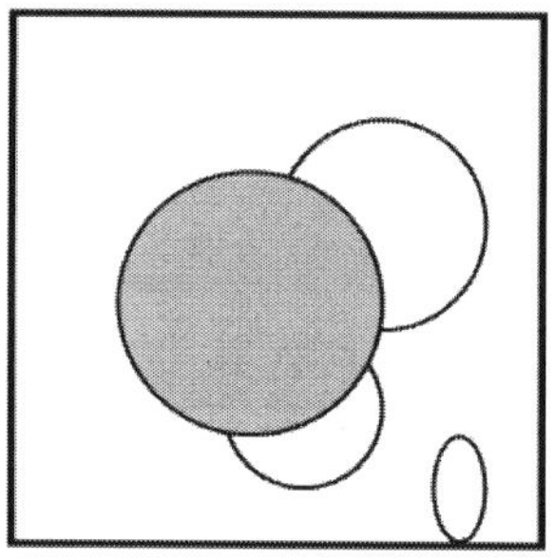

Likewise we can see two whole circular shapes in this picture so know that it must fit into set B.

And this shape has three whole visible circular shapes. That doesn't fit into set A or set B so the correct answer must be neither.

Place: This doesn't play a role in this panel.

Other: It may be sensible to see if you can see any other rules but as the one already found explains every picture it isn't necessary on this occasion.

Direction: There are no lines or arrows

Picture 1: Set A

Picture 2: Set B

Picture 3: Neither

Picture 4: Set B

Picture 5: Set A

Worked answer - Abstract Reasoning Type 1 sample 2

First impressions...There is always three shapes in total and two of them are circles or ovals. Some shapes are white, others are shaded. Some back grounds are white and others are shaded.

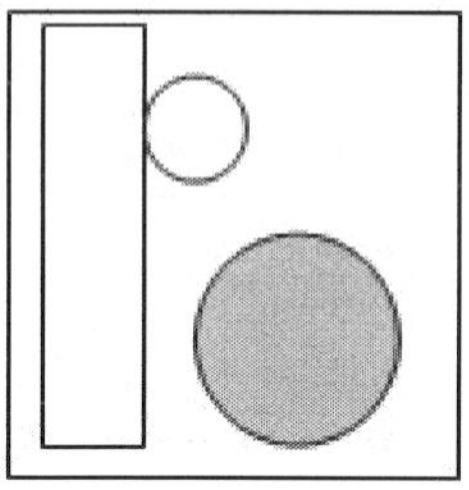

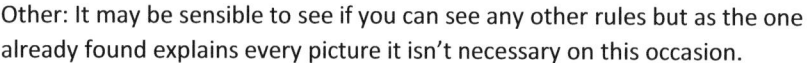

Pattern: There doesn't seem to be any pattern to the arrangement of shapes

Count: There are always three shapes including two circles and ovals. The other shape must be the crucial point. The other shape has between three and eight edges. All of the shapes in Set B have at least one right angle. This picture therefore seems to fit in Set B.

None of the larger shapes in Set A have any right angles meaning this shape might fit in Set A. However the next consideration may change that.

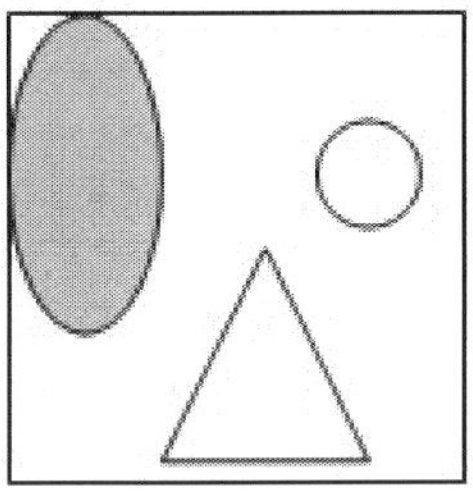

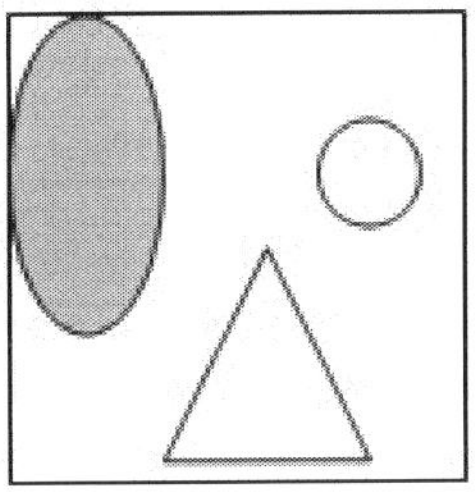

Place: In Set B there is **always a circle touching either the edge or the larger shape** and this is not the case in Set A. Consequently we can see that this picture is Set A whereas the previous one wasn't.

Other: The shading doesn't seem to contribute to the rule at all.

Direction: There are not any lines and only one arrow in the whole set of pictures – it seems unlikely this has a role.

The rule is: In Set A there are two free floating circles and no right angles. In Set B there are two circles but one of them is touching the edge of the box or another shape and the bigger shape has at least one right angle.

Picture 6: Set B

Picture 7: Set A

Picture 8: Set A

Picture 9: Set B

Picture 10: Neither

<u>Worked answer - Abstract Reasoning Type 1 sample 3</u>

First impressions...There are always four lines – of varying length, weight, design and direction.

Pattern: The lines in Set A are placed in pairs with each pair running parallel to each other – albeit sometimes they are not adjacent nor the same length. This picture might be in Set A.

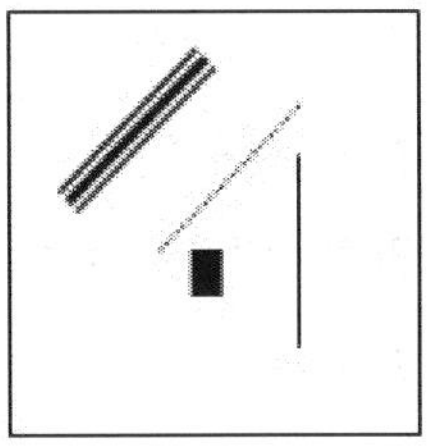

Count: There are always four lines – this can't be relevant to the rule.

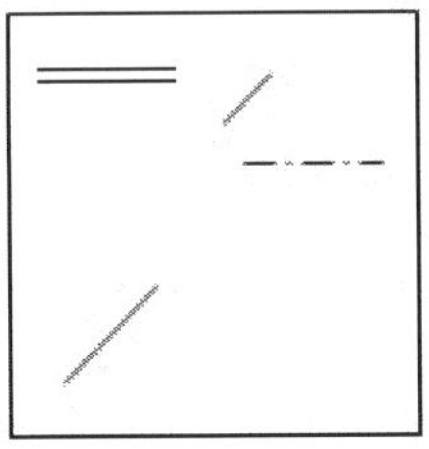

Place: The lines placement in Set A places them in parallel pairs.
In Set B there are not any parallel pairs. This picture looks like it belongs in Set B.

Other: The weight and pattern of the lines doesn't follow any pattern.

Direction: In Set A and Set B the lines are in pairs pointing in the same direction. This picture doesn't belong in either set.

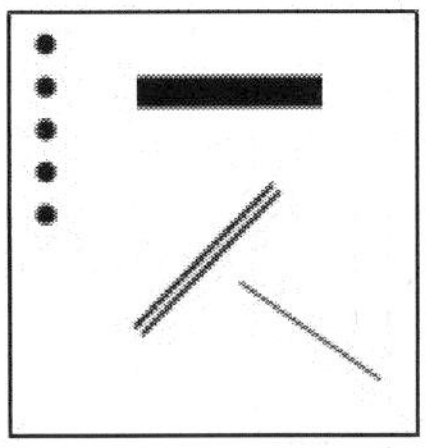

The rule is: In Set A there are two sets of parallel lines. In Set B there are two sets of lines of identical orientation which are not parallel.

Picture 11: Set B

Picture 12: Neither

Picture 13: Set A

Picture 14: Set A

Picture 15: Neither

Worked answer - Abstract Reasoning Type 2

First impressions...This is a Type 2 question and there is a lot going on!

With the sequence question type you have to notice small changes in the pictures as they change from left to right. The PC Plod acronym can still be useful.

Pattern: The elements move around the square and there doesn't seem to be a pattern.

Count: This seems very significant as the number of different shapes in each picture changes each time. Breaking the task down makes it quite straightforward

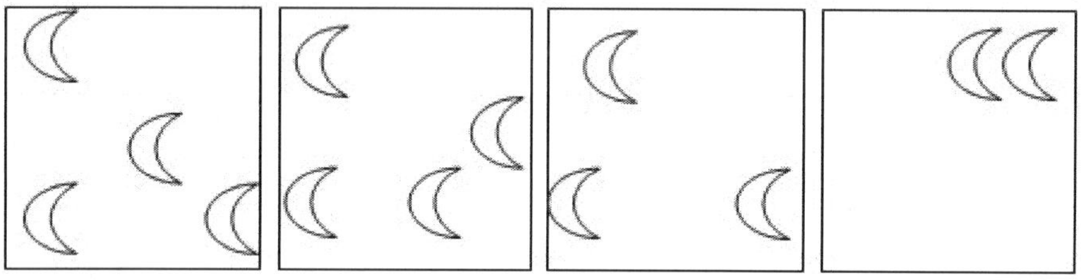

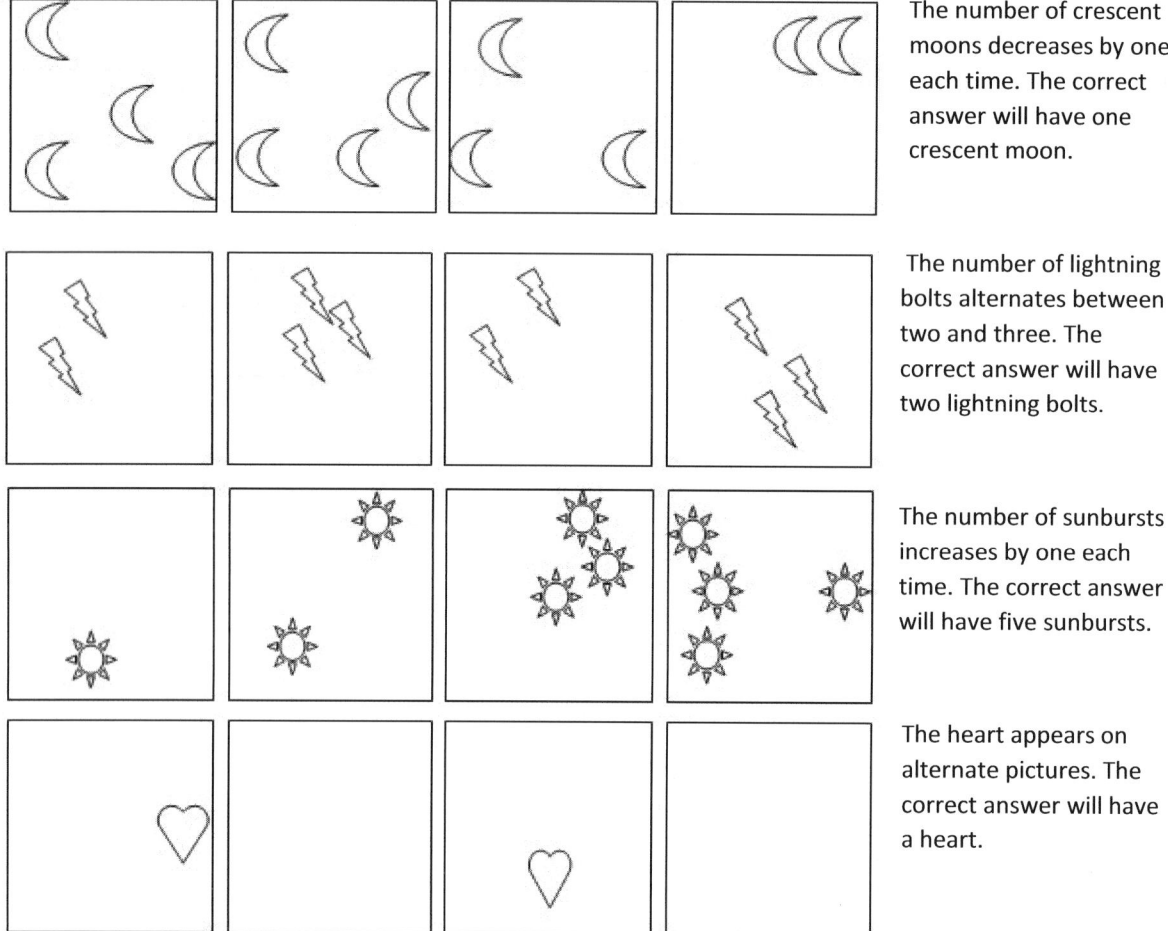

The number of crescent moons decreases by one each time. The correct answer will have one crescent moon.

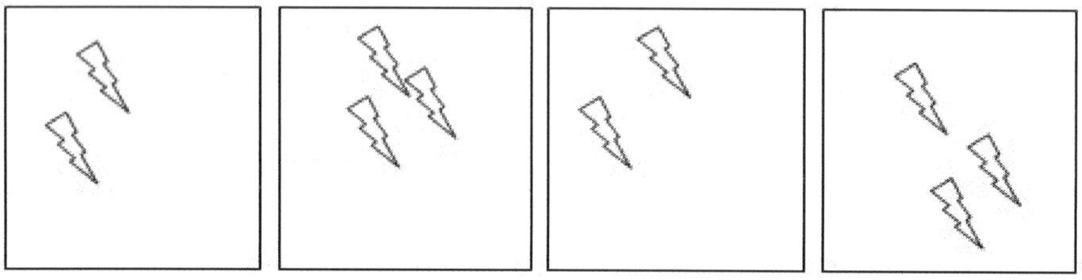

The number of lightning bolts alternates between two and three. The correct answer will have two lightning bolts.

The number of sunbursts increases by one each time. The correct answer will have five sunbursts.

The heart appears on alternate pictures. The correct answer will have a heart.

The only answer which fits all of the rules is C

Worked answer - Abstract Reasoning Type 3

First impressions...This is a Type 3 question and there is some ambiguity.

Here you're being asked to observe what has happened between the first and second box on the top row and see what would happen in the second box in the second row if the same rule were applied.

In this example we can see that there has been some rotation either of the whole circle including the central cross or just of the cross – we can't tell because a circle doesn't change appearance when rotated. We also know that the small outer shapes have moved within the quadrants and that some of them have become shaded. As we don't know which way the outer shape and cross within it have altered it is best to concentrate on how the smaller shapes behave.

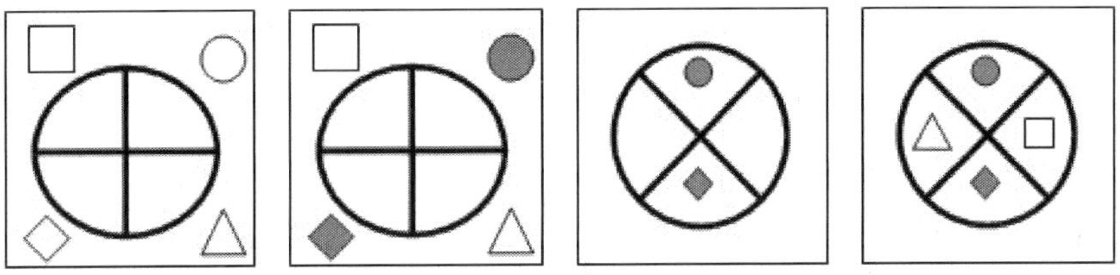

The pattern followed in the first set can be systematically applied to the second to find the correct answer. Applying the more obvious pattern first may allow you to arrive quickly at the correct answer – the shaded shapes are easy to spot and track.

However – in this question it is necessary to spot what happens with the un-shaded shapes as well to discern between options B and D.

The correct answer is option B.

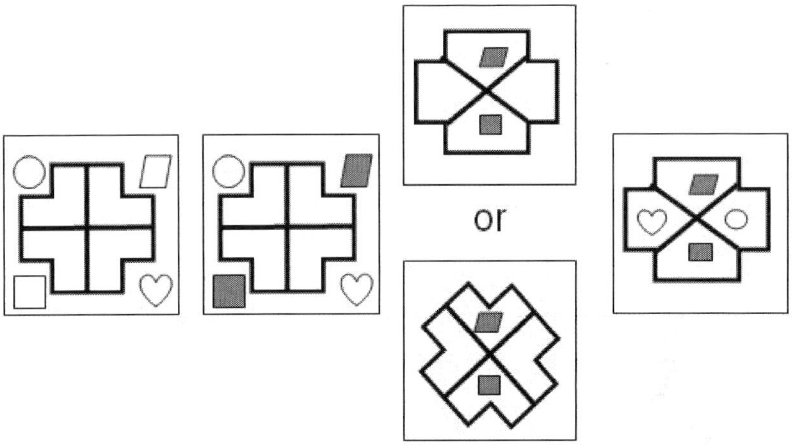

Worked answer - Abstract Reasoning Type 4

First impressions...This is a Type 4 question which looks a lot like a Type 1 question. The boxes are all shaded and have a number of overlapping, identical shapes within them. The white shapes touch the side of the box in every picture in both sets.

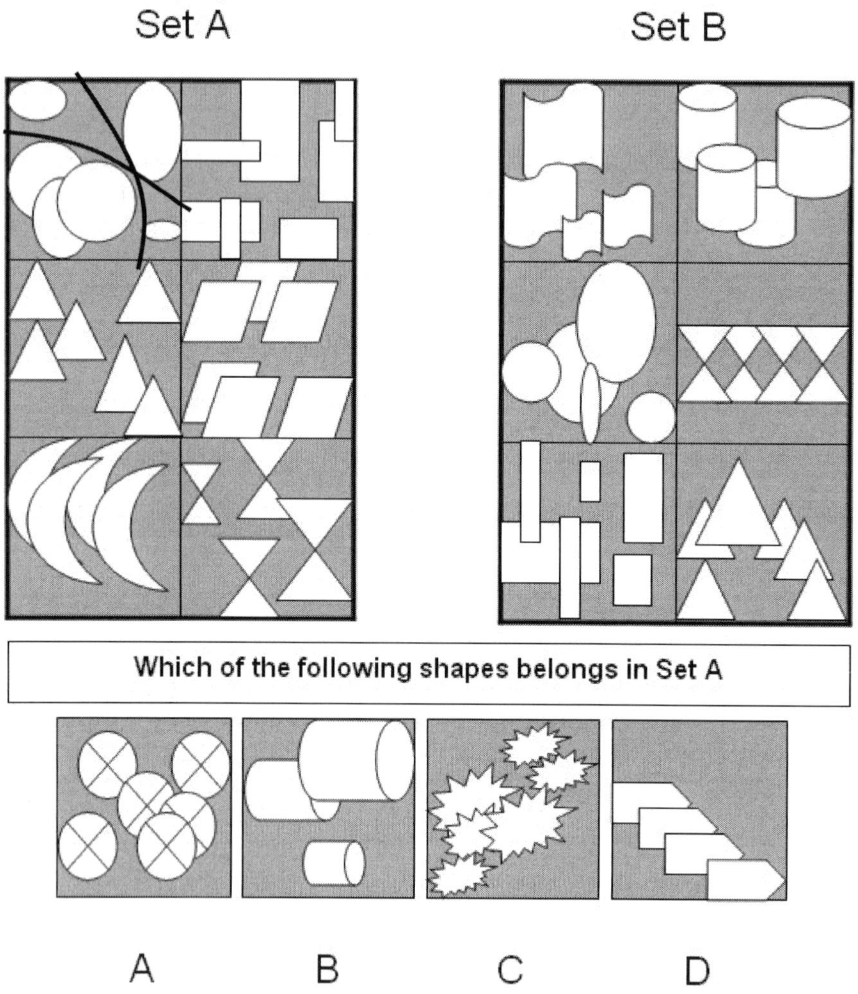

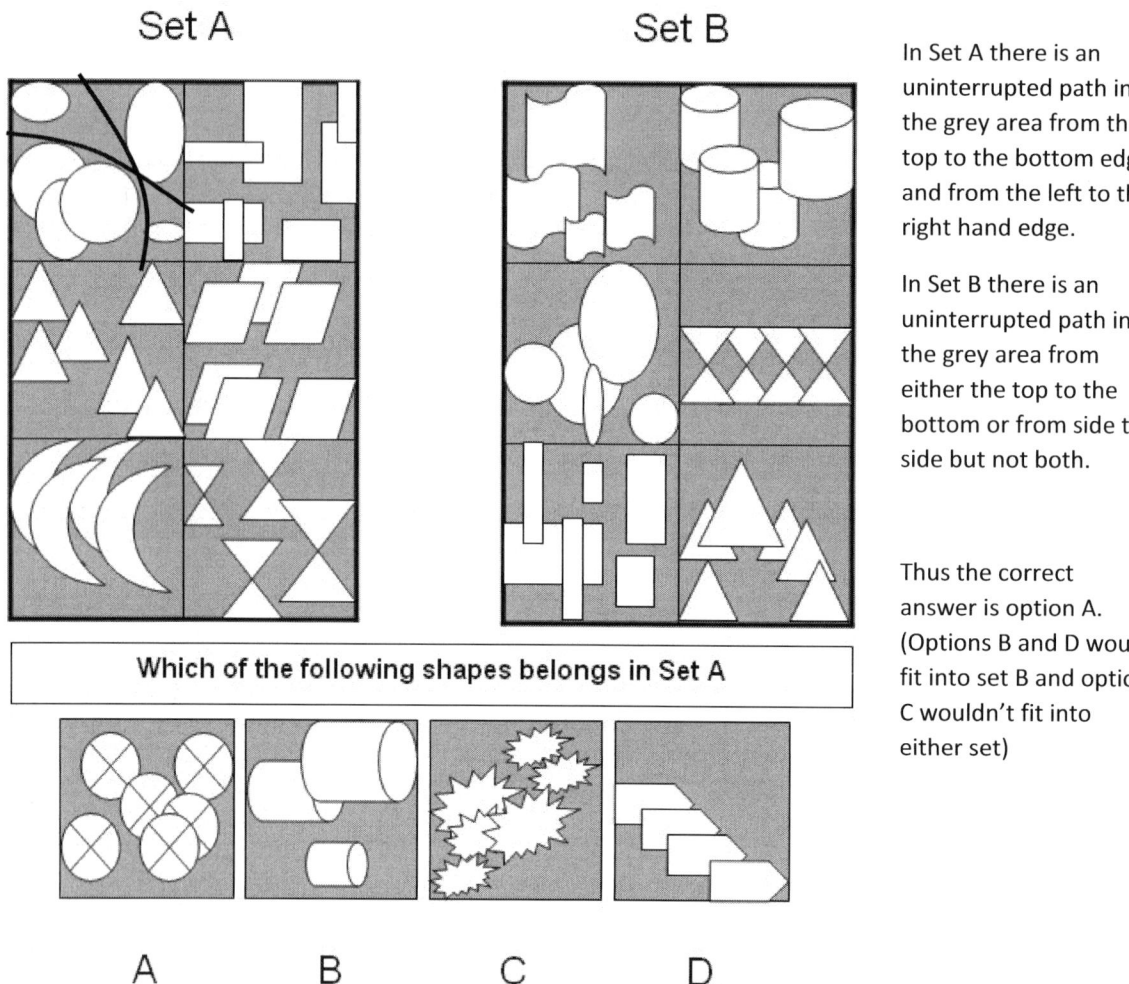

In Set A there is an uninterrupted path in the grey area from the top to the bottom edge and from the left to the right hand edge.

In Set B there is an uninterrupted path in the grey area from either the top to the bottom or from side to side but not both.

Thus the correct answer is option A. (Options B and D would fit into set B and option C wouldn't fit into either set)

Introduction to Situational Judgement

More than any other this section feels like it's testing your aptitude for being a doctor! Situational Judgement is used regularly in medical training – from UCAT right up to experienced doctors embarking on further training. An instinctive understanding of good practice regarding ethics is highly prized in many fields – not least medicine – and few professional people will succeed without having to sit at least a few of these kinds of tests.

In this section you will be presented with a hypothetical situation. It will usually have some sort of medical content but not always. For each scenario presented there will be between four and six further statements. The statement will either be an action or a consideration regarding the scenario. You have to judge the appropriateness of the action or the importance of that statement.

This section of the UCAT is marked differently. Although there is always a 'best answer' you will receive marks for getting close to the best answer even if you miss it. The clue is in the name – it's about making a judgement regarding a situation.

Within Situational Judgement you must consider each option entirely separately. You are not being asked to rank them as better than, or worse than, each other – there may be three 'very appropriate' actions or none at all related to a scenario. It may be that the response you feel is most appropriate is not one of the options – this doesn't matter as you're simply being asked to judge the options.

Techniques for Situational Judgement

Things to take into account when answering these questions include:

- A response should NOT be judged as if it were the ONLY thing you would do. There are often many appropriate responses to a situation, some of which may seem small and unimportant compared to the others. If you have a scenario about having to cross a road to provide first aid in an accident it is very appropriate to ensure you're safe when crossing the road for example; but it's also important you DO cross the road to treat the casualties.

- The response options need to be treated independently – you're not being asked to rank them or compare them. If all four suggestions seem 'very appropriate' to you then mark all four as 'very appropriate'.

- Response options should be considered in both the short and long term. Therefore, it is very important to treat a patient who has been hit by a car, and also very important to investigate if a new pedestrian crossing should be implemented.

The issues you should consider when approaching a Situational Judgment question include:

- Patient safety – the health and wellbeing of the patient is always the first consideration. Be aware that 'wellbeing' will encompass more than their physical health.

- Confidentiality – this is a key consideration. It is almost always inappropriate to breach confidentiality – unless patient safety is at stake. Young people are entitled to confidentiality regarding their health and medical care.

- Respect and dignity – treating others with proper respect is a common courtesy which professionalism demands. 'Others' includes patients, other doctors and other colleagues (nurses, midwives, physiotherapists etc), and other people such as the relatives of the patient

- Integrity – this is to do with behaving properly yourself – this main pertain to accepting gifts, making sure your own health is cared for, knowing your own limits and asking for help when required.

- The 'Doctor Pepper' Principle – always consider what the very worst outcome might be of any particular action.

SJT Worked Sample 1: Answers on page 40

A businessman visits his GP as he has been suffering from vomiting and diarrhoea for the last three days. He says he is feeling a bit better but hasn't eaten for two days and looks quite dehydrated. There is no significant medical history and the GP has no reason, after an examination, to suspect it's anything other than a viral infection. He is due to fly to China the following day for a two week work trip.

How appropriate are the following actions?

1. The GP should give the man some advice about re-hydrating himself before he flies

   A. A very appropriate thing to do
   B. Appropriate but not ideal
   C. Inappropriate but not awful
   D. A very inappropriate thing to do

2. The GP should tell the man to delay his trip until he is fully recovered

   A. A very appropriate thing to do
   B. Appropriate but not ideal
   C. Inappropriate but not awful
   D. A very inappropriate thing to do

3. The GP should ask which airline he is flying with and warn them to protect the health of other passengers

   A. A very appropriate thing to do
   B. Appropriate but not ideal
   C. Inappropriate but not awful
   D. A very inappropriate thing to do

4. The GP should check the man has the relevant inoculations for a trip of this nature

   A. A very appropriate thing to do
   B. Appropriate but not ideal
   C. Inappropriate but not awful
   D. A very inappropriate thing to do

SJT Worked sample 2: Answers on page 41

A patient on a surgical ward receives gifts of chocolate and biscuits at every visiting time. This patient is due to go to surgery later that day and needs to be nil by mouth until after the operation. There is concern that he may eat some of the snacks and put himself at risk.

How important is it to consider:

5. The patient already knows he shouldn't eat and telling him again would patronise and annoy him

A. Very important
B. Important
C. Of minor importance
D. Not important

6. The nurses are very busy and are unlikely to be able to 'police' this patient

A. Very important
B. Important
C. Of minor importance
D. Not important

7. The snacks are the patient's personal property and cannot be confiscated

A. Very important
B. Important
C. Of minor importance
D. Not important

8. If the patient eats before his surgery then the risks could be significant or even fatal

A. Very important
B. Important
C. Of minor importance
D. Not important

9. The snacks aren't healthy

A. Very important
B. Important
C. Of minor importance
D. Not important

Situational Judgement Worked sample 1 – Answer

1. The GP should give the man some advice about re-hydrating himself before he flies

This would be a **very appropriate** thing for the GP to do. If the man is unwell, but not dangerously so (which is the GP's diagnosis) then any advice which will make him more comfortable on a long flight would be helpful.

2. The GP should tell the man to delay his trip until he is fully recovered

This would be **inappropriate, but not awful**. Although the GP is acting out of concern both for his patient and other passengers, we know that the GP is not concerned that this is a serious condition. This suggestion may have professional and financial ramifications which are not warranted for a simple stomach bug.

3. The GP should ask which airline he is flying with and warn them to protect the health of other passengers

This would be **very inappropriate**. The patient's confidentiality is compromised where there is no major public health risk. If the patient wanted to fly with a confirmed serious health issue then this may be necessary but we know the GP does not think this is the case.

4. The GP should check the man has the relevant inoculations for a trip of this nature

This would be **very appropriate**. Although any inoculation at this late stage may well be pointless and ineffective – if the patient knew that he was not protected against a particular disease then he could take steps to minimise his possibility of being exposed. Additionally it is possible that some inoculations are a legal requirement.

What you're thinking.... But what if there is an immune-suppressed patient on the plane for whom a stomach bug may be deadly? What if it isn't a simple stomach bug but something far more serious? Don't GPs have a responsibility for public health as well as patient health? Surely health should come before business?

And the answers are.... There MAY be a passenger for whom a stomach bug would prove deadly – however, even if this patient is prevented from boarding the plane there may well be another patient who hasn't bothered to visit his GP and has just taken some medicine and plans to sweat it out. Severely ill patients have to take responsibility for minimising their exposure to infection, as avoiding infection entirely whilst continuing with normal life is impossible.

It is possible that it is more than a simple stomach bug but if the GP has arrived at that diagnosis after an examination and with the benefit of that patient's medical history it is likely to be just that. Although GPs probably do occasionally miss more serious conditions but it can't be assumed that this one has in this instance.

GPs do have a responsibility to public health – when a notifiable disease crops up they must report it, if an epidemic of some sort begins they will be involved in collecting and reporting date – however this really doesn't fall into that category. If GPs tried to prevent all people with a viral infection from continuing with normal life then they would have a much harder job (and people with minor conditions would stop visiting them!)

Of course it's easy to blithely pronounce that health comes before business... which in the grand scheme of things it does. If the GP had pronounced a terminal disease then the businessman may have had no objection to cancelling his trip. However, people have complex lives and it is not the place of a GP to judge their decisions.

Situational Judgement Worked sample 2 – Answer

5. The patient already knows he shouldn't eat and telling him again would patronise and annoy him. This is of **minor importance** – just because the patient has had it explained already does not mean he shouldn't have it explained again. If there are genuine reasons to think he may not be compliant with instructions then repeating them may be necessary and sensible. Irritation to the patient is of little importance compared to their safety.

6. The nurses are very busy and are unlikely to be able to 'police' this patient. This is **important**. The nurses may do all they can to 'police' this patient but given the busy nature of their job the responsibility cannot be reasonably placed solely on them.

7: The snacks are the patient's personal property and cannot be confiscated. This is **important** – a patient cannot have their property taken away without very good reason. However, if there is good reason, and the patient has those reasons fully explained, then this may be an appropriate course of action.

8: If the patient eats before his surgery then the risks could be significant or even fatal. This is **very important**. Patient safety is always the most important consideration.

9: The snacks aren't healthy. This is, in this context, **not important**. If he had a bowl of fruit the risks would be identical.

Mini Mocks

The next few pages are a 'mini mock' for you to put into practice some of the techniques you have learned. We suggest you do this in timed, exam conditions.

Section	Number of questions	Time allowed
Verbal Reasoning	3 passages of text – 12 questions	6 minutes
Decision Making	10 questions	10 minutes 30 seconds
Quantitative Reasoning	3 data sets – 12 questions	8 minutes
Abstract Reasoning	18 questions	4 minutes 30 seconds
Situational Judgement	5 scenarios – 20 questions	8 minutes
	72 questions	37 minutes

Before you start you will need to get:

- Paper, pencil and pen
- A simple calculator
- A stopwatch or timer

Make sure:

- Your mobile phone is on silent or notifications are switched off
- The people around you know not to disturb you for an hour
- You're ready for an hour's work and won't need to stop for a drink or to use the bathroom

Verbal Reasoning Mini Mock 6 minutes - answers on page 62

Lake Taupo

Lake Taupo in the centre of New Zealand's North Island is actually the caldera of a large volcano - which produced two of the most significant volcanic eruptions in recent geological times. A caldera forms when the land mass above an active volcanic area under the surface literally collapses to leave a basin, or cauldron above.

The Taupo began erupting about 300,000 years ago but the main eruptions which still affect the surrounding landscape occurred about 26,500 years ago and are responsible for the shape of the modern caldera. Also significant was the Taupo eruption about 1,800 years ago. However, there have been many more eruptions - averaging about one every thousand years.

The Taupo volcano erupts rhyolite, a viscous magma with high silica content. If the magma does not contain much gas the volcano tends to form a lava dome. However, when mixed with gas or steam a rhyolitic eruption can be very violent as the magma froths to form pumice and ash which can be thrown out with great force.

The Orunanui eruption of the Taupo volcano was the world's largest known volcanic eruption for the last 70,000 years. It occurred around 26,500 years ago and generated approximately 430 cubic kilometres of pyroclastic fall deposits. Lake Taupo partially fills the caldera generated in this eruption. The ash from this eruption profoundly affected most of New Zealand, and the Chatham Islands (1000km away) experienced an 18cm ash layer.

The Taupo eruption (also known as the Hatepe eruption) represents the latest eruption from Taupo and occurred about 1,800 years ago. It was the largest volcanic eruption in the world in the last 5,000 years. The eruption further expanded the lake as the previous outlet was blocked and the water level rose to 35 metres above its present level. However the outlet then broke and caused a huge flood causing the Waikato River to flow at 200 times its usual rate for over a week.

At the time of this eruption there was no human presence in New Zealand and the nearest humans would have been in Australia - 2000 km to the east well outside visible range.

1. Which of the following is not an impact of Taupo volcano's activities over the years?

A. The variation of river flows

B. Ash fall affecting most of a country

C. Alterations in the depth of a lake

D. Alterations in the shape of a landmass

2. Which of the following is a correct sequence of events?

A. Orunanui eruption, Taupo eruption, Hatepe eruption

B. Taupo began erupting, main eruption which continues to affect landscape, Orunanui eruption

C. Taupo began erupting, Hatepe eruption, humans populate New Zealand

D. Orunanui eruption, humans populate Australia, Taupo eruption

3. Which of the following is likely to be true?

A. Ash from the Orunanui eruption travelled 1000 miles

B. Taupo has erupted around 300 times

C. If the magma contains a lot of gas then a lava dome tends to form

D. Hatepe was around 5000 years ago

4. Which of the following statements is true?

A. The Orunanui eruption of Taupo occurred approximately 70,000 years ago

B. No human has ever seen Taupo erupt

C. New Zealand's North Island is a highly volcanic area

D. A rhyolitic eruption always causes the formation of pumice as magma froths with gas

Six-wheel drive, 6WD or 6x6 is a drivetrain configuration of six wheels, all of which are driven simultaneously by the vehicle's engine. Unlike four-wheel drive drivetrains, the configuration is largely confined to off-road and military vehicles, particularly heavy-duty ones. Six-wheel drive vehicles may have two wheels at the front and four at the rear (with only the front pair steering), or three evenly spaced axles, where the front and middle pair may both steer (as in the Alvis Saladin). Drive may be limited to the rear two axles for on-road use.

T815, M35 2-1/2 ton cargo truck (aka "Deuce and a half") and the Pinzgauer High Mobility All-Terrain Vehicle are production examples of vehicles using this type of drive system.

The Alvis Stalwart is an amphibious 6x6 military truck built by Alvis that served with the British Army.

Six-wheeled conversions of four-wheel drive trucks are widely made. These may be six-wheel drive (such as the 6x6 version of the Australian Army's Perentie Land Rover Defender), but are commonly 6x4 (with only front and rear or front and middle axles driven), a technically simpler construction with stock components. Polaris Industries has produced a number of 6 wheel drive ATVs and UTVs for many years, they are based on a standard Magnum, Sportsman or Ranger with an extra axle and a Cargo Box over the rear wheels. John Deere also produced a 6 wheel Gator model, but only the rear wheels have power. There are also a number of companies who produce 6x6 and 8x8 amphibious ATVs.

5. Which of the following is probably not a manufacturer with a 6WD model in existence?

A. Pinzgauer

B. Polaris Industries

C. John Deere

D. Alvis Saladin

6. What is a main difference between production 6WD vehicles and conversions?

A. Conversions are not used in a military context

B. Production vehicles are more likely to be amphibious

C. Conversions are much more common

D. Conversions are less complex in construction

7. What advantage seems likely to be gained by a six wheel drive vehicle?

A. Better control

B. Can perform in water and on land

C. Better performance on rugged terrain and off road

D. Extra storage space for cargo

8. Which of the following statements is untrue?

A. The British Army have used an amphibious 6x6 vehicle

B. For on-road use the Alvis Saladin may be limited to use of the forward two axles only

C. Steering in a 6x6 vehicle is operated by the wheels on the front axle where the three axles are evenly spaced

D. A true 6x6 will have capacity for all six wheels to be driven simultaneously by the engine

Tobacco use commonly leads to diseases affecting the heart and lungs, with smoking being a major risk factor for heart attacks, strokes, chronic obstructive pulmonary disease (COPD), emphysema, and cancer (particularly lung cancer, cancers of the larynx and mouth, and pancreatic cancer).

The World Health Organization estimates that tobacco caused 5.4 million deaths in 2004 and 100 million deaths over the course of the 20th century. Similarly, the United States Centre for Disease Control and Prevention describes tobacco use as "the single most important preventable risk to human health in developed countries and an important cause of premature death worldwide."

Rates of smoking have levelled off or declined in the developed world. Smoking rates in the United States have dropped by half from 1965 to 2006, falling from 42% to 20.8% in adults. In the developing world, tobacco consumption is rising by 3.4% per year.

9. Which of the following statements seems likely to be false?

A. Tobacco consumption causes both morbidity and mortality

B. People in the developed world are less likely to die as a result of tobacco use

C. Tobacco use is the main cause of premature death worldwide

D. Tobacco use is associated with illnesses other than cancer

10. Which of the following is unlikely based on current trends?

A. There will be more deaths in 21st century from tobacco use than in the 20th

B. Smoking could be eradicated in the US within 20 years

C. Tobacco use in the developing world will double in around 20 years

D. The population of the developing world is greater than that of the developed world

11. What is unlikely to be contributing to a change in the number of deaths in the world from tobacco use related disease?

A. Increasing tobacco consumption

B. Reducing tobacco consumption

C. A change in the location and resources of tobacco using people

D. Health education and health care

12. Which of the following statements is definitely true?

A. Tobacco usually causes cancer lung cancer, cancers of the larynx and mouth, and pancreatic cancer

B. Tobacco use causes premature death.

C. Tobacco caused around 5.4 million deaths in the 20th Century.

D. In 2006, 42% of adults in the United States smoked.

8/12 verbal

Decision Making Mini Mock 10.5 minutes. Answers on page 64

1. Not all members of a football team also play golf but members who play golf are married and some of these golfers also play cricket.

Place 'Yes' if the conclusion does follow. Place 'No' if the conclusion does not follow.

Some cricketers who are members of the football team also play golf.	Yes / No
Some golfers who are members of the football team are both married and play cricket.	Yes / No
All married members of the football team are either golfers or cricketers.	Yes / No
Not all married members of the football team who are golfers are cricketers.	Yes / No
All the cricketers who are members of the football team that are married also play golf.	Yes / No

all golf = married
some golf = cricket
some football = golf

2. Priya, Martin, Joe, Umar and Alice sat a maths test gaining scores of 34, 46, 58, 20 and 43.

- Joe got a lower score than Alice.
- Umar got a higher score than Martin.
- Priya got a higher score than Umar but a lower score than Joe.
- Umar got a lower score than Joe and Alice.

Which of the following statements is true?

A. Alice got a score of 46 in the test.
B. There were 12 marks difference between Joe and Umar's test scores.
C. Martin got the highest score on the test.
D. Priya got the second highest test score.

3. The government should produce legislation to limit the meat consumption of individuals in order to decrease the ecological damage caused by industrial farming?

Select the strongest argument from the statements below

A. Yes, the government should do everything they can to limit environmental damage
B. Yes, livestock production may be responsible a large proportion of greenhouse gas emissions, lessening the demand might reduce the amount of emissions.
C. No, it would be more effective to work to reduce the impact of industrial farming and offer clear information and guidelines to consumers
D. No, the government has no right to decide what people can and cannot eat.

4. Yoga is a form of exercise growing in popularity for people seeking to stay healthy in both body and mind. Improving balance, flexibility and strength, it can also be beneficial to people with high blood pressure or heart disease; not to mention the benefits to mental health. Yoga is a non-strenuous activity suitable for people of all ages and ability due to the large variety of classes available. Although it has been specifically recommended to older adults to help prevent falls.

Place 'Yes' if the conclusion does follow. Place 'No' if the conclusion does not follow.

Yoga has so many benefits, it should be used instead of some medicines.	Yes / No
Performing Yoga as part of a healthy active lifestyle can bring about many health improvements.	Yes / No
Only the elderly can benefit from the effects of yoga.	Yes / No
Yoga has gained popularity due to people wanting more natural treatment for ailments.	Yes / No
Practicing Yoga will stop an elderly person having falls.	Yes / No

5. Starting the school day at 10.30 or 11am and finishing later would enable teenagers to benefit more from school as the biological circadian rhythms in adolescence make concentration in the morning difficult.

A. Yes – a small change in school hours may make education more effective for teenagers
B. Yes – this would take traffic off the roads in the morning rush hour and save students and teachers time
C. No – flexible study hours do not prepare teenagers for the very fixed working hours of adult life
D. No – pandering to teenagers wanting a lie in will not teach them discipline

6. The diagram shows features amongst various cars which are for sale.

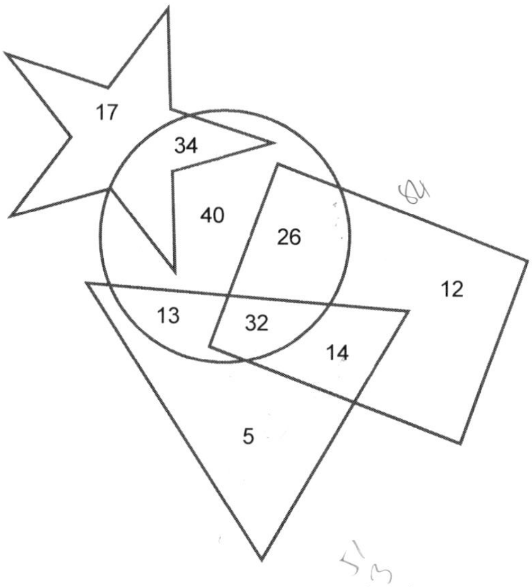

- The star represents cars on sale for <£2000.
- The triangle represents cars with in-built satnav.
- The rectangle represents cars with parking sensors.
- The circle represents cars with CD players.

Which of the following statements is true?

A. There are fewer cars with parking sensors than inbuilt satnav.
B. Exactly half of the cars have more than one of the specified features.
C. The number of cars with only one feature is equal to that of cars with exactly two features.
D. There are 27 cars with inbuilt satnav and exactly one additional feature.

7. Corner Shop A has 25 varieties of chocolate bar. Corner Shop B has 20 varieties of chocolate bar. Each day 20% of Corner Shop A's chocolate bars are out of stock and 10% of Corner Shop B's chocolate bars are out of stock. The chance that any particular chocolate bar will go out of stock on any given day is 2 in 20 in Corner Shop A and 1 in 10 in Corner Shop B.

Considering only the number of chocolate bar varieties in each shop and the chance of varieties going out of stock, is Corner Shop B the better Shop to buy a chocolate bar from?

A. Yes, Corner Shop B has a lower chance of a chocolate bar going out of stock.
B. Yes, Corner Shop B has 20 varieties of chocolate bar in stock on any given day
C. No, Corner Shop A has more varieties of chocolate bar in stock each day
D. No, Corner shop A has a higher chance of a chocolate bar going out of stock.

8. Nancy is making tea for her four colleagues – Olivia, Peter, Rachel and Steve. She does so quite carefully as they all like their tea made differently – extra strong, extra weak, without milk or with sugar. And they each like their tea served in a specific mug.

- Nancy always pours the water into the pink mug first so that the tea will be extra strong as requested
- Nancy always pours Steve's drink last as he likes it extra weak, but not in the green mug
- Nancy fills the black mug fuller as she won't be adding milk to it
- Olivia has 2 sugars in her tea but doesn't use a blue mug

Which of the following must be true?

A. Rachel likes her tea extra strong
B. Peter drinks from a black mug
C. The green mug contains tea with sugar
D. Olivia has a pink mug

9. The shopping mall has thirty shops which all sell one kind of product. Half of the shops sell clothing of some sort. A third of the shops are independent and not part of a larger chain of shops. One tenth of the shops sell food and more than half of these are restaurants or cafes.

There are two restaurants	Yes / No
There are no independent food outlets	Yes / No
Two thirds of the shops are part of chains	Yes / No
There are some chain stores selling clothes in the mall	Yes / No
Half of the independent shops sell clothes	Yes / No

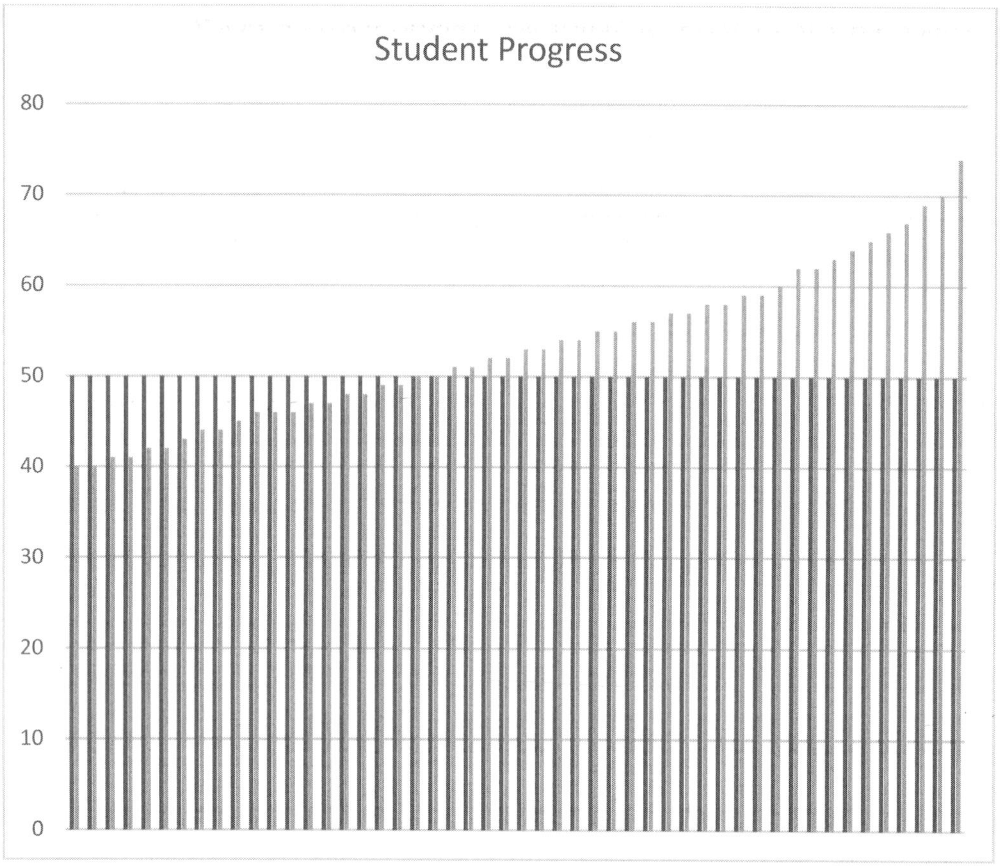

10. 50 students were selected for a small-scale longitudinal study based on performance percentile when leaving primary school (dark bars) versus performance percentile three years later (light bars).

All the students selected for this study were on the 50th centile in performance at the end of primary school — Yes / No

Fewer than half of students made failed to progress in their studies — Yes / No

More than half of the students made better progress than their peer group — Yes / No

The most highly achieving student here moved from the 50th to the 75th centile. — Yes / No

Around a third of students moved down in the centile scale — Yes / No

Quantitative Reasoning Mini Mock 8 Minutes. Answers on page 67

Marks

	Assignment 1 15% of total	Assignment 2 25% of total	Exam 60%
Aman	70%	57%	50%
Bryony	66%	70%	60%
Cody	60%	65%	75%
Daljit	50%	58%	62%
Ellis	68%	75%	63%

Grade Boundaries	
9	70%
8	65%
7	60%
6	55%
5	50%

1. Which student got the highest grade?

A. Aman
B. Bryony
C. Cody
D. Daljit
E. Ellis

2. One student had their exam and assignments re-marked and gained 0.5% which brought their grade up to the next level. Which student was this?

A. Aman
B. Bryony
C. Cody
D. Daljit
E. Ellis

3. Bryony was ill on the day of the exam and under-performed. What did she need to get in the exam to secure an 9?

A. 6.6%
B. 67%
C. 71%
D. 74%
E. 78%

4. The exam board announced that they had made an error and that the two assignments should have accounted for 20% each. How would this have altered the grade spread for these students?

A. Two grades worse
B. One grade worse
C. No change
D. One grade better
E. Two grades better

Quantitative Reasoning Mini Mock – Fish Tank

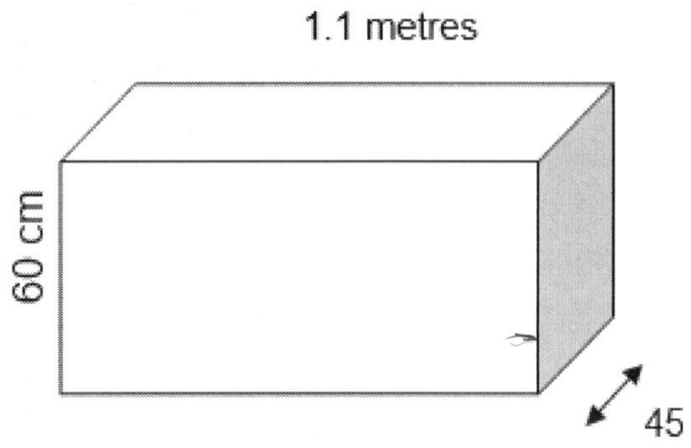

Kian's fish tank has 5cm of gravel in the base. The gravel displaces all the water.

It is full to 5cm below the rim.

Each cubic centimetre of water weighs 1g. Each cubic centimetre of water is 1 ml

5. The tank itself weighs 20kg and the gravel in the tank weighs 30kg. Kian has filled his tank with water as described and will be adding accessories and fish weighing a few kg. What strength display cabinet should Kian buy as a minimum?

A. Up to 200kg
B. Up to 250kg
C. Up to 300kg
D. Up to 350kg
E. Up to 400 kg

6. The fish shop told Kian that he should allow 2 litres per small fish, 4 litres per medium fish and 10 litres per large fish. What's the maximum number of fish Kian could have in his tank?

A. 24
B. 62
C. 123
D. 123.75
E. 124

7. Kian buys a heater which can heat 100 litres of water up by 1 degree centigrade every hour. It will take 15 hours for this tank to reach 25 degrees. What is its current temperature?

A. 6 degrees
B. 10 degrees
C. 19 degrees
D. 21 degrees
E. 24 degrees

8. Kian must allow 4 litres of water per medium fish and 10 litres per large fish. He wants equal numbers of just medium and large fish. What number of each will he have?

A. 17
B. 20
C. 34
D. 17 and 19
E. 18 and 16

Quantitative Reasoning Mini Mock – Revision

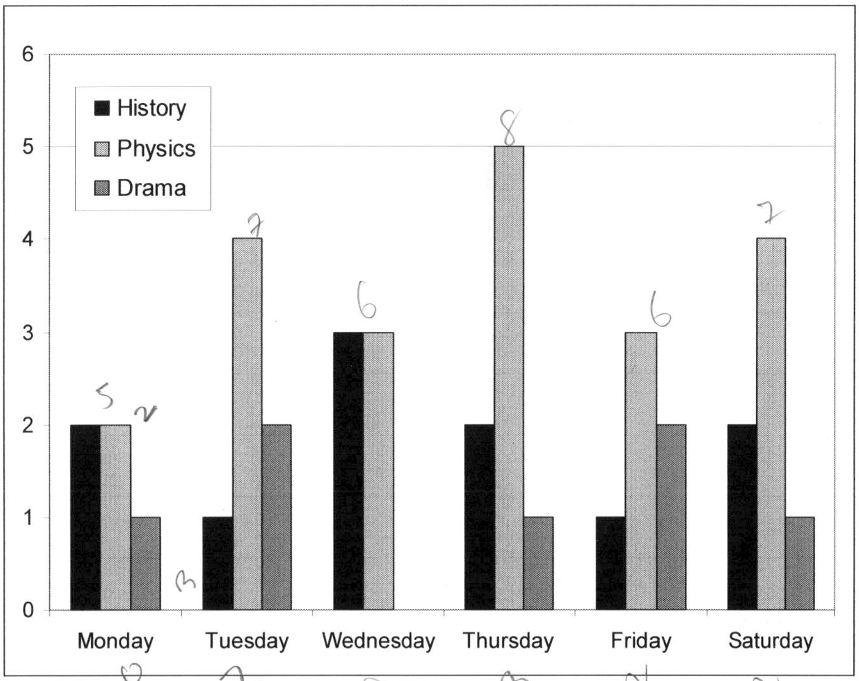

Ethan is revising for his A level exams.

This graph shows the number of hours he revises, in each subject, during one week of study leave.

He does his drama revision at school with his classmates and the other subjects at home.

9. What is the mean number of hours per day Ethan spends revising during the time period shown?

A. 5.6 hours
B. 6 hours
C. 6.5 hours
D. 7 hours
E. 8 hours

10. Ethan's school is a 45-minute journey away. Whilst travelling he listens to drama podcasts in addition to the revision time shown on the graph. How many hours drama revision has Ethan done?

A. 7 hours
B. 10 hours, 45 minutes
C. 14 hours, 30 minutes
D. 14 hours, 50 minutes
E. 16 hours

11. On Wednesday Ethan starts revising at 10am. He works in one-hour time slots. He wants to finish work at 8pm. How long is his average break between revision hours?

A. 48 minutes
B. 40 minutes
C. 30 minutes
D. 24 minutes
E. 20 minutes

12. How much more time does Ethan spend revising Physics compared to History?

A. 60%
B. 70%
C. 80%
D. 90%
E. 100%

Abstract Reasoning Mini Mock – 4 ½ minutes Answers on page 69

Set A

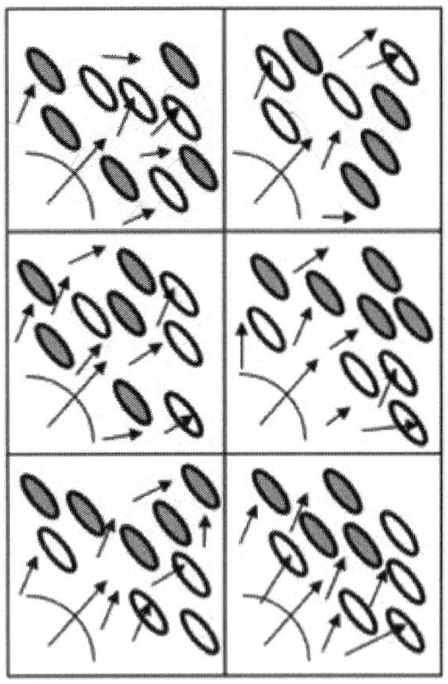

Set B

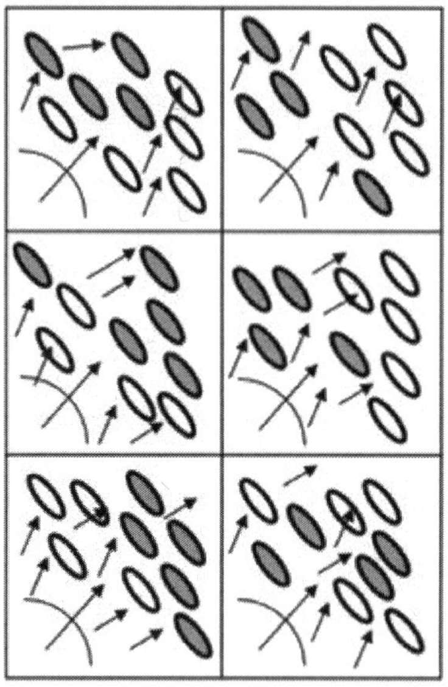

1 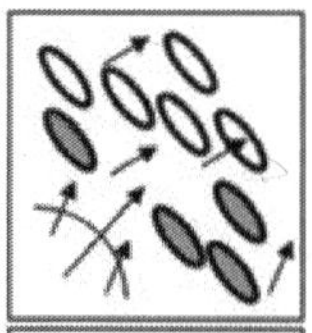
Set A
Set B
Neither

2 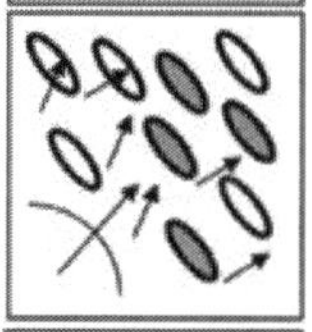
Set A
Set B
Neither

3 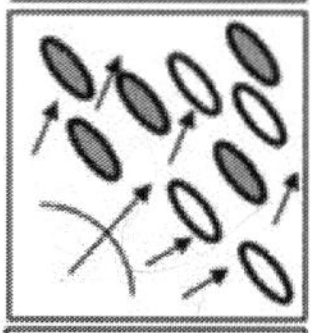
Set A
Set B
Neither

4 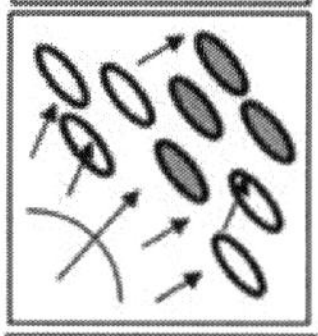
Set A
Set B
Neither

5 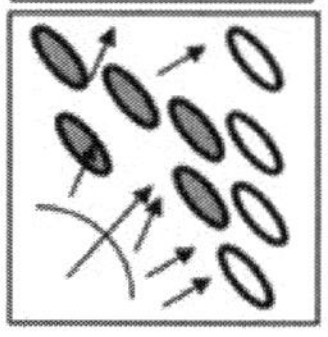
Set A
Set B
Neither

To which of the two sets do the following shapes belong?

6 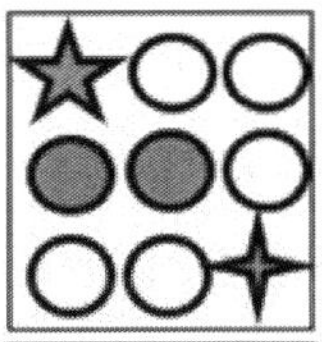
Set A
Set B
Neither

7 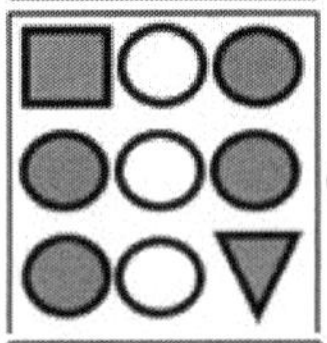
Set A
Set B
Neither

8 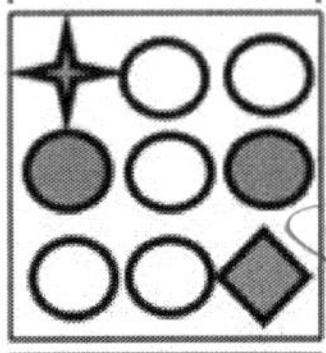
Set A
Set B
Neither

9 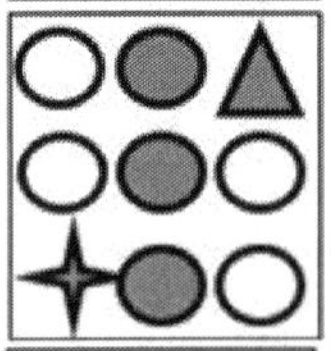
Set A
Set B
Neither

10 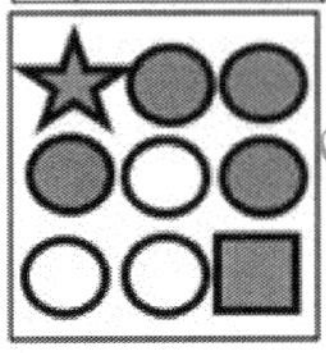
Set A
Set B
Neither

Set A

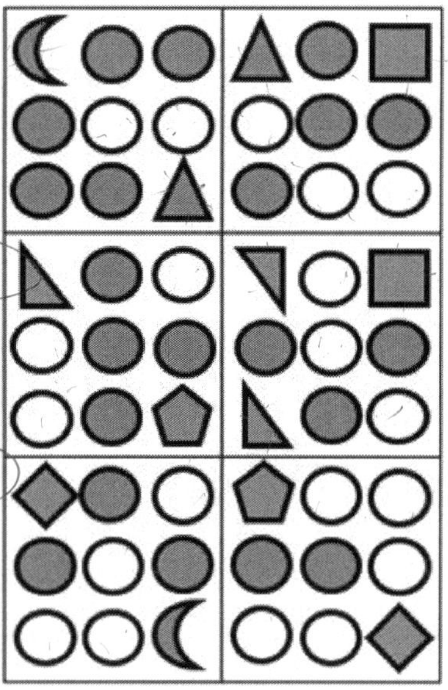

Set B

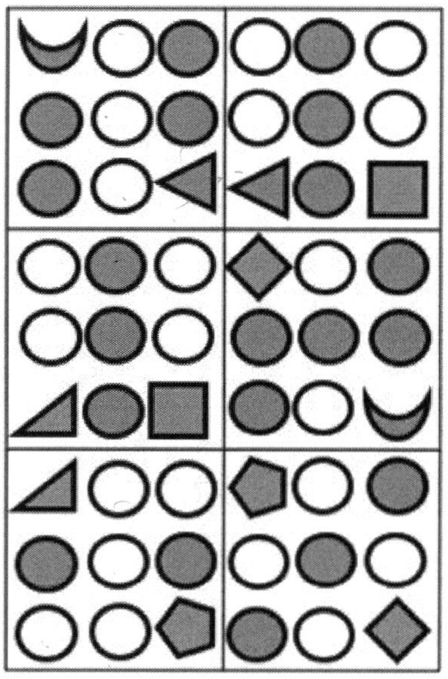

Set A | Set B

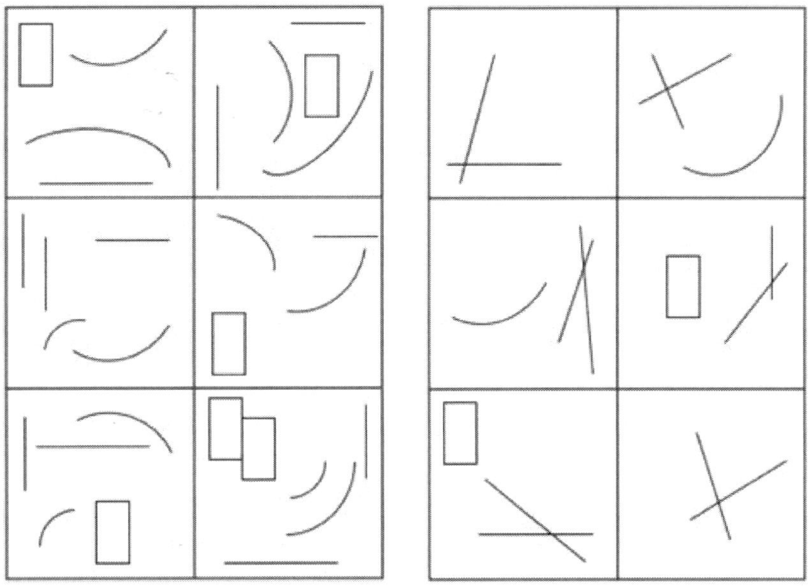

To which of the two sets do the following shapes belong?

11

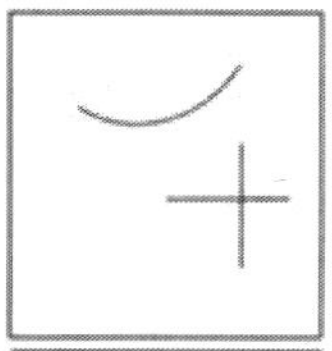

Set A
Set B
Neither

12

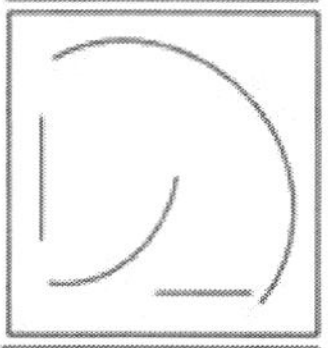

Set A
Set B
Neither

13

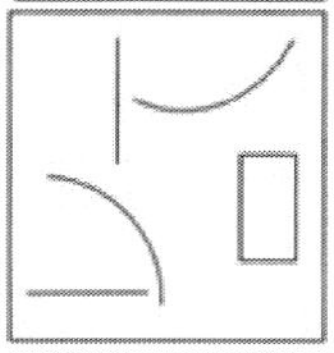

Set A
Set B
Neither

14

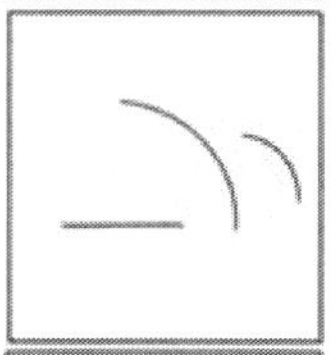

Set A
Set B
Neither

15

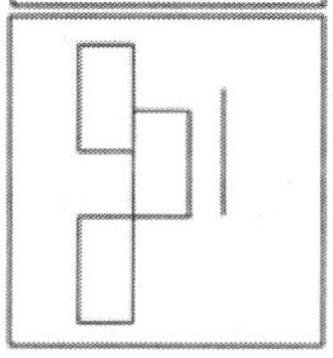

Set A
Set B
Neither

16

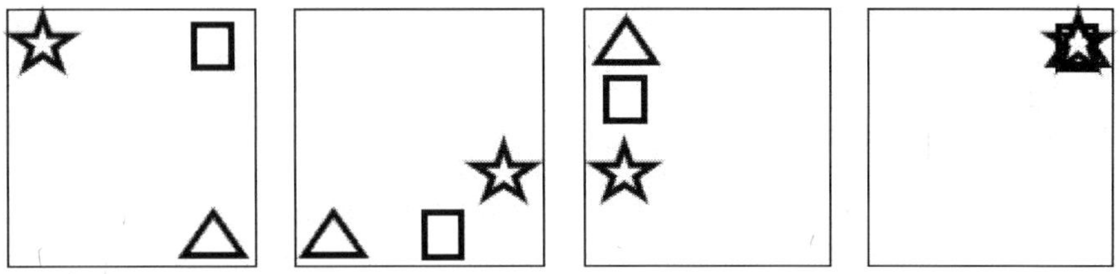

Which figure completes the series?

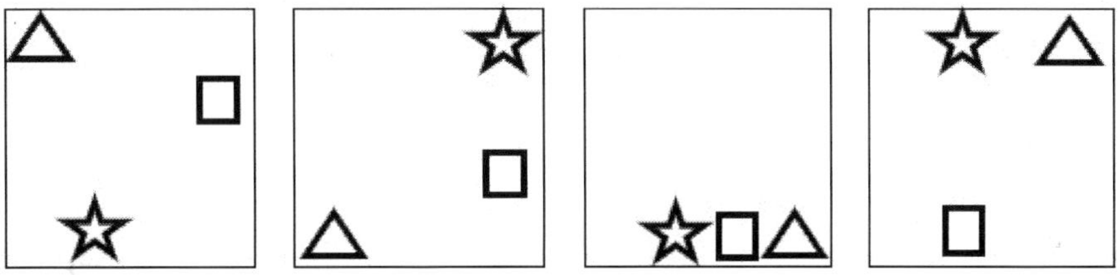

A | B | C | D

17

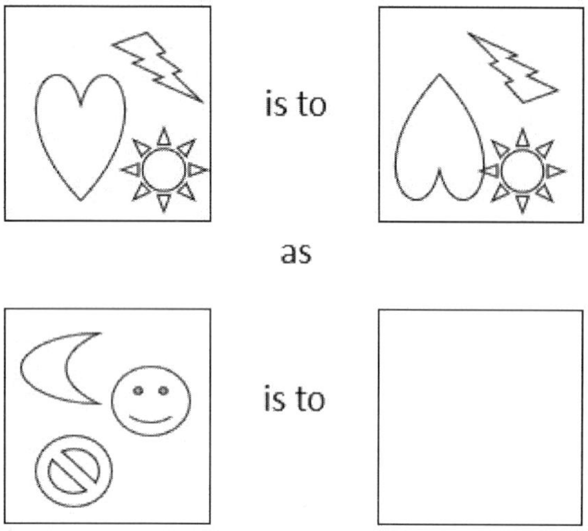

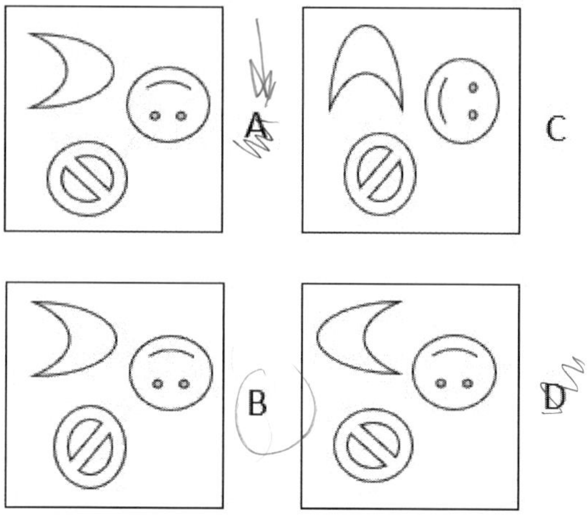

18

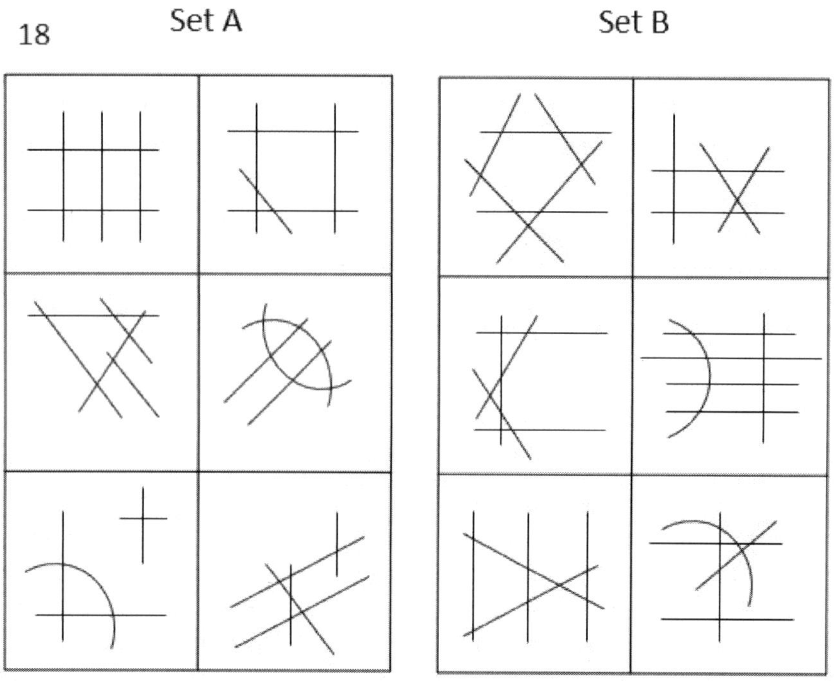

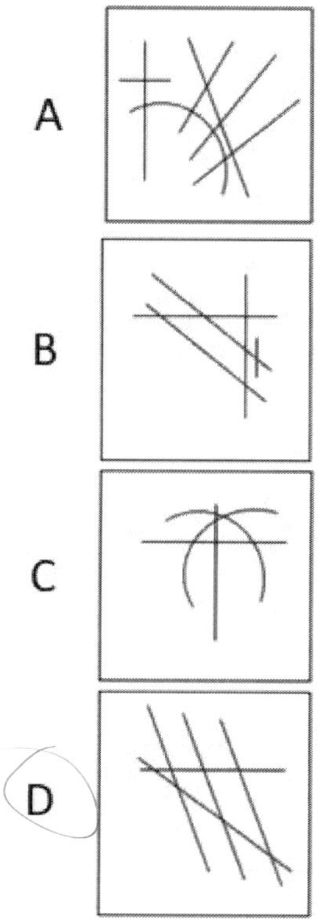

Which of the shapes belongs in Set B?

Situational Judgement Mini Mock – 8 minutes. Answers on page 70

Naomi is doing work experience in a nursery. She spends the day caring for a child with severe physical disabilities. When the child is collected from nursery at the end of the day she realises that it is the daughter of her former Maths teacher who left the school last year.

How important are the following considerations?

1. Naomi has not signed any confidentiality agreement as a nursery worker

   A. Very important
   B. Important
   C. Of minor importance
   D. Not important at all

2. Some of Naomi's friends would be interested to know how their old teacher is getting on

   A. Very important
   B. Important
   C. Of minor importance
   D. Not important at all

3. The teacher may feel awkward

   A. Very important
   B. Important
   C. Of minor importance
   D. Not important at all

4. Naomi needs to write a post placement report which will be circulated at school

   A. Very important
   B. Important
   C. Of minor importance
   D. Not important at all

Edward is working in a paediatric ward. He gets to know long term patient, an 8-year-old boy – Finley - who is very keen on football. He supports the traditional rival team to Edward and the two enjoy a great deal of 'banter' regarding football. There is a big match one weekend and Edward's team win convincingly. Edward goes into work on the Monday.

How appropriate are the following actions by Edward?

5. Make some cheering noises when he sees Finley.

   A. Very appropriate
   B. Appropriate but not ideal
   C. Inappropriate but not awful
   D. Very inappropriate

6. Remark that it was a good game and that his team were lucky

   A. Very appropriate
   B. Appropriate but not ideal
   C. Inappropriate but not awful
   D. Very inappropriate

7. Don't mention football at all for a few days

A. Very appropriate
B. Appropriate but not ideal
C. Inappropriate but not awful
D. Very inappropriate

8. Wait for Finley to mention the match first

A. Very appropriate
B. Appropriate but not ideal
C. Inappropriate but not awful
D. Very inappropriate

Faiz is a med student. He has received a disappointing mark for his last exam and has to re-sit. He worked hard for the exam and doesn't know exactly where he should concentrate his efforts.

How important are the following considerations?

9. If you work hard and still fail it may be evidence that you're not up for the task

A. Very important
B. Important
C. Of minor importance
D. Not important at all

10. University staff will be able to direct students for good exam preparation

A. Very important
B. Important
C. Of minor importance
D. Not important at all

11. Effective study is a lifelong skill

A. Very important
B. Important
C. Of minor importance
D. Not important at all

12. Not many other people failed this exam

A. Very important
B. Important
C. Of minor importance
D. Not important at all

Susie is a student doctor. She has to hand in an assignment the following morning and plans to buy printer ink on the way home from a shift in hospital. The shift becomes very busy and she ends up staying a lot later than planned and knows she will not be able to buy her cartridge and thus not be able to print out her assignment. She has the assignment on a memory stick.

How appropriate are the following courses of action for Susie?

13. Quietly print out her assignment using a hospital computer and printer

A. Very appropriate
B. Appropriate but not ideal
C. Inappropriate but not awful
D. Very inappropriate

14. Ask a senior staff member if she can print her assignment as she has stayed late

A. Very appropriate
B. Appropriate but not ideal
C. Inappropriate but not awful
D. Very inappropriate

15. Get up early the following morning and go and buy a printer cartridge

A. Very appropriate
B. Appropriate but not ideal
C. Inappropriate but not awful
D. Very inappropriate

16. Call a friend and ask if she can drop in and use her printer

A. Very appropriate
B. Appropriate but not ideal
C. Inappropriate but not awful
D. Very inappropriate

Luca is a junior doctor and a keen user of Twitter. He has set his account to be as anonymous as possible and has not included his doctor status in his bio, nor does he have a personal photograph on the site. One evening, he has a long Twitter conversation with someone. He suddenly realises that it is one of his current patients.

How important are the following considerations?

17. This interaction was entirely coincidental

A. Very important
B. Important
C. Of minor importance
D. Not important at all

18. It would be impolite and unkind to abruptly terminate the conversation

A. Very important
B. Important
C. Of minor importance
D. Not important at all

19. Luca has enjoyed the interaction

A. Very important
B. Important
C. Of minor importance
D. Not important at all

20. It is wise for doctors to be careful with their presence on online media sites

A. Very important
B. Important
C. Of minor importance
D. Not important at all

After the UCAT

Results

At the test centre you will receive a printed copy of your results immediately after completing the test.

Once you have submitted your UCAS application you need to give Pearson Vue the following information to allow your result to correctly be delivered to your chosen universities:

- 10-digit UCAS Personal Identification Number (PID)
- The university name and UCAS course code (e.g. A100) of all your choices that require the UCAT.

Pearson Vue will email you in mid-September asking you to provide this information. You will need your Pearson Vue account details to login and submit the information.

Pearson Vue will expect you to take responsibility for providing the correct and relevant details by the 16 October 2015 – the day after the deadline for submitting your UCAS form. If you fail to supply this information correctly it may delay the processing of your application to your chosen UCAT Universities. Results are sent only to universities in the UCAT consortium and usually go out in November.

You may only sit the UCAT once each year. If you try to sit it twice in the same test cycle, the later sitting will be automatically invalidated and the first result will be used.

Your result is valid for one year only, this means that if you end up reapplying in a subsequent year you will re-sit the UCAT in the next admissions year along with all your fellow applicants in that cycle.

When you present yourself for your test you declare that you are fit and well to take it and neither the UCAT Consortium nor Pearson VUE will make any adjustments to your scores for adverse circumstances, distress or illness. Adjustments or consideration of this kind is at the discretion of the university to which you have applied.

Before you apply to UCAS

Check the UCAT policies carefully for every institution which you're interested in. They often change – both in small and large ways – between, and even within, cycles and the only way to be absolutely sure your information is up to date is to look at their websites or telephone them.

The UCAT publish preliminary 'decile' information in September. If you take your test in the summer this enables you to get a rough idea of where your UCAT score places you amongst your cohort. If you haven't taken you test yet it gives you a definite target to aim for! Full decile information is published quite soon after the end of testing and often shows a slight decrease in scores as people who take the test earlier get slightly higher scores.

UCAT scores vary from season to season by a significant margin so 'thresholds' and 'cut offs' do as well. Your decile range is a better indicator than your actual score.

Apply to UCAS wisely – making the most of your academic scores, your UCAT, and your additional skills. Different institutions want different things – find the ones which want what you have!

Always double check but this is a snapshot of different universities:

Kings College London, Newcastle University and St Andrew's University have all had very high thresholds for UCAT – usually the top decile.

Candidates with a high UCAT may also want to consider Barts (Queen Mary), Nottingham University, Southampton University, Plymouth University and Warwick University. In recent years the average UCAT of their successful applicants has been high.

If your UCAT is slightly above average then institutions such as Dundee University, Sheffield University, St George's University, Leicester University, Manchester University, Exeter University, Glasgow University or Queen's College Belfast may be good places to consider. Each of them places some weight on the UCAT but other factors are also more highly weighted.

If your UCAT is broadly average then Aberdeen University, University of East Anglia, Hull York University and Edinburgh University all have previously only asked for a modest UCAT.

If your UCAT is below average, then it's worth remembering that Cardiff University only use UCAT in a tie break situation and Keele University only reject the lowest two deciles.

Alternatively, you can apply to universities which use an alternative entrance exam (BMAT or GAMSAT) which are Brighton and Sussex, Cambridge, Imperial, Leeds, Oxford, Swansea and UCL.

There are further universities which use no entrance exam at all – they are Buckingham, Lancaster and the London School of Hygiene.

And finally

The UCAT is hard work and it's a significant step on the road to becoming a doctor or a dentist. However, it is important to keep it in perspective! Finding the UCAT challenging is the norm. A poor (below average) UCAT score is the experience of 50% of those who enter it. Not getting a brilliant score on your UCAT is not the end of the world... it may not even be the end of your medical aspirations. It certainly is only a blip in the grand scheme of your life.

By all means prepare well and take it seriously – everything worthwhile in life requires this – but once you've done all you can do, accept that you have done all you could have done.

We at UCATprep.com wish you all the very best in your UCAT preparation, your test, your applications and your future careers. Please keep in touch – it's great to hear how people get on and makes our job very rewarding.

Mini Mock Answers Verbal Reasoning

Lake Taupo

1. Which of the following is not an impact of Taupo volcano's activities over the years?

The correct answer is D. Alterations in the shape of a landmass

There is nothing in the text to suggest the overall shape of any landmass has been affected by Taupo. All of the others are cited as effects of different eruptions and activities.

2. Which of the following represents a correct sequence of events?

The correct answer is C. Taupo began erupting, Hatepe eruption, humans populate New Zealand

We know Taupo began erupting around 300,000 years ago, the Hatepe eruption happened around 1,800 years ago before there were humans in New Zealand. Thus the population must have arrived since then. Option A is incorrect as the Taupo and Hatepe eruption are the same event. Option B is incorrect as the main eruption which continues to affect the landscape is the same as the Orunanui eruption. Option D is incorrect as we don't know when Australia first was populated by humans.

3. Which of the following is likely to be true?

The correct answer is B. Taupo has erupted around 300 times

We know that Taupo began erupting around 300,000 years ago and that there has been an average of an eruption every 1000 years. Option A is likely to be false as the figure given in the text is in km, not miles. Option C is false as the exact opposite is described in the text – if the magma didn't contain much gas a lava dome would form. Option D is incorrect – the Hatepe eruption was around 1800 years ago.

4. Which of the following statements is true?

The correct answer is B. No human has ever seen Taupo erupt

The latest eruption is stated as being 1800 years ago and the nearest human presence at that time is stated as having been in Australia which it turn is described as being well outside of visible range. Option A is false because the Orunanui eruption of the Taupo volcano was the world's largest known volcanic eruption for the last 70,000 years. It occurred around 26,500 years ago. Option C is an unknown as this statement only mentions Taupo and no inference of other volcanic activity can be drawn. Option D is false because a rhyolitic eruption will only cause the formation of pumice if gas is also present. The summary states that sometimes rhyolitic eruptions form a lava dome in the absence of gas.

Six Wheel Drive

5. Which of the following is probably not a manufacturer with a 6WD model in existence?

The correct answer is D. Alvis Saladin

It seems, from the text, that this is a model rather than a manufacturer. The others are clearly manufacturers. Pinzgauer is mentioned alongside what appears to be a model name (option A). Polaris Industries has a list of 6WD models mentioned in the text (option B). John Deere is described as having produced a 6WD model.

6. What is a main difference between production 6WD vehicles and conversions?

The correct answer is D. Conversions less complex in construction

The text states that conversions are a technically simpler construction. Option A is untrue – there is reference to the Australian army using Land Rover Defender conversions. Option B cannot be known – production vehicles with amphibious qualities are referred to but there is nothing to imply that conversions cannot also have these. Option C is also unknown – conversions are described as being 'widely made' but there is no information about the numbers of either type of 6WD vehicle nor of the proportions of each compared to the other.

7. What advantage seems likely to be gained by a six wheel drive vehicle?

The correct answer is C. Better performance on rugged terrain and off road

This is the only factor which can generally be deduced from the text – as the vehicles are described as being largely confined to off road and head-duty military vehicles. Option A cannot be supported by the text. Option B is only definitely true of one model of six wheel drive vehicle as described in the text. Similarly – option D is described as a feature in a few vehicles rather than an advantage generally.

8. Which of the following statements is untrue?

The correct answer is B. For on-road use the Alvis Saladin may be limited to use of the forward two axles only

Drive may be limited to the rear two axles for on-road use, not the forward two axles. Option A is true – the Alvis is described as having served with the British Army. Option C cannot be known as there are no definite rules referred to in the text. In vehicles with non evenly spaced axles it is said that steering may be done by the front pair of wheels, and in evenly spaced axle vehicles that steering may be done by two sets of axles. Option D is true as referred to at the beginning of the text.

Tobacco

9. Which of the following statements seems likely to be false?

The correct answer is C. Tobacco use is the main cause of premature death worldwide

The passage describes tobacco use as an important case of premature death worldwide, and the single most important preventable risk to human health in developed countries. The fact it is described as 'an' important rather than 'the most' important issue makes this statement likely to be false. Option A is true – both illness (morbidity) and death (mortality) are cited in the text. Option B seems likely to be true given that the United States Centre for Disease Control and Prevention emphasise health risk specifically to people in the developed world who use tobacco, rather than death which is a global problem. Option D is true – there are a number of diseases other than cancer mentioned in the text.

10. Which of the following is unlikely based on current trends?

The correct answer is B. Smoking could be eradicated in the US within 20 years

It took around 40 years for smoking to drop from 42% to 20.8%. It seems more likely that it will take another 40 years for either the percentage to halve again to around 10% or for a a further drop in use of around 20% of the population to zero. Option A seems likely given that the WHO estimate that in the 20th century there were 100 million tobacco caused deaths, and 5.4 million in 2004 alone. If the figures were static you would expect around 1 million deaths per year. Option C seems likely – an annual increase of 3.4% leads to doubling in 20-21 years. Option D also seems likely – if the number of deaths is going up but smoking levels are dropping in the developed world whilst rising in the developing world it is logical to deduce that the 3.4% annual increase in the developing world is greater than the drop / levelling in the developed world.

11. What is unlikely to be contributing to a change in the number of deaths in the world from tobacco use related disease?

The correct answer is C. A change in the location and resources of tobacco using people

We don't have information about the total numbers of people using tobacco – just that it's reducing in the developed world and increasing in the developing world – meaning that neither A or B can be known. Option D may have an impact but there is nothing about it in the text.

12. Which of the following statements is definitely true?

The correct answer is B. Tobacco use causes premature death.

Tobacco use is described as "an important cause of premature death worldwide." Option A cannot be known – there is mention of smoking being a major risk for the diseases but there is no warrant for saying it 'usually' leads to such diseases. Option C is also unknown, but likely to be false – the WHO estimates put tobacco related deaths at 5.4 million in 2004 alone and at 100 million over the course of the 20th century. Option D is false – the adult smoking rates in the United States were 42% in 1965 and 20.8% in 2006.

Decision Making

1. Not all members of a football team also play golf but members who play golf are married and some of these golfers also play cricket.

Square – married
Triangle – golf
Arrow - cricket

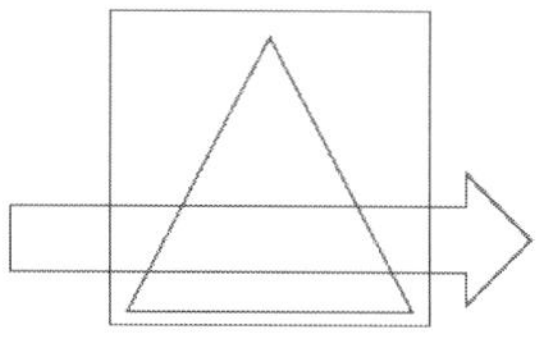

Some cricketers who are members of the football team also play golf.	**Yes**
Some golfers who are members of the football team are both married and play cricket.	**Yes**
All married members of the football team are either golfers or cricketers.	**No**
Not all married members of the football team who are golfers are cricketers.	**Yes**
All the cricketers who are members of the football team that are married also play golf.	**No**

2. E. There were 12 marks difference between Joe and Umar's test scores.

20	Martin
34	Umar
43	Priya
46	Joe
58	Alice

3. The government should produce legislation to limit the meat consumption of individuals in order to decrease the ecological damage caused by industrial farming?

Option C is the strongest argument as it addresses the supply and demand sides of the problem. Option A suggests 'everything they can' which does not stand up to scrutiny – executing half of the population would limit environmental damage but few governments or activists would suggest it as a strategy. Option B describes lessening demand but is vague about the scale of the problem and the potential impact of this solution. Option D is incorrect – the government already has food standards and regulations which are law.

4. Yoga is a form of exercise growing in popularity for people seeking to stay healthy in both body and mind. Improving balance, flexibility and strength, it can also be beneficial to people with high blood pressure or heart disease; not to mention the benefits to mental health. Yoga is a non-strenuous activity suitable for people of all ages and ability due to the large variety of classes available. Although it has been specifically recommended to older adults to help prevent falls.

Place 'Yes' if the conclusion does follow. Place 'No' if the conclusion does not follow.

Yoga has so many benefits, it should be used instead of some medicines. There is no suggestion that Yoga should replace anything else	No
Performing Yoga as part of a healthy active lifestyle can bring about many health improvements. This is clearly stated in the text	Yes
Only the elderly can benefit from the effects of yoga. The elderly are mentioned as a group who could benefit but not as the only group.	No
Yoga has gained popularity due to people wanting more natural treatment for ailments. The reasons mentioned are people seeking to stay healthy. The word 'natural' is not used at all.	No
Practicing Yoga will stop an elderly person having falls. There is a specific recommendation as it may help prevent falls – there is no guarantee.	No

5. Starting the school day at 10.30 or 11am and finishing later would enable teenagers to benefit more from school as the biological circadian rhythms in adolescence make concentration in the morning difficult.

A. Yes – a small change in school hours may make education more effective for teenagers

The best answer is option A. The preposition makes it clear that the aim is to enable teenagers to benefit more from their education and whilst option B may be true it does not answer the main point of the proposition. Option C assumes that all working roles have very fixed working hours. Option D says that a move like this would be 'pandering' whereas the proposition clearly states that the cause is biological.

6. The diagram shows features amongst various cars which are for sale.

Which of the following statements is true?

A. There are 27 cars with inbuilt satnav and exactly one additional feature.

7. Corner Shop A has 25 varieties of chocolate bar. Corner Shop B has 20 varieties of chocolate bar. Each day 20% of Corner Shop A's chocolate bars are out of stock and 10% of Corner Shop B's chocolate bars are out of

stock. The chance that any specific chocolate bar will go out of stock on any given day is 2 in 20 in Corner Shop A and 1 in 10 in Corner Shop B.

Considering only the number of chocolate bar varieties in each shop and the chance of varieties going out of stock, is Corner Shop B the better Shop to buy a chocolate bar from?

The correct answer is C as Corner Shop A has more variety of chocolate bar in stock each day and the chance of a specific chocolate bar going out of stock is the same in both corner shops.

8. Nancy is making tea for her four colleagues – Olivia, Peter, Rachel and Steve. She does so quite carefully as they all like their tea made differently – extra strong, extra weak, without milk or with sugar. And they each like their tea served in a specific mug.

C. The green mug contains tea with sugar

Peter or Rachel	Extra strong	Pink
Steve	Extra weak	Blue
Peter or Rachel	No milk	Black
Olivia	With sugar	Green

9. The shopping mall has thirty shops which all sell one kind of product. Half of the shops sell clothing of some sort. A third of the shops are independent and not part of a larger chain of shops. One tenth of the shops sell food and more than half of these are restaurants or cafes.

There are two restaurants Yes
There are three food outlets (10% of 30) and more than half are restaurants

There are no independent food outlets No
We don't know if any of the food outlets are part of the 10 independent shops

Two thirds of the shops are part of chains Yes
We know a third are independent so the other two thirds must be part of a chain

There are some chain stores selling clothes in the mall Yes
There are 20/30 chain stores in the mall and 15/30 clothes shops. There must be an overlap of at least 5 shops.

Half of the independent shops sell clothes No
We can't assume the ratio of independent shops is the same as the ratio of shop types.

All the students selected for this study were on the 50th centile in performance at the end of primary school All 50 students started on the 50th centile	Yes
Fewer than half of students made failed to progress in their studies Progress is not measured in centile level. A student making exactly average progress would remain on the same centile line.	No
More than half of the students made better progress than their peer group In this group more than half of the students moved up centile lines meaning they made better progress than the population they were being compared to.	Yes
The most highly achieving student here moved from the 50th to the 75th centile. They did not quite reach the 75th centile but got close.	No
Around a third of students moved down in the centile scale A minority of students were on a lower centile line at the end of the study	Yes

Quantitative Reasoning

	Assignment 1 15% of total	**Assignment 2 25% of total**	**Exam 60%**	**Total**	**Grade Boundaries**
Aman	70% 10.5%	57% 14.25%	50% 30%	**54.75% - 5**	9 **70%**
Bryony	66% 9.9%	70% 17.5%	60% 36%	**63.4% - 7**	8 **65%**
Cody	60% 9%	65% 16.25%	75% 45%	**70.25% - 9**	7 **60%**
Daljit	50% 7.5%	58% 14.5%	62% 37.2%	**59.2% - 6**	6 **55%**
Ellis	68% 10.2%	75% 18.75%	63% 37.8%	**66.75% - 8**	5 **50%**

1. The correct answer is C. Cody

The table above shows the marks per assessment once the weightings have been taken into account.

This question can also be estimated as Cody has a significantly higher scores than any other candidate in the exam which also has the highest weighting. The two assignments together still have a lower weighting than the exam and none of the other candidates scored so well in the assignments to counteract Cody's advantage in the exam.

2. The correct answer is A. Aman

Aman was only 0.25% off a grade 6. He is the only student where 0.5% would made a difference to their grade.

3. The correct answer is C. 71%

Bryony needed an extra 6.6% in total to reach the grade boundary of 70%. The exam has a weighting of 60% so every 1% increase in the exam score translates to an increase of 0.6% in the grading score. 6.6 divided by 0.6 = 11 so her raw exam score will need to be 11% higher to change her grading score by 6.6%.

Her original exam score was 60% and her she will have needed a score of 71% to be graded with an 9.

This is a question where you can again make an estimate. We can see Bryony's second assignment was at 9 level and her first assignment was at 8 grade level. We can guess, therefore, that she will need to get slightly above the 9 grade boundary to pull up her average. As the first assignment only counted for 15% of her total grade we can also guess that it will only have to be slightly above the grade boundary level. This means that it must be either options C or D.

4. The correct answer is D. One grade better

Aman would have got a 6 instead of a 5. All of the other students would have still got the same grade.

	Assignment 1 20% of total	**Assignment 2 20% of total**	**Exam 60%**	**Total**	**Grade Boundaries**
Aman	70% 14%	57% 11.4%	50% 30%	**55.4% - 6**	**9 70%**
Bryony	66% 13.2%	70% 14%	60% 36%	**63.2% - 7**	**8 65%**
Cody	60% 12%	65% 13%	75% 45%	**70.25% - 9**	**7 60%**
Daljit	50% 10%	58% 11.6%	62% 37.2%	**58.8% - 6**	**6 55%**
Ellis	68% 13.6%	75% 15%	63% 37.8%	**66.4% - 8**	**5 50%**

This is another question where applying some logic before doing any maths would be appropriate – it's clear that this change of policy would favour people who did better in the first assignment than the second. Aman was the only candidate for whom this was the case and you already know that he was close to the grade boundary from question 2 in this set. It would be detrimental to any candidate who did a lot better in assignment 2 than 1, but none of the others have a large difference – max 8%.

5. The correct answer is D. Up to 350kg

The tank and gravel weigh 50kg. Taking away the 5cm taken up by the gravel and the 5cm of empty space at the top the height of the water is 50cm. The water's volume can be calculated as 50cm x 110cm x 45cm = 247500cm3

Each cubic centimetre of water weighs 1gram, so the water will weigh 247.5kg.

247.5 + 50 = 297.5kg. The additional, but small, weights are likely to take it over 300kg so the 'up to 350kg' cabinet is likely to be a better option.

6. The correct answer is C. 123 fish.

The total amount of water in the tank equals 247.5 litres. Allowing for two litres per fish this means there could be 123.75 fish – but of course there's no such thing as 0.75 of a fish!

7. The correct answer is C. 19 degrees

We have already calculated that there is 247.5 litres of water in the tank and therefore the heater will take just under 2.5 hours to heat the whole tank up by 1 degree. In 15 hours the heater will heat the water 6 degrees meaning it must currently be 19 degrees.

8. The correct answer is A. 17

Kian will be able to fit in 17 large fish (170 litres) and 17 medium fish (68 litres). 170 + 68 = 238. This is less than the 247.5 litres of water in the tank.

Note that Kian wants equal numbers of medium and large fish so options D and E can immediately be excluded.

9. The correct answer is C. 6.5 hours

Ethan revised for 5, 7, 6, 8, 6 and 7 hours. The total hours are 39, which divided by the period shown (which is six days, not a full week) is 6.5 hours.

10. The correct answer is D. 14 hours, 30 minutes

Ethan spends 7 hours doing drama revision which we know takes places at school. His school is 45 minute journey away – 1.5 hours for both journeys. Ethan does not do any drama on Wednesday. 1.5 hours x 5 days = 7.5 hours. 7 hours + 7.5 hours = 14.5 hours (which is equal to 14 hours and 30 minutes).

11. The correct answer is A. 48 minutes.

Ethan revises for six hours on Wednesday and therefore has five breaks. His available work time is 10 hours, during which he will be working for six. The remaining four hours, when divided into five breaks, is 48 minutes.

12. The correct answer is D. 90%

Ethan spends 11 hours revising History and 21 revising Physics. This is approximately 90% more.

Abstract Reasoning

Question Set 1:

Set A: Two arrows have penetrated a white oval

Set B: One arrow has penetrated a white oval

1. Set B
2. Set A
3. Neither
4. Set A
5. Neither

Question Set 2:

Set A: The number of white spots matches the number of points on the top left hand shape

Set B: The number of white spots matches the number of points on the bottom right hand shape

6. Set A
7. Set B
8. Neither
9. Neither
10. Set B

Question Set 3:

Set A: There is always one horizontal line and two curved lines

Set B: There is always an intersection of two straight lines

11. Set B
12. Set A
13. Neither
14. Set A
15. Neither

Question 16:

The correct answer is C

Imagine there are twelve points around the edge of the square. All of the shapes are moving in a clockwise direction. The triangle moves three spaces, the square moves four and the star moves five spaces each time.

Question 17:

The correct answer is A.

All three shapes have done a 180 degree turn.

Question 18:

The correct answer is D

In Set A there are 6 intersections, in Set B there are 7 intersections

Situational Judgement

1. Naomi has not signed any confidentiality agreement as a nursery worker

The correct answer is D: Not important at all

Even if Naomi hasn't signed anything to say she agrees to keep the details of the children and families private it is common courtesy to do so

2. Some of Naomi's friends would be interested to know how their old teacher is getting on

The correct answer is C: Of minor importance

This consideration might help Naomi to make some small talk and put her old teacher at ease. Naomi can mention her friend's interest in her teacher's general wellbeing to gauge how the teacher might feel about her passing on details of their conversation. A more importance consideration might be how the teacher feels about sharing any details about her life.

3. The teacher may feel awkward

The correct answer is A: Very Important

Naomi has an opportunity to demonstrate her ability to act in a professional manner and put the teacher at ease. She could reassure them that this won't become playground gossip in a frank and polite manner and as a nursery worker she has responsibility for the wellbeing of the children and their families.

4. Naomi needs to write a post placement report which will be circulated at school

The correct answer is A: Very important

Naomi will need to be a more careful that her post placement report doesn't divulge unnecessary personal information given the previous relationship between the family and the school.

5. Make some cheering noises when he sees Finley.

The correct answer is D: A very inappropriate thing to do

It is important to remember this is an 8 year old boy and Edward is much older. Therefore any 'banter' between them must remain kind and respectful. It is likely Finley is upset about the result and Edward shouldn't try to make it worse.

6. Remark that it was a good game and that his team were lucky

The correct answer is A: A very appropriate thing to do

In softening the blow of a bad result Edward will build further rapport Finley which can only be a good thing.

7. Don't mention football at all for a few days

The correct answer is B: Appropriate but not ideal

Whilst this course of action avoids any potential upset it also will stall their rapport and good relationship.

8. Wait for the boy to mention the match first

The correct answer is A: A very appropriate thing to do

This is very patient centred and respectful. They can still chat about football more generally but it protects Finley from upset about his team's loss.

9. If you work hard and still fail it may be evidence that you're not up for the task

The correct answer is C: Somewhat important

A sober assessment of your capabilities is sometimes appropriate when you've tried your best and still failed. However – determination and resilience are key skills necessary for anyone who wants to pursue a challenging academic path and consequent career so giving up after one failure is a poor choice.

10. University staff will be able to direct students for good exam preparation

The correct answer is A: Very Important

Lecturers, professors and teachers all have lots of experience and knowledge and are likely to be very happy, and skilled, in helping students best realise their potential.

11. Effective study is a lifelong skill

The correct answer is A: Very important

Hard work is not always effective work. Learning to work effectively will be invaluable through all study, work and life.

12. Not many other people failed this exam

The correct answer is D: Not important at all

Faiz is only responsible for his own progress and should not compare himself to his colleagues. He may have done better in another exam which they struggled with.

13. Quietly print out her assignment using a hospital computer and printer

The correct answer is D: A very inappropriate thing to do

Susie has not asked anyone about this and is just going ahead. Whilst a bit of printer ink and some sheets of paper may seem like small things it is still inappropriate to use these things as they don't belong to her.

14. Ask a senior staff member if she can print her assignment as she has stayed late

The correct answer is C: Inappropriate but not awful

Susie has put her senior colleague in an awkward situation by asking if she can do this, particularly as she has phrased it the way she has. The senior colleague is likely to be grateful for Susie's help but may still not wish to allow her the use of hospital resources this way. However – at least Susie has asked rather than just helping herself.

15. Get up early the following morning and go and buy a printer cartridge

The correct answer is A: Very appropriate

This might inconvenience Susie a little but at least it means that she is not utilising anyone else's resources.

16. Call a friend and ask if she can drop in a use her printer

The correct answer is A: Very appropriate

Although this would mean Susie using someone else's paper and ink, because it is a friend rather than the hospital, it is far more likely she will be able to reciprocate at some point.

17. This interaction was entirely coincidental

The correct answer is A: Very important

As Luca has taken steps to keep his Twitter account anonymous it seems unlikely the patient could have deliberately sought him out so he need not feel guilty that this has happened.

18. It would be impolite and unkind to abruptly terminate the conversation

The correct answer is C: Somewhat important

What is most important is that Luca terminates the conversation one way or another. It might be hard to do this in a polite or kind way though, of course, it would be good to try.

19. Luca has enjoyed the interaction

The correct answer is D: Not important at all

As soon as Luca realised who he was in conversation with the enjoyment became irrelevant and Luca needs to take a professional position.

20. It is wise for doctors to be careful with their presence on online media sites

The correct answer is A: Very important

Naturally doctors are allowed to have a Facebook page, Twitter feed and Instagram account if they wish. They must, however, realise that their patients will also have these things and may seek them out. It is therefore wise for them to manage their privacy settings (and similar) quite carefully.

100 Verbal Reasoning Questions **(answers begin on page 96)**

Operation Arctic Fox was the codename given to a campaign by German and Finnish forces during World War II against Soviet Northern Front defences at Salla, Finland in July 1941. This Operation was part of a larger Operation called Operation Silver Fox (Silberfuchs) which aimed to capture the vital port of Murmansk. Artic Fox was conducted parallel to Operation Platinum Fox (Platinfuchs) in the far north of Lappland. The principal goal of Operation Arctic Fox was to capture the town of Salla and then to advance in direction of Kandalaksha, to block the route to Murmansk.

The offensive commenced on 1 July 1941 with the Finnish 6th Division crossing the border at midnight. Several hours later the 6th SS Mountain Division Nord started its frontal assault against the Soviet line. In the next days the SS Division tried repeatedly to break through the Soviet lines, but all attempts failed. It was not until the 169th Division supported the attack, that the Germans broke through the Soviet defences on 6 July and captured Salla. A heavy Soviet counterattack drove them back out of the town, but on 8 July a general Soviet retreat of the 122nd Rifle Division allowed the Germans to capture the town again. The Soviets had to leave most of their artillery behind and in the heavy fighting some 50 Soviet tanks were destroyed. Afterwards, the SS Division Nord pursued the 122nd Rifle Division toward Lampela, while the 169th Division turned toward Apa and the Lake Kuola.

During the successful advance of the Finnish forces in the south, XXXVI Corps also prepared for a new attack. At the beginning of August 1941, the Finnish 6th Division headed the renewed drive of the XXXVI Corps. The 169th Division followed. In the face of the new German thrust, the Soviets retreated to the Tuutsa River, lost Alakurtti and later withdrew to the Voyta River, where the old 1939 Soviet border fortifications were situated.

On 6 September XXXVI Corps made a frontal assault against the Soviet lines but made only slow progress. The Soviets now formed a strong defence line from Lake Verkhneye Verman to Tolvand. The German casualties were heavy, and the attack was finally called off at the end of September. With the Finns stopping their offensive in the south on 17 November 1941 too, this marked the end of Operation Arctic Fox.

1. Which of the following statements is most likely to be true?

   A. Operation Artic Fox was terminated after four months.
   B. The XXXVI Corps was unsuited, ill-trained and unprepared for arctic warfare and therefore made only small progress while suffering heavy casualties.
   C. The main objective of the operation Artic Fox was to capture the vital port of Murmansk.
   D. A total of three divisions played a part in Operation Artic Fox

2. According to the text, which of the following statements is false?

   A. The German 6th Division initiated the attack by crossing the border at midnight.
   B. During the Soviet retreat of the 122nd Rifle Division they had to leave most of their artillery behind
   C. With many attempts the SS division finally managed to break through the Soviet defences with no aid or support.
   D. The Soviets formed a strong defence along the Tuutsa River

3. Which of the following statements is mostly likely to be false?

   A. Salla was captured on the 6th July by the German troops.
   B. Two rivers were associated with the attack.
   C. The new attack in August 1941 was initiated by the Finnish 6th division.
   D. Operation Platinum Fox was known as (Silberfuchs)

4. Which of the following statements is true?

A. XXXVI Corps denotes to being six more than thirty
B. The German casualties were heavy so the attack was called off because of this.
C. Operation Platinum Fox (Platinfuchs) took place in Salla, Finland.
D. During the heavy fighting some 50 Soviet tanks were destroyed

Chocolate comprises a number of raw and processed foods including cacao from the seed of the tropical Theobroma cacao tree. Cacao has been cultivated for at least three millennia in Mexico, Central and South America, with its earliest documented use around 1100 BC. The majority of the Mesoamerican peoples made chocolate beverages, including the Aztecs, who made it into a beverage known as xocolatl, a Nahuatl word meaning "bitter water". The seeds of the cacao tree have an intense bitter taste and must be fermented to develop the flavour.

After fermentation, the beans are dried, cleaned, and roasted, and the shell is removed to produce cacao nibs. The nibs are then ground to cocoa mass, pure chocolate in rough form. Because this cocoa mass usually is liquefied then moulded with or without other ingredients, it is called chocolate liquor. The liquor also may be processed into two components: cocoa solids and cocoa butter. Unsweetened baking chocolate (bitter chocolate) contains primarily cocoa solids and cocoa butter in varying proportions. Much of the chocolate consumed today is in the form of sweet chocolate, combining cocoa solids, cocoa butter or other fat, and sugar. Milk chocolate is sweet chocolate that additionally contains milk powder or condensed milk. White chocolate contains cocoa butter, sugar, and milk but no cocoa solids (and thus does not qualify to be considered true chocolate).

5. Cacao is only grown in the Americas.

A. True
B. False
C. Can't tell

6. The Aztecs drank chocolate

A. True
B. False
C. Can't tell

7. Chocolate grows on trees.

A. True
B. False
C. Can't tell

8. White chocolate is not considered to be true chocolate because it contains cocoa butter.

A. True
B. False
C. Can't tell

Rapid ascent can lead to altitude sickness. The best treatment is to descend immediately. The climber's motto at high altitude is "climb high, sleep low", referring to the regimen of climbing higher to acclimatise but returning to lower elevation to sleep. In the South American Andes, the chewing of coca leaves has been traditionally used to treat altitude sickness symptoms.

Common symptoms of altitude sickness include severe headache, sleep problems, nausea, lack of appetite, lethargy and body ache. Mountain sickness may progress to HACE (High Altitude Cerebral Edema) and HAPE (High Altitude Pulmonary Edema), both of which can be fatal within 24 hours.

In high mountains, atmospheric pressure is lower and this means that less oxygen is available to breathe. This is the underlying cause of altitude sickness. Everyone needs to acclimatise, even exceptional mountaineers that have been to high altitude before. Generally speaking, mountaineers start using bottled oxygen when they climb above 7,000 metres. Exceptional mountaineers have climbed 8000m peaks (including Everest) without oxygen, almost always with a carefully planned program of acclimatisation.

Attempts to treat or stabilise the climber in situ can be dangerous unless highly controlled and with good medical facilities. For serious cases, or where rapid descent is impractical, a portable plastic hyperbaric chamber inflated with a foot pump can be used as an aid to evacuate. Pharmaceuticals such as acetazolamide may assist in acclimatization but is not a reliable treatment for altitude sickness and steroids can help with pulmonary edema, but again only to buy time to descend by treating a symptom.

9. Which of the following statements is not true:

A. Oxygen deprivation can cause headaches
B. Bottled oxygen can be used to help with altitude sickness
C. Exceptional climbers can climb without needing to acclimatise
D. HAPE can be fatal

10. Which of the following statements is not true:

A. Mild symptoms of altitude sickness may be confused with general physical tiredness on a difficult climb
B. Traditional remedies may mask some of the symptoms of altitude sickness
C. Acclimatisation must be achieved by all climbers
D. The 'climb high, sleep low' regimen will always prevent altitude sickness

11. Which of the following statements best describes altitude sickness

A. A mild series of symptoms that can be alleviated by descending down the mountain
B. Less oxygen is available resulting in a varied range of symptoms
C. Is caused by climbers being ill-prepared and not carrying bottled oxygen
D. Is caused by higher atmospheric pressure meaning less oxygen is available to breathe

12. Which of the following statements is most likely to be true:

A. Descending safely and quickly is the only treatment for altitude sickness
B. Treating the patient in situ is safer than trying to move them while they are suffering from the symptoms of altitude sickness
C. The use a portable hyperbaric chamber increases the oxygen levels and allows the climber to continue on
D. Steroids treat the underlying cause of altitude sickness

The Himalayas are among the youngest mountain ranges on the planet and consist mostly of uplifted sedimentary and metamorphic rock. According to the modern theory of plate tectonics, their formation is a result of a continental collision or orogeny along the convergent boundary between the Indo-Australian Plate and the Eurasian Plate. The Arakan Yoma highlands in Myanmar and the Andaman and Nicobar Islands in the Bay of Bengal were also formed as a result of this collision.

During the Upper Cretaceous, about 70 million years ago, the north-moving Indo-Australian Plate was moving at about 15 cm per year. About 50 million years ago, this fast moving Indo-Australian plate had completely closed the Tethys Ocean, the existence of which has been determined by sedimentary rocks settled on the ocean floor, and the volcanoes that fringed its edges. Since both plates were composed of low density continental crust, they were thrust faulted and folded into mountain ranges rather than subducting into the mantle along an oceanic trench. An often-cited fact used to illustrate this process is that the summit of Mount Everest is made of marine limestone from this ancient ocean.

Today, the Indo-Australian plate continues to be driven horizontally below the Tibetan plateau, which forces the plateau to continue to move upwards. The Indo-Australian plate is still moving at 67 mm per year, and over the next 10 million years it will travel about 1,500 km into Asia. About 20 mm per year of the India-Asia convergence is absorbed by thrusting along the Himalaya southern front. This leads to the Himalayas rising by about 5 mm per year, making them geologically active. The movement of the Indian plate into the Asian plate also makes this region seismically active, leading to earthquakes from time to time.

During the last ice age, there was a connected ice stream of glaciers between Kangchenjunga in the east and Nanga Parbat in the west. In the west, the glaciers joined with the ice stream network in the Karakoram, and in the north, joined with the former Tibetan inland ice. To the south, outflow glaciers came to an end below an elevation of 1,000-2,000 metres (3,300-6,600 ft). While the current valley glaciers of the Himalaya reach at most 20 to 32 kilometres (12 to 20 mi) in length, several of the main valley glaciers were 60 to 112 kilometres (37 to 70 mi) long during the ice age. The glacier snowline (the altitude where accumulation and ablation of a glacier are balanced) was about 1,400-1,660 metres (4,590-5,450 ft) lower than it is today. Thus, the climate was at least 7.0 to 8.3 °C (12.6 to 14.9 °F) colder than it is today.

13. Which of the following statements is true?

A. The mountain was formed along the convergent boundary, with the Indo-Australian Plate subducting below the Eurasian Plate
B. Sedimentary rocks settled on the ocean floor can determine that the Indo-Australian plate had completely closed the Tethys Ocean
C. The climate was at least 7.0 to 8.3 °C warmer than it is today
D. Nanga Parbat is in the North of Asia

14. Which of the following statements is most likely to be false?

A. The Himalayas are the youngest mountain ranges on the planet
B. During the Ice age, there was a connected ice stream of glaciers between Kangchenjunga and Nanga Parbat
C. Twenty to thirty-two kilometres is equivalent to twelve to twenty miles
D. As of the Himalayas rising by around 5 mm per year the area is geologically active

15. Which of the following statements is false?

A. The Arakan Yoma highlands were formed during the collision that created the Himalayas
B. Glaciers during the ice age were much longer in length than the ones of today
C. Three mountains are mentioned throughout the passage
D. The first recorded mountain formation was over 100 million years ago

16. Which of the following statements is most likely to be true?

A. The Himalayas are 10 km higher than any other recorded mountain
B. The Tibetan plateau plate continues to be driven horizontally below the Indo-Australian
C. The glacier snowline is the altitude where accumulation and ablation of a glacier are completely balanced
D. An oceanic trench is a long but narrow depression of the sea floor

Schistosomiasis (also known as bilharzia, bilharziosis or snail fever) is a parasitic disease caused by several species of fluke of the genus Schistosoma. Among human parasitic diseases, schistosomiasis ranks second behind malaria in terms of socio-economic and public health importance in tropical and subtropical areas. The disease is endemic in 74-76 developing countries, infecting more than 200 million people living in rural agricultural and peri-urban areas, half of whom live in Africa.

Of the infected patients, 20 million suffer severe consequences from the disease. Some estimate that there are approximately 20,000 deaths related to schistosomiasis yearly. In many areas, schistosomiasis infects a large proportion of children under 14 years of age. An estimated 600 million people worldwide are at risk from the disease.

A few countries have eradicated the disease, and many more are working toward it. The World Health Organization is promoting these efforts. In some cases, urbanization, pollution, and/or consequent destruction of snail habitat has reduced exposure, with a subsequent decrease in new infections. The most common way of getting schistosomiasis in developing countries is by wading or swimming in lakes, ponds and other bodies of water that are infested with the snails that are the natural reservoirs of the Schistosoma pathogen.

17. The Schistosoma genus contains several fluke species

A. True
B. False
C. Can't tell

18. Schistosomiasis is endemic in half the population of Africa

A. True
B. False
C. Can't tell

19. 20 million people in the world are infected with schistosomiasis

A. True
B. False
C. Can't tell

20. A few countries have eradicated schistosomiasis because of the World Health Organisation's efforts

A. True
B. False
C. Can't tell

All study designs involve some implicit (descriptive) or explicit (analytic) type of comparison of exposure and disease status. In a case report where a clinician observes a particular feature of a single case, a hypothesis is formulated based on an implicit comparison with the 'expected' or usual experience. In analytic study designs the comparison is explicit, since the investigator assembles groups of individuals for the specific purpose of systematically determining whether or not the risk of disease is different for individuals exposed or not exposed to a factor of interest. It is the use of an appropriate comparison group that allows testing of epidemiologic hypotheses in analytic study designs.

There are a number of specific analytic study design options that can be employed. These can be divided into two broad design strategies: observational and intervention. The major difference between the two lies in the role played by the investigator. In observational studies, the investigator simply observes the national course of events, noting who is exposed and not exposed and who has and has not developed the outcome of interest. In intervention studies, the investigator themselves allocates the exposure and then follows the subjects for the subsequent development of disease.

Taken from: Epidemiology in Medicine (1987) Hennekens, C.H. and Buring, J.E.

21. Which of the following is an interventional study?

A. A group of patients who have a disease are compared to a similar group of patients who do not have the disease
B. A group of people who are exposed to a factor are compared to a group of people who are not exposed to that factor
C. A group of people are allocated to an exposure or non-exposure group and followed up to see if that exposure causes a disease.
D. A group of patients with a disease are studied and the investigator looks at their previous exposure

22. Which of the following statements is false?

A. A comparison group is always needed for interventional study designs
B. Observational analytic studies may need to be carried out over a long period of time
C. A comparison group is always needed for analytic study designs
D. Analytic studies are based on an implicit comparison

23. Which of the following would be classed as an analytic study?

A. A case report on a patient who has developed a new type of cancer previously unseen in the group the patient belongs to
B. A comparison between per capita meat consumption and colon cancer among females in various countries
C. A survey that collects information about people's exposures and health status at certain points in time
D. A group of patients with bladder cancer and a group of patients without are interviewed to obtain information about artificial sweetener consumption in food and drink

24. Which of the following statements is true?

A. Descriptive studies test hypotheses
B. Descriptive studies help to develop hypotheses
C. Investigators always observe the natural course of events in analytic studies
D. Comparison groups are required for all types of descriptive studies

The Tanzanian economy is mostly based on agriculture, which accounts for more than half of the GDP, provides approximately 85 percent of exports, and employs approximately 80 percent of the workforce. Topography and climate, though, limit cultivated crops to only 4 percent of the land area.

Recent public sector and banking reforms, and revamped and new legislative frameworks have all helped increase private-sector growth and investment. Short-term economic progress also depends on curbing corruption.

25. 80% of people in Tanzania work in the export industry

A. True
B. False
C. Can't tell

26. 85% of agricultural produce is exported from Tanzania

A. True
B. False
C. Can't tell

27. An increase in cultivatable land would lead to an increase in exports

A. True
B. False
C. Can't tell

28. The recent banking and legislative reforms have helped curb corruption and hence helped increase private-sector growth and investment.

A. True
B. False
C. Can't tell

Antimicrobial Chemotherapy

The study of antimicrobial agents embraces not only antibacterial compounds but also antiviral, antifungal, antiprotozoal and even anthelminthic agents. The term chemotherapy is usually used more generally to include the use of anti-tumour drugs.

The term antibiotic strictly refers to naturally occurring products of one organism that are inhibitory to others. According to this definition, chemical compounds such as sulphonamides, quinolones, nitrofurans and imidazoles should be referred to as chemotherapeutic agents. However, since some antibiotics can be manufactured synthetically while others are the products of chemical manipulation of naturally occurring antibiotics (semi-synthetic antibiotics) the distinction has become blurred and of doubtful value.

Antimicrobial substances that are too toxic to be used other than in topical therapy or for environmental decontamination are referred to as antiseptics or disinfectants.

29. Which of the following statements is false?

A. Antimicrobial agents is a term that encompasses a variety of compounds
B. Antimicrobial chemotherapy is the term given to the use of chemical agents to treat microbial pathogens
C. The term antibiotic used appropriately refers to naturally occurring compounds
D. Antimicrobials are always used internally

30. Which of the following statements is true?

A. Antimicrobials can be made by chemically altering natural compounds
B. Antimicrobials are all synthetically produced
C. Antibiotics are all synthetically produced
D. Antiseptics are used to treat tumours

31. Which of the following can antimicrobial chemotherapy not treat?

A. Viral disease
B. Bacteria
C. Cancerous tumours
D. Protozoal infection

32. Which of the below best describes antimicrobial agents?

A. A group of manufactured agents which inhibit bacteria
B. A group of naturally occurring agents which are inhibitory to infective organisms
C. A group of agents which inhibit viruses and bacteria
D. A group of synthetic agents which can be used to treat viruses and bacteria

The tiger (*Panthera tigris*) is a member of the Felidae family; the largest of the four "big cats" in the genus Panthera. Native to much of eastern and southern Asia, the tiger is an apex predator and an obligate carnivore. Reaching up to 3.3 metres (11 ft) in total length and weighing up to 300 kilograms (660 pounds), the larger tiger subspecies are comparable in size to the biggest extinct felids. Aside from their great bulk and power, their most recognisable feature is a pattern of dark vertical stripes that overlays near-white to reddish-orange fur, with lighter underparts. The most numerous tiger subspecies is the Bengal tiger while the largest subspecies is the Siberian tiger.

Highly adaptable, tiger habitats range from the Siberian taiga, to open grasslands, to tropical mangrove swamps. They are territorial and generally solitary animals, often requiring large contiguous areas of habitat that support their prey demands. This coupled with the fact that they are endemic to some of the more densely populated places on earth, has caused significant conflicts with humans. Of the nine subspecies of modern tiger, three are extinct and the remaining six are classified as endangered, some critically so. The primary direct causes are habitat destruction and fragmentation, and hunting.

Tigers are among the most recognisable and popular of the world's charismatic mega-fauna. They have featured prominently in ancient mythology and folklore and continue to be depicted in modern films and literature. Tigers appear on many flags and coats of arms, as mascots for sporting teams, and as the national animal of several Asian nations, including India.

33. All 'big cats' mentioned in the text belong to the genus *Panthera*

A. True
B. False
C. Can't tell

34. Siberian tigers are generally larger in size than Bengal tigers

A. True
B. False
C. Can't tell

35. In the natural world tigers can only survive in large open areas

A. True
B. False
C. Can't tell

36. Tigers have been popular mega-fauna since ancient times

A. True
B. False
C. Can't tell

HMAS Flinders named for Matthew Flinders (1774-1814), was a hydrographic survey ship of the Royal Australian Navy (RAN).

The ship was ordered in 1970 to replace the light survey vessel HMAS Paluma. Flinders was 161 feet (49 m) in length overall, with a beam of 33 feet (10 m), a draught of 12 feet (3.7 m), and a full load displacement of 740 tons. Propulsion was provided by two Paxman Ventura diesel motors connected to twin screws, providing a top speed of 13.5 knots (25.0 km/h; 15.5 mph) and a range of 5,000 nautical miles (9,300 km; 5,800 mi) at 9 knots (17 km/h; 10 mph). The hull was all-welded and designed to Australian Shipping Board standards for coastal operations. Increased seakeeping ability was imparted through a bulbous bow, high forecastle, and a stabilising system. Most operations were intended to be in the waters of Australia and Papua New Guinea, although Flinders was also capable of limited oceanographic work. The ship's company consisted of 38 personnel, and Flinders carried light-calibre weapons for self-defence. Flinders was laid down by HMA Naval Dockyard at Williamstown, Victoria on 11 June 1971. She was launched on 29 July 1972 and commissioned into the RAN on 27 April 1973. On commissioning, the ship was based in Cairns.

Following the destruction of Darwin by Cyclone Tracy during the night of 24-25 December 1974, Flinders was deployed as part of the relief effort; Operation Navy Help Darwin. She sailed from Cairns on 26 December, and as the first ship to arrive, Flinders was tasked with surveying the harbour to work out the position of wrecks and the safest areas for the other RAN ships to anchor.

Flinders was decommissioned in 1998. In October 1999, the ship was sold at auction for A$518,460 to a New Zealand consortium. She was remodelled into a private yacht, and now operates at MY Plan B, registered in the Cayman Islands.

37. Which of these statements is most likely to be true?

A. Flinders was launched 27 April 1972 and commissioned 29 July 1972
B. Her first base after commissioning was Darwin
C. Flinders was built at Williamstown, NSW
D. Flinders carried a crew of 38

38. Which of these statements is true?

A. Flinders replaced HMS Paluma
B. The hull was welded in line with international standards for coastal operations
C. 13.5 knots is more than 12 knots
D. Flinders was part of the relief force sent to Darwin after Cyclone Theresa

39. Which of these statements is false?

A. Flinders was decommissioned in October 1999
B. She was sold for over half a million Australian dollars to a New Zealand group
C. She is now registered in the Cayman Islands as a private yacht
D. She was in service with RAN for approx. 25 years

40. Which of these statements is likely to be false?

A. Flinders was not expected to work outside Australian coastal areas
B. Flinders conducted a survey of Darwin harbour in December 1974
C. A nautical mile is longer than a land mile
D. By keeping to a speed of 9 knots, Flinders could extend her range to 5,000 nautical miles

Space is the boundless three-dimensional extent in which objects and events have relative position and direction. Physical space is often conceived in three linear dimensions, although modern physicists usually consider it, with time, to be part of a boundless four-dimensional continuum known as space time. In mathematics, "spaces" are examined with different numbers of dimensions and with different underlying structures. The concept of space is considered to be of fundamental importance to an understanding of the physical universe. However, disagreement continues between philosophers over whether it is itself an entity, a relationship between entities, or part of a conceptual framework.

Debates concerning the nature, essence and the mode of existence of space date back to antiquity; namely, to treatises like the Timaeus of Plato, or Socrates in his reflections on what the Greeks called khora (i.e. "space"), or in the Physics of Aristotle (Book IV, Delta) in the definition of topos (i.e. place), or even in the later "geometrical conception of place" as "space qua extension" in the Discourse on Place (Qawl fi al-Makan) of the 11th-century Arab polymath Alhazen. Many of these classical philosophical questions were discussed in the Renaissance and then reformulated in the 17th century, particularly during the early development of classical mechanics. In Isaac Newton's view, space was absolute-in the sense that it existed permanently and independently of whether there were any matter in the space. Other natural philosophers, notably Gottfried Leibniz, thought instead that space was in fact a collection of relations between objects, given by their distance and direction from one another. In the 18th century, the philosopher and theologian George Berkeley attempted to refute the "visibility of spatial depth" in his Essay Towards a New Theory of Vision. Later, the metaphysician Immanuel Kant said neither space nor time can be empirically perceived, they are elements of a systematic framework that humans use to structure all experiences. Kant referred to "space" in his Critique of Pure Reason as being: a subjective "pure a priori form of intuition", hence it is an unavoidable contribution of our human faculties.

In the 19th and 20th centuries mathematicians began to examine non-Euclidean geometries, in which space can be said to be curved, rather than flat. According to Albert Einstein's theory of general relativity, space around gravitational fields deviates from Euclidean space. Experimental tests of general relativity have confirmed that non-Euclidean space provides a better model for the shape of space.

41. Which of the following statements is false?

A. Physical space is often conceived in four linear dimensions
B. Space existed permanently and independently of whether there were any matters in the space through the eyes of Isaac Newton
C. George Berkeley was an established philosopher
D. Tests have confirmed that non-Euclidean space is a better model than Euclidean space for the shape of space

42. Which of the following statements is most likely to be true?

A. George Berkeley Essay on Towards a New Theory of Vision was his most famous work to date
B. Space can only be seen as subjective
C. Five treaties are mentioned in the passage
D. Albert Einstein completed a theory of general relativity

43. Which of the following statements are true?

A. Physical space is always conceived in three linear dimensions
B. Greeks knew space as khora
C. There was no evidence of space before the 10th century
D. Two entities make up space as we know it

44. Which of the following statements is most likely to be false?

A. Philosophers have found more evidence about space than mathematicians
B. Gottfried Leibniz was a natural philosopher
C. In mathematics, "spaces" are examined with different numbers of dimensions and with different underlying structures
D. Immanuel Kant was a metaphysician

Retroviruses are an important group of RNA viruses with single-stranded positive sense RNA (ssRNA) genomes. The group includes human immunodeficiency virus (HIV). Retroviruses contain two copies of the genome in each viral particles. On infection of a host cell, the ssRNA enters the cell, is converted to a double-stranded DNA copy by reverse transcriptase and is integrated into the host cell genome by a viral integrase enzyme. The integrated form is known as a provirus and acts as the template for replication of the viral genome and expression of the viral genes. The genomes of retroviruses have structural similarities and some sequence homology with sequence elements present in the human genome called retrotransposons. Retroviruses vary in complexity. Some are extremely simple and differ from retrotransposons essentially only by having an env gene that encodes envelope glycoproteins required for infectivity. Others, such as HIV, have larger genomes with more complex life cycles, encode proteins that are active at different stages of the replication cycle and are involved in regulating both viral and cellular functions.

Some retroviruses are known to cause cancer in animals although they are linked only rarely to human cancers. These retroviruses are said to be oncogenic and frequently carry a gene called an oncogene which was originally acquired from the host cell genome by recombination with the viral genome. Oncogenes encode proteins involved in regulating cell growth and have cellular counterparts called proto-oncogenes. Expression of the oncogene following viral infection results in uncontrolled cell division associated with the formation of a tumour.

45. Identify the true statement below:

A. Retroviruses are a type of virus that have double stranded DNA genomes
B. Retroviruses are a type of virus that have double-stranded RNA genomes
C. Retroviruses are a type of viruses that have single-stranded RNA genomes
D. Retroviruses have a single copy of their genome in their cells.

46. Which of the following sequences is correct?

A. ssRNA is converted into dsRNA by reverse transcriptase and combined into the host genome by integrase
B. ssRNA is converted into dsDNA by reverse transcriptase and combined into the host genome by integrase
C. ssDNA is combined into the host genome by integrase after being converted from ssRNA by reverse transcriptase
D. dsDNA is combined into the host genome by integrase after being converted from dsRNA by reverse transcriptase

47. All of the following statements are true except:

A. Retroviruses carry two copies of their genome in their cells
B. Retroviruses can cause cancer
C. Retroviruses contain their own enzymes
D. Retroviruses only use the host cell enzymes

48. Retroviruses can cause cancer:

A. By encoding proteins involved in regulating cell growth, infection results in unrestrained cell death
B. By encoding proteins involved in regulating cell growth, infection results in unrestrained cell division
C. By recombining with the host cell genome and causing uncontrolled cell death
D. By recombining with the host cell genome and multiplying in the host cell causing a tumour

Language is the human capacity for acquiring and using complex systems of communication, and a language is any specific example of such a system. The scientific study of language is called linguistics.

Estimates of the number of languages in the world vary between 6,000 and 7,000. However, any precise estimate depends on a partly arbitrary distinction between languages and dialects. Natural languages are spoken or signed, but any language can be encoded into secondary media using auditory, visual, or tactile stimuli - for example, in graphic writing, braille, or whistling. This is because human language is modality-independent. When used as a general concept, "language" may refer to the cognitive ability to learn and use systems of complex communication, or to describe the set of rules that makes up these systems, or the set of utterances that can be produced from those rules. All languages rely on the process of semiosis to relate signs with particular meanings. Oral and sign languages contain aphonological system that governs how symbols are used to form sequences known as words ormorphemes, and a syntactic system that governs how words and morphemes are combined to form phrases and utterances.

Human language has the properties of productivity, recursivity, and displacement, and relies entirely on social convention and learning. Its complex structure affords a much wider range of expressions than any known system of animal communication. Language is thought to have originated when early hominins started gradually changing their primate communication systems, acquiring the ability to form a theory of other minds and a shared intentionality. This development is sometimes thought to have coincided with an increase in brain volume, and many linguists see the structures of language as having evolved to serve specific communicative and social functions. Language is processed in many different locations in the human brain, but especially in Broca's and Wernicke's areas. Humans acquire language through social interaction in early childhood, and children generally speak fluently when they are approximately three years old. The use of language is deeply entrenched in human culture. Therefore, in addition to its strictly communicative uses, language also has many social and cultural uses, such as signifying group identity, social stratification, as well as social grooming and entertainment.

Languages evolve and diversify over time, and the history of their evolution can be reconstructed by comparing modern languages to determine which traits their ancestral languages must have had in order for the later developmental stages to occur. A group of languages that descend from a common ancestor is known as a language family.

49. All of the following are true except:

A. There are more than 10,000 different languages
B. Language is a form of communication
C. Evolution has played a part in the changes seen in language
D. Human language relies entirely on social convention and learning

50. According to the text which of the statements is true?

A. Only humans can communicate
B. Language originated when early hominins started gradually changing their primate communication systems
C. All languages rely on aphonological systems
D. Social grooming and entertainment lead to humans communicating between each other more

51. All of the statements are true except:

A. The scientific study of language is called linguistics
B. Language is processed in many different locations in the human brain, but especially The Broca's and Wernicke's areas of the brain process language
C. A group of languages that descend from a common ancestor is known as a barrier family
D. Linguists see the structures of language as having evolved to serve specific communicative and social functions

52. All of the statements are true except:

A. Natural language can be transformed into secondary media
B. Children generally speak fluently when they are approximately two years old
C. Language has uses in group identity and social stratification
D. Language is the human capacity for acquiring and using complex systems of communication

Cyprus elects at national level a head of state - the president - and a legislature. The election of the President is direct, by universal suffrage and secret ballot. Voting is compulsory and every citizen over the age of eighteen must vote, by law. The president is elected for a five year term by the people. The election of a new President takes place before the expiration of the five-year period of office of the outgoing President so as to enable the newly-elected President to be invested on the date that period expires.

Candidates for election must be citizens of the Republic of Cyprus and over thirty five years of age. If there is only one candidate for election, he is declared elected. For a candidate to be elected he or she needs more than 50% of the votes validly cast. If none of the candidates attains the required majority the election is repeated on the corresponding day of the following week between the two candidates who received the greater number of votes. The candidate who receives the greatest number of votes at these repeated elections is deemed elected.

If there is a vacancy in the office of President, the vacancy is filled by a by-election taking place within a period not exceeding 45 days of the occurrence of such a vacancy. In the event of a temporary absence or incapacity of the President to perform his duties, the President of the House of Representatives acts for him.

53. Cyprus cannot be without a President or acting President for more than 45 days.

A. True
B. False
C. Can't tell

54. A thirty-four-year-old woman cannot run for President in Cyprus.

A. True
B. False
C. Can't tell

55. There is no Vice President in Cyprus

A. True
B. False
C. Can't tell

56. In Cyprus the presidential term is 6 years

A. True
B. False
C. Can't tell

To make bread, water is mixed with flour, salt and the leavening agent (usually baker's yeast). Other additions (spices, herbs, fats, seeds, fruit, etc.) are not needed to bake bread, but are often used. The mixed dough is then allowed to rise one or more times. A longer rising time results in more flavour, so bakers often "punch down" the dough and let it rise again. Then loaves are formed, and the bread is baked in an oven.

Many breads are made from a "straight dough", which means that all of the ingredients are combined in one step, and the dough is baked after the rising time. Also, dough can be made using a "pre-ferment", when the leavening is combined with some of the flour and water a day or so ahead of baking and allowed to ferment overnight. On the day of the baking, the rest of the ingredients are added, and the rest of the process is the same as that for straight dough. This produces a more flavourful bread with better texture. Many bakers see the starter method as a compromise between the highly reliable results of baker's yeast and the flavour and complexity of a longer fermentation. It also allows the baker to use only a minimal amount of baker's yeast, which was scarce and expensive when it first became available.

57. All of the following statements are true except:

A. To make bread, water, flour, salt and yeast are the minimum requirements
B. Sometimes the leaving agent and flour are combined in advance
C. Allowing part of the dough to ferment overnight effects the texture of the bread
D. Dough is always made by combining all the ingredients at the same time

58. According to the text what is the 'starter method'?

A. The method of adding extra ingredients to the original mix
B. The process of mixing dough, letting it rise, and then punching the dough down again
C. The process of making a 'pre-ferment' of yeast and flour
D. The method of using baker's yeast to make the bread rise

59. Which of the reasons below is not why is a pre-ferment used?

A. It makes the bread rise higher
B. It provides the bread with a better texture
C. It is less complex than using the traditional method of fermentation
D. It saves the bakers using too much baker's yeast

60. The following statements are all true except:

A. Other ingredients can be added to bread to produce different flavours
B. Baker's yeast is a reliable method of making bread rise
C. The straight dough method will be quicker than the 'starter method'
D. The longer the rising time of the dough, the less flavour is produced in the bread

Revesby Abbey was a Cistercian monastery located near the village of Revesby in Lincolnshire, England. When the monks arrived there was a pre-existing village on the site. The population was moved and the village was demolished save for the church of St. Laurence, which the monks initially retained for their own use. Over the latter part of the twelfth century a stone monastery was constructed on the site. There was a large church with a nave of seven bays, an aisled presbytery and numerous chapels. South of this stood the domestic buildings, arranged around two cloisters. This core was surrounded by gardens, fishponds, orchards, barns, guesthouses, stables, a farmyard and industrial buildings. A wall protected the monastic grounds and entry was controlled by gatehouses.

Very little is known of the internal history of the abbey, which seems to have been uneventful. Revesby had been given a fairly substantial endowment and hence had a comfortable income. In the thirteenth century the house was fairly prosperous, however, in the fourteenth century the monks were hit hard by government exactions, unpaid debts from the king, animal plagues that killed all the stock and barrenness of the abbey lands. In 1382 the abbey received an additional grant of property which may have gone some way towards alleviating the situation, but it is likely that the decline (not helped by mismanagement) continued though the fifteenth century.

In 1535 the abbey had an income of £287 (placing it among the middle ranks of its order). No records survive as to exactly how or when Revesby Abbey fell, but it is likely that the monks were compelled to give their house to the king in 1538 and compensated with pensions.

Very little of the abbey is visible today, though archaeologists have investigated some parts of the site. Earthworks show where the abbey buildings lie buried and the site also has fishponds and moated enclosures that may be gardens. The remains are on farmland and are not open to the public.

61. The monks were given pensions when the abbey fell in 1538.

A. True
B. False
C. Can't tell

62. Revesby Abbey had domestic buildings arranged around three cloisters

A. True
B. False
C. Can't tell

63. At one time the Abbey had an income of £287

A. True
B. False
C. Can't tell

64. The stone monastery was constructed in the twelfth century

A. True
B. False
C. Can't tell

A collision avoidance system is an automobile safety system designed to reduce the severity of an accident. Also known as precrash system, forward collision warning system or collision mitigating system, it uses radar and sometimes laser and camera sensors to detect an imminent crash. Once the detection is done, these systems either provide a warning to the driver when there is an imminent collision or take action autonomously without any driver input (by braking or steering or both)

In 2009, the U.S. National Highway Traffic Safety Administration (NHTSA) began studying whether to make frontal collision warning systems and lane departure warning systems mandatory.

In 2011, a question was submitted to the European Commission regarding stimulation of these "collision mitigation by braking" systems. The mandatory fitting of Advanced Emergency Braking Systems in commercial vehicles will be implemented on 1 November 2013 for new vehicle types and on 1 November 2015 for all new vehicles in the European Union. This could, according to the impact assessment, ultimately prevent around 5,000 fatalities and 50,000 serious injuries per year across the EU.

In an important 2012 study by the nonprofit research organization Insurance Institute for Highway Safety, researchers examined how particular features of crash-avoidance systems affected the number of claims under various forms of insurance coverage. They found that two crash-avoidance features provide the biggest benefits: (a) autonomous braking that would brake on its own, if the driver does not, to avoid a forward collision, and (b) adaptive headlights that would shift the headlights in the direction the driver steers. Unexpectedly, they found lane departure systems to be not helpful, and perhaps harmful, at the circa 2012 stage of development.

Collision avoidance features are rapidly making their way into the new vehicle fleet.

65. A collision avoidance system is not designed to:

A. Prevent an accident
B. Minimise death and injury on the roads
C. Take action when a crash is imminently detected
D. Reduce the number of insurance claims

66. Based on the text what is the most likely assumption, from the following list, you could draw?

A. Many accidents are caused by driver error
B. American roads are safer than European roads
C. Commercial vehicles are involved in more accidents than private vehicles
D. The automotive industry is developing anti-collision technologies

67. Which of the following has been found to be the least helpful form of collision avoidance systems?

A. Warning the driver
B. Autonomous action by the car
C. Lane departure systems
D. Adaptive headlights

68. Which of the following is a true statement?

A. All vehicles sold in Europe from November 2015 will have Advanced Emergency Braking Systems
B. The US study regarding warning systems is still ongoing
C. There are around 5,000 road fatalities per year across the EU
D. The Insurance Institute for Highway Safety is a non-profit organisation

The Killer Whale or Orca, or less commonly, Blackfish, is the largest species of the dolphin family. It is found in all the world's oceans, from the frigid Arctic and Antarctic regions to warm, tropical seas. Some killer whale populations feed mostly on fish while others hunt sharks and marine mammals, including sea lions, seals, walruses and even large whales.

There are up to five distinct killer whale types distinguished by geographical range, preferred prey items and physical appearance. Some of these may be separate races, subspecies or even species. Killer whales are highly social; some populations are composed of matrilineal family groups, which are the most stable of any animal species. The sophisticated social behaviour, hunting techniques, and vocal behaviour of killer whales have been described as manifestations of culture.

Although the killer whale is not considered to be an internationally endangered species, some local populations are considered threatened or endangered due to depletion of prey species, habitat loss, pollution, captures for marine mammal parks, and conflicts with fisheries.

Wild killer whales are usually not considered a threat to humans. There have, however, been isolated reports of captive killer whales attacking and, in some instances, killing their handlers at marine theme parks.

69. Orcas can be found in the Pacific Ocean

A. True
B. False
C. Can't tell

70. Despite their name - killer whales do not actually kill people.

A. True
B. False
C. Can't tell

71. The number of killer whales worldwide is in decline.

A. True
B. False
C. Can't tell

72. There are six distinct killer whale types.

A. True
B. False
C. Can't tell

The spores formed by Clostridium difficile are highly resilient and can persist on surfaces after basic cleaning. Spores of these bacteria can remain viable outside of the human body for very long periods of time, and this means that patients in a medical facility are often exposed to situations where they end up accidentally ingesting spores from an infected patient. Extremely rigorous infection protocols are required in order to decrease or eliminate this risk.

C. difficile infection (CDI) can range in severity from asymptomatic to severe and life-threatening, especially among the elderly. People are most often infected in hospitals, nursing homes, or other medical institutions, although CDI in the community setting is increasing.

C. difficile-associated diarrhoea (CDAD) is most strongly associated with fluoroquinolones, although other antibiotics including clindamycin, 3rd generation cephalosporins and beta-lactamase inhibitors are also associated. In addition to previous use of antimicrobials, use of proton pump inhibitors [PPIs] is associated with an increase in risk for CDI.

The European Centre for Disease Prevention and Control recommend that fluoroquinolones and clindamycin be avoided in clinical practice due to their high association with subsequent CDI. Immunocompromised status and delayed diagnosis appear to result in elevated risk of death. Early intervention and aggressive management are key factors to recovery. There are highly toxic strains of C. difficile emerging which show resistance to fluroquinolones such as ciprofloxacin and levofloxacin.

Some recent research suggests that the overuse of antibiotics in the raising of livestock for meat consumption is contributing to outbreaks of bacterial infections such as C. difficile.

73. According to the text which of the following statements is true?

A. C. difficile bacteria can survive outside their host
B. Cleaning will remove all traces of c. difficile
C. Patients are usually infected by an oral route
D. Antibiotics should be used to prevent c. difficile infection

74. All of the following statements are true except:

A. Infection control policies must be adhered to
B. Care must be taken when cleaning surfaces
C. Overuse of antibiotics may be contributing to the rise in CDI
D. CDI only affects patients in healthcare settings

75. All of the following statements are true except:

A. CDAD is associated with previous use of antibiotics
B. CDAD can also be associated with other medications
C. CDAD is associated with overuse of antibiotics in the farming industry
D. CDAD only affects patients on antibiotics

76. Identify which method below will not help reduce rate of infection:

A. Early diagnosis and treatment of patients with CDI
B. Adherence to infection control policies
C. Appropriate use of antibiotics and other medications
D. Basic cleaning of all surfaces when a patient is identified as having CDI

The Emperor Penguin is the tallest and heaviest of all living penguin species and is endemic to Antarctica. Its diet consists primarily of fish, but can also include crustaceans, such as krill, and cephalopods, such as squid. In hunting, the species can remain submerged up to 18 minutes, diving to a depth of 535 m (1,755 ft). It has several adaptations to facilitate this, including an unusually structured haemoglobin to allow it to function at low oxygen levels, solid bones to reduce barotrauma, and the ability to reduce its metabolism and shut down non-essential organ functions.

The Emperor Penguin is perhaps best known for the sequence of journeys adults make each year in order to mate and to feed their offspring. The only penguin species that breeds during the Antarctic winter, it treks 50-120 km (31-75 mi) over the ice to breeding colonies which may include thousands of individuals. The female lays a single egg, which is incubated by the male while the female returns to the sea to feed; parents subsequently take turns foraging at sea and caring for their chick in the colony. The lifespan is typically 20 years in the wild, although observations suggest that some individuals may live to 50 years of age.

77. The Emperor Penguin is the only animal that breeds during the Antarctic Winter

A. True
B. False
C. Can't tell

78. Emperor Penguins only eat fish and crustaceans.

A. True
B. False
C. Can't tell

79. Emperor Penguins can dive to 1,755m.

A. True
B. False
C. Can't tell

80. Emperor Penguins have solid bones.

A. True
B. False
C. Can't tell

The stock of a corporation is partitioned into shares, the total of which are stated at the time of business formation. Additional shares may subsequently be authorized by the existing shareholders and issued by the company. In some jurisdictions, each share of stock has a certain declared par value, which is a nominal accounting value used to represent the equity on the balance sheet of the corporation. In other jurisdictions, however, shares of stock may be issued without associated par value.

Shares represent a fraction of ownership in a business. A business may declare different types (classes) of shares, each having distinctive ownership rules, privileges, or share values. Ownership of shares may be documented by issuance of a stock certificate. A stock certificate is a legal document that specifies the amount of shares owned by the shareholder, and other specifics of the shares, such as the par value, if any, or the class of the shares.

Stock typically takes the form of shares of either common stock or preferred stock. As a unit of ownership, common stock typically carries voting rights that can be exercised in corporate decisions.

Preferred stock differs from common stock in that it typically does not carry voting rights but is legally entitled to receive a certain level of dividend payments before any dividends can be issued to other shareholders. Convertible preferred stock is preferred stock that includes an option for the holder to convert the preferred shares into a fixed number of common shares, usually any time after a predetermined date. Shares of such stock are called "convertible preferred shares" (or "convertible preference shares" in the UK).

Preferred stock may be hybrid by having the qualities of bonds of fixed returns and common stock voting rights. They also have preference in the payment of dividends over common stock and also have been given preference at the time of liquidation over common stock. They have other features of accumulation in dividend. In addition, preferred stock usually comes with a letter designation at the end of the security; for example, Berkshire-Hathaway Class "B" shares sell under stock ticker BRK.B, whereas Class "A" shares of ORION DHC, Inc will sell under ticker OODHA until the company drops the "A" creating ticker OODH for its "Common" shares only designation. This extra letter does not mean that any exclusive rights exist for the shareholders but it does let investors know that the shares are considered for such, however, these rights or privileges may change based on the decisions made by the underlying company.

81. According to the text which of the following statements are true?

A. Berkshire-Hathaway Class "B" shares sell under stock ticker OODHA
B. Ownership of shares may be documented by issuance of a stock certificate
C. Preferred stock and common stock both carry voting rights but is legally entitled to receive a certain level of dividend payments before any dividends can be issued to other shareholders
D. There are three types of stock

82. Which of the following is likely to be false?

A. As a unit of ownership, common stock typically carries voting rights that can be exercised in corporate decisions
B. Stocks are controlled by the government in each country
C. The extra letter A does not mean that any exclusive rights exist for the shareholders, but it does let investors know that the shares are considered for such, however, these rights or privileges may change based on the decisions made by the underlying company
D. Stocks represent a fraction of ownership in a business

83. All of the following are true except:

A. At the time of business formation the total stock of a corporation is partitioned into shares
B. A stock certificate is a legal document that specifies the amount of shares owned by the shareholder
C. All shares of stock may be issued without associated par value
D. Preferred stock includes an option for the holder to convert the preferred shares into a fixed number of common shares, usually any time after a predetermined date

84. Which of the following statements are most likely to be true?

A. As a unit of ownership, common stock typically carries voting rights that can be exercised in corporate decisions
B. Additional shares may subsequently be authorized by the company
C. ORION DHC is an internal capital allocation and asset management corporation for its various subsidiary businesses
D. The corporate decision is the most important type of decision in stocks

School uniforms in England were first introduced on a large scale during the reign of King Henry VIII. The uniforms of the time were referred as "bluecoats", as they consisted of long trench-coat-style jackets dyed blue. Blue was the cheapest available dye and showed humility amongst all children. The first school to introduce this uniform was Christ's Hospital and it is the oldest uniform of any school.

In 1870, the Elementary Education Act 1870 made elementary education available for all children in England and Wales. The popularity of uniforms increased and eventually most schools had a uniform. During this period most uniforms reflected the trends of the age, with boys wearing short trousers and blazers until roughly the age of puberty and then long trousers from about 14 or 15. Girls mainly wore blouse, tunic dress and pinafore later progressing towards the beginning of the 20th century to gymslips.

These uniforms continued until the 1950s when after the Butler reforms secondary education was made free and the school leaving age was raised to 15. These reforms encouraged schools to implement uniform codes which were similar to other schools. Distinct "summer" and "winter" uniforms were sometimes required, particularly for girls where dresses were mandated for summer and gymslip for winter.

Today, the Government believes that school uniforms play a valuable role in contributing to the ethos of schools: The Department for Children, Schools and Families strongly encourages schools to have a uniform as it can instil pride; support positive behaviour and discipline; encourage identity with, and support for, school ethos; ensure pupils of all races and backgrounds feel welcome; protect children from social pressures to dress in a particular way; nurture cohesion and promote good relations between different groups of pupils.

School uniforms are required to be fair for both genders, be available at a reasonably low cost and tolerate religious freedoms e.g. allowing Sikhs to wear turbans.

85. Which of the following is a historical fact based on the text?

A. The Elementary Education Act of 1870 made education available to all British children
B. Uniforms remained broadly unchanged from the Elementary Education Act until the 1950s
C. The Butler reforms made secondary education free
D. Seasonal uniforms were often required for all pupils

86. Based on the text which of the following rules does it seem unlikely that the government would enforce regarding school uniform?

A. School uniform should be flexible enough to allow for religious differences
B. Schools should ensure that school uniform isn't unduly expensive
C. School uniform should be broadly similar for both genders
D. Most schools should have a school uniform

87. All of the following are cited as benefits of school uniforms except:

A. It can instil pride
B. It showed humility
C. It changed according to season
D. It protects children from social pressure

88. Which of the following may be false?

A. Blue was selected because it was the cheapest dye
B. Contemporary Government policy is supportive of school uniform
C. School uniforms must be affordable
D. Christ's Hospital was the first English school to introduce uniform

Gorillas constitute the eponymous genus *Gorilla*, the largest extant genus of primates by physical size. They are ground-dwelling, predominantly herbivorous apes that inhabit the forests of central Africa. The genus is divided into two species and either four or five subspecies. The DNA of gorillas is highly similar to that of a human, from 95-99% depending on what is counted, and they are the next closest living relatives to humans after the bonobo and common chimpanzee.

Gorillas' natural habitats cover tropical or subtropical forests in Africa. Although their range covers a small percentage of Africa, gorillas cover a wide range of elevations. The mountain gorilla inhabits the Albertine Rift montane cloud forests of the Virunga Volcanoes, ranging in altitude from 2,200-4,300 metres (7,200-14,100 ft). Lowland gorillas live in dense forests and lowland swamps and marshes as low as sea level, with western lowland gorillas living in Central West African countries and eastern lowland gorillas living in the Democratic Republic of the Congo near its border with Rwanda.

The closest relatives of gorillas are chimpanzees and humans, all of the Hominidae having diverged from a common ancestor about 7 million years ago. Human gene sequences differ only 1.6% on average from the sequences of corresponding gorilla genes, but there is further difference in how many copies each gene has. Until recently, gorillas were considered to be a single species, with three subspecies: the western lowland gorilla, the eastern lowland gorilla and the mountain gorilla. There is now agreement that there are two species with two subspecies each. More recently, a third subspecies has been claimed to exist in one of the species. The separate species and subspecies developed from a single type of gorilla during the Ice Age, when their forest habitats shrank and became isolated from each other.

Primatologists continue to explore the relationships between various gorilla populations. The species and subspecies listed here are the ones upon which most scientists agree.

The proposed third subspecies of *Gorilla beringei*, which has not yet received a trinomen, is the Bwindi population of the mountain gorilla, sometimes called the Bwindi gorilla.

Some variations that distinguish the classifications of gorilla include varying density, size, hair colour, length, culture, and facial widths. Now, over 100,000 western lowland gorillas are thought to exist in the wild, with 4,000 in zoos; eastern lowland gorillas have a population of 4,000 in the wild and 24 in zoos. Mountain gorillas are the most severely endangered, with an estimated population of about 620 left in the wild and none in zoos.

89. According to the text which of the following statements is true?

A. Under 100,000 western lowland gorillas are thought to exist in the wild
B. 95-99% of DNA from gorillas is the same DNA as humans
C. There are three types of gorilla species
D. There are more eastern lowland gorillas than western lowland gorillas

90. All of the following statements are true except:

A. Gorillas live in a wide variety of terrains
B. Other animals are closer relatives of humans
C. Two species came from the same ancestral species when the forest habitats shrank and became isolated from each other
D. Mountain gorillas cannot survive in zoos

91. Which of the following is most likely to be true?

A. The Virunga Volcanoes reach a maximum of 14,100 ft in height
B. Gorillas are entirely vegetarian
C. Over 95% of living gorillas are western lowland gorillas
D. Human and gorilla genes only differ by 1.6%

92. With regard to species and subspecies classifications:

A. The third subspecies is called the *Gorilla beringei* will be official when a trinomen is received
B. Gorilla species began to diverge from one another 7 million years ago
C. All scientists agree on the species and subspecies listed in the passage
D. Appearance features are key in distinguishing between species and subspecies of gorilla

Surfing is a surface water sport in which the wave rider, referred to as a surfer, rides on the forward or deep face of a moving wave, which is usually carrying the surfer towards the shore. Waves suitable for surfing are primarily found in the ocean but can also be found in lakes or in rivers in the form of a standing wave or tidal bore. However, surfers can also utilize man-made waves such as those from boat wakes and the waves created in artificial wave pools.

The term surfing refers to the act of riding a wave, regardless of whether the wave is ridden with a board or without a board, and regardless of the stance used (goofy or regular stance). The native peoples of the Pacific, for instance, surfed waves on alaia, paipo, and other such craft, and did so on their bellies and knees. The modern-day definition of surfing, however, most often refers to a surfer riding a wave standing up on a surfboard; this is also referred to as stand-up surfing. One variety of stand-up surfing is paddle boarding.

Another prominent form of surfing in the ocean today is body boarding, when a surfer rides a wave either on the belly, drop knee, or sometimes standing-up on a body board. Other types of surfing include knee boarding, surf matting (riding inflatable mats), foils. Body surfing, where the wave is surfed without a board, using the surfer's own body to catch and ride the wave, is very common and is considered by some to be the purest form of surfing.

Three major subdivisions within standing-up surfing are long boarding, short boarding, and stand up paddle surfing (SUP), and these three have several major differences, including the board design and length, the riding style, and the kind of wave that is ridden.

In tow-in surfing (most often, but not exclusively, associated with big wave surfing), a motorized water vehicle, such as a personal watercraft, tows the surfer into the wave front, helping the surfer match a large wave's higher speed, which is generally a higher speed than a self-propelled surfer can obtain. Surfing-related sports such as paddle boarding and sea kayaking do not require waves, and other derivative sports such as kite surfing and wind surfing rely primarily on wind for power, yet all of these platforms may also be used to ride waves. Recently with the use of V-drive boats, wake surfing, in which one surfs on the wake of a boat, has emerged. The Guinness Book of World Records recognized at 78 feet (23.8 m) wave ride by Garrett McNamara at Nazaré, Portugal as the largest wave ever surfed.

93. Which of the following statements are most likely to be true

A. The Guinness Book of World Records recognised a 22.8m wave ride
B. Competitive surfing always requires a board
C. In tow-in surfing is always associated with big wave surfing
D. Surfing waves are only found in the ocean

94. All of the following statements may be true except:

A. Surfing without a board is the most common type of surfing
B. There are three types of standing up surfing
C. The native people of the Pacific were the first to surf
D. Waves are required for surfing-related sports

95. All of the following statements are true except:

A. Surfing is a surface water sport
B. With the use of U-drive boats, wake surfing has emerged
C. Body surfing does not involve a board
D. One main difference between different standing up surfing styles are the board design and length

96. According to the text which of the statements is true?

A. A personal watercraft tows the surfer away from the wave front in some surf activities
B. Garret McNamara is Portuguese
C. The modern-day definition of surfing refers to a surfer riding a wave sitting on a surfboard
D. Surfers can utilize man-made waves

Jiaozi, the world's first paper-printed currency, was an innovation of the Song Dynasty.

The Song Dynasty (960-1279 CE) also provided some of the most significant technological advances in Chinese history, many of which came from talented statesmen drafted by the government through imperial examinations.

The ingenuity of advanced mechanical engineering had a long tradition in China. The Song Dynasty engineer Su Song admitted that he and his contemporaries were building upon the achievements of the ancients such as Zhang Heng (78-139 CE), an astronomer, inventor, and early master of mechanical gears. The application of movable type printing advanced the already widespread use of woodblock printing to educate and amuse Confucian students and the masses. The application of weapons employing the use of gunpowder enabled the Song Dynasty to ward off its militant enemies (the Liao, Western Xia, and Jin) with weapons such as cannons until its collapse to the Mongol forces of Kublai Khan in the late 13th century.

Notable advances in civil engineering, nautics, and metallurgy were made in Song China, as well as the introduction of the windmill to China during the thirteenth century. These advances, along with the introduction of printed currency, helped revolutionize and sustain the economy of the Song Dynasty.

97. Jiaozi is the Chinese word for banknotes

A. True
B. False
C. Can't tell

98. Cannons were invented by the Song Dynasty

A. True
B. False
C. Can't tell

99. Zhang Heng was a Song Dynasty engineer

A. True
B. False
C. Can't tell

100. The Dutch introduced windmills to China in the thirteenth century

A. True
B. False
C. Can't tell

100 Verbal Reasoning Question Answers

1. The correct answer is A. Operation Artic Fox was terminated after four months.

The passage states both the start and end date of the operation - the operation began on July 1 and is stated as ending on November 17. This is slightly over four months. There is no information about the XXXVI Corps level of training or preparedness in the text so whilst option B may be true it cannot be shown using the information given. Operation Artic Fox was part of a larger operation - Operation Silver Fox. The larger operation is stated as having the capture of Murmansk as its primary aim but it is incorrect to say that the main objective of operation Artic Fox was this as it is stated as being the recapture of the town Salla. There are three military divisions named in the text - the 6th, 122nd and 169th but there is nothing to suggest that they were the only ones.

2. The correct answer is B. During the Soviet retreat of the 122nd Rifle Division they had to leave most of their artillery behind

The passage states that the 122nd Rifle Division had to retreat and whilst doing so had to "leave most of their artillery behind". Option A is false as the passages clearly states that the Finnish 6th Division crossed the border at midnight not the German 6th division. Option C is false as the SS division did break the Soviet defences however, "it was not until the 169th Division supported the attack". Option D was false as the Soviets formed a strong defence from "Lake Verkhneye Verman to Tolvand" not the Tuutsa River.

3. The correct answer is D. Operation Platinum Fox was known as (Silberfuchs)

This is was as Operation Platinum Fox was known "Platinfuchs" and Operation Silver Fox was known as "Silberfuchs". Option A is incorrect as Salla was captured on the "6 July". Option B is incorrect as two rivers are mentioned in the passage Tuutsa and the Voyta river. Option C is incorrect as the beginning of August 1941, the Finnish 6th Division headed the renewed drive of the XXXVI Corps.

4. The correct answer is D. During the heavy fighting some 5 Soviet tanks were destroyed.

Option C is false as Operation Platinum Fox took place in the far north of Lappland. Option A is incorrect as there is no mention as to what the XXXVI Corps means in the passage. Option B is incorrect as the German casualties were heavy but it does not state in the text that this was the only cause as to why the attack was called off.

5. Cacao is only grown in the Americas – Can't tell

Although cacao has been cultivated for at least 3000 years in the Americas, it is not clear whether it has been grown elsewhere.

6. The Aztecs drank chocolate - True

The majority of Mesoamerican peoples (including Aztecs) made chocolate beverages. The Aztec version of this was known as xocolatl.

7. Chocolate grows on trees - False

Cacao seeds/beans grow on the Theobroma cacao tree. Chocolate only comes into being after the seeds/beans are processed.

8. White chocolate is not considered to be true chocolate because it contains cocoa butter - False

White chocolate does not contain cocoa solids and therefore is not considered to be true chocolate.

9. The correct answer is C. Exceptional climbers can climb without needing to acclimatize.

The passage states in the third paragraph that 'everyone needs to acclimatise' The statement "Exceptional mountaineers have climbed 8000 metre peaks (including Everest) without oxygen, almost always with a carefully planned program of acclimatisation." may appear to imply that it is possible to climb without acclimatisation but as this would contradict the previous statement that everyone needs to acclimatise, this sentence would be interpreted as meaning that the acclimatisation, which logically must take place, does not have to be carefully planned.

10. The correct answer is D. The 'climb high, sleep low' regimen will always prevent altitude sickness

While the first paragraph states that the 'climb high, sleep low' regimen is used to allow climbers to acclimatise and will help to prevent altitude sickness, it does not mean that altitude sickness will always be prevented by this regimen.

11. The correct answer is B. Less oxygen is available resulting in a varied range of symptoms.

The third paragraph states that the underlying cause of altitude sickness is less oxygen being available and the second paragraph indicates the wide range of symptoms that can be cause.

12. The correct answer is A. Descending safely and quickly is the only treatment for altitude sickness

Rapid but safe descent is the only way to treat altitude sickness. The final paragraph states a few ways in which climbers' symptoms can be treated, allowing them to descend to a lower height. Treating the patient in situ is not a safer option unless there are medical facilities present to alleviate the symptoms and treat the underlying cause. The portable hyperbaric chamber can be used to increase oxygen levels but is only used to allow the climber to descend safely. Steroids can be used to treat pulmonary edemas but will not treat the altitude sickness itself.

13. The correct answer is B. Sedimentary rocks settled on the ocean floor can determine that the Indo-Australian plate had completely closed the Tethys Ocean.

Option B is correct as in the second paragraph it clearly states that "the existence of" the Indo-Australian plate had completely closed the Tethys Ocean "which has been determined by sedimentary rocks settled on the ocean floor". Option A is incorrect as the mountain was formed continental collision or orogeny along the convergent boundary between the Indo-Australian Plate and the Eurasian Plate not through subduction. Option C is incorrect as the climate was at least 7.0 to 8.3 °C colder than it is today. Option D is incorrect as Nanga Parbat is in the west.

14. The correct answer is A. The Himalayas are the youngest mountain ranges on the planet.

This is as the first sentence states how the Himalayas are among the youngest mountain ranges on the planet but does not say the youngest. Option B is incorrect as the statement is found in the text so is correct. Option C is incorrect as Himalaya reach at most 20 to 32 kilometres (12 to 20 mi) in length so the ratios of length are correct. Option D is incorrect as The Himalayas are rising by "5 mm per year, making them geologically active".

15. The correct answer is C. Three mountains are mentioned throughout the passage

Throughout the text only one mountain is mentioned, Mount Everest. Option A was incorrect as the answer is true as The Arakan Yoma highlands "were also formed as a result of this collision". Option B can also be found in the text as the glaciers length during the Ice Age were 60 to 112 kilometres but the "current valley glaciers of the Himalaya reach at most 20 to 32 kilometres". Option D is incorrect as the passage does not clarify when the first recorded mountains were formed.

16. The correct answer is C. The glacier snowline is the altitude where accumulation and ablation of a glacier are completely balanced.

The definition is stated in the 4th paragraph. Option A is incorrect as the passage does not state which mountain has the highest peak. Option B is incorrect as the Indo-Australian plate continues to be driven horizontally below the Tibetan Plateau. Option D is incorrect as the definition of oceanic trench is not stated in the text only that it exists.

17. The Schistosoma genus contains several fluke species - True

"Schistosomiasis (also known as bilharzia, bilharziosis or snail fever) is a parasitic disease caused by several species of fluke of the genus Schistosoma"

18. Schistosomiasis is endemic in half the population of Africa – Can't tell

Half of the 200 million people who are infected with schistosomiasis in the world reside in Africa, as no population data is given for Africa it is impossible to tell what proportion of the African Population this equates to.

19. 20 million people in the world are infected with schistosomiasis - False

Of the infected patients 20 million people suffer severe consequences due to the disease but the disease is stated to be infecting more than 200 million people

20. A few countries have eradicated schistosomiasis because of the World Health Organisation's efforts – Can't tell

Although a few countries have eradicated schistosomiasis and the World Health Organisation is promoting those efforts, it is unclear whether the World Health Organisation's efforts are the cause of the eradication of schistosomiasis.

21. The correct answer is C. A group of people are allocated to an exposure or non-exposure group and followed up to see if that exposure causes a disease.

This is the only study where the investigator allocated people to an exposure group or non-exposure group. They are causing the exposure and then waiting for a result. Answers a, b and d all describe observational studies of different types.

22. The correct answer is D. Analytic studies are based on an implicit comparison

Analytic studies as the name suggests are explicit in nature. They involve the investigator comparing two groups of individuals systematically to determine risk for disease. A comparison group is needed for all analytic study designs (and interventional study designs are analytic) and observational analytic studies may take a long time as they are observing the natural course of events after an exposure (which depending on the exposure and disease may mean years)

23. The correct answer is D. A group of patients with bladder cancer and a group of patients without are interviewed to obtain information about artificial sweetener consumption in food and drink

Two groups (one with and one without the disease of interest) are being compared for differences in an exposure (in this case artificial sweeteners) Answer a) refers to a case report which may provide a suggestion of a link to exposure, it does not provide any analytic data about the link to exposure. Answer b) refers to whole populations. Any link between exposure and disease is not possible as they do not necessarily occur in the same person. This is still a descriptive study. Answer c) is also descriptive as it cannot always be determined that the exposure pre-dated the disease.

24. The correct answer is B. Descriptive studies help with the development of hypotheses.

The first paragraph states that 'a hypothesis is formulated based on an implicit comparison with the 'expected' or normal'. They cannot test hypotheses as there is no comparison group (therefore answer a is false). Comparison groups are needed for all analytic studies but not descriptive studies so d) is false and observers in interventional studies will expose certain groups to an exposure therefore altering the natural course of events.

25. 80% of people in Tanzania work in the export industry - False

80% of working people work in agriculture. 85% of exports are from agriculture. There is no information which would enable you to deduce the proportion of people who work in exports.

26. 85% of agricultural produce is exported from Tanzania – Can't tell

85% of Tanzania's total exports are of agricultural origin but as numbers are not provided it is impossible to tell if this also equates to 85% of the total agricultural produce in Tanzania

27. An increase in cultivatable land would lead to an increase in exports – Can't tell

There is no suggestion of a link between cultivatable land and export. Exports may currently be limited by law or by market forces.

28. The recent banking and legislative reforms have helped curb corruption and hence helped increase private-sector growth and investment – Can't tell

Economic progress depends on curbing corruption. Economic progress post reforms suggest lower levels of corruption. However, it is unclear if the lower levels of corruption were down to the reforms or other variables.

29. The correct answer is D. Antimicrobials are always used internally

The last paragraph states that antimicrobial substances that are too toxic to be used other than in topical therapy or for environmental decontamination are referred to as antiseptics or disinfectants. Therefore, not all antimicrobials are used internally.

30. The correct answer is A. Antimicrobials can be made by chemically altering natural compounds

Antimicrobials can consist of naturally occurring compounds, chemically altered naturally occurring compounds or manufactured synthetic compounds.

31. The answer is C. Cancerous tumours

The first paragraph states 'The term chemotherapy is usually used more generally to include the use of anti-tumour drug' however, antimicrobial chemotherapy is the term given to the use of chemical agents to treat microbial pathogens. Therefore, antimicrobial chemotherapy is not used to treat cancerous tumours.

32. The correct answer is C. A group of agents which inhibit viruses and bacteria

Although antimicrobial agents can treat a wider range of microbes than viruses and bacteria, the other statements are not correct. Antimicrobials can be naturally occurring, manufactured or synthetic (or a combination of these) therefore answers a, b and d are incorrect.

33. All 'big cats' mentioned in the text belong to the genus *Panthera* – True

34. Siberian tigers are generally larger in size than Bengal tigers - True

Siberian tigers are the largest subspecies therefore they are generally larger than any other tiger subspecies.

35. In the natural world tigers can only survive in large open areas - False

Tigers are described as highly adaptable and as living in various habitats including mangrove swamps.

36. Tigers have been popular mega-fauna since ancient times - True

Tigers are mega-fauna and have featured prominently in ancient mythology and folklore.

37. The correct answer is D. Flinders carried a crew of 38

Option A has the wrong dates. They should be 29 July 1972 and 27 April 1973.

Option B confuses the base. It should read Cairns.

Option C puts Williamstown in New South Wales instead of Victoria.

38. The correct answer is C. 13.5 knots is more than 12 knots

Option A supposes that Paluma was part of the Royal Navy. The 'A' is missing from her title.

Option B. Presumably Australian standards are as good as international standards but the text only mentions Australian.

Option D. Just the name of the cyclone is faulty.

39. The correct answer is A. Flinders was decommissioned in October 1999

She was decommissioned in 1998 and sold in 1999. Option B is true - the figure in the text is A$518,460 which is over half a million. The final position of the ship as described in the text is as a private yacht in the Cayman Islands (option C). The dates of commissioning for the RAN and the date of decommission are 1973 and 1998 respectively - a period of 25 years (option D).

40. The correct answer is A. Flinders was not expected to work outside Australian coastal areas

Option A is a false statement. She was also expected to sail to Papua New Guinea. The survey of Darwin Harbour (option B) is described in the text. The text shows that option C is actually true in more than one place. Option D is also described in the text.

41. The correct answer is A. Physical space is often conceived in four linear dimensions.

The passage states that physical space is often conceived in three linear dimensions. Option B is incorrect as in Isaac Newton's view, space existed permanently and independently of whether there were any matter in the space. Option C is incorrect as from the passage it states that George Berkeley was named a philosopher and theologian. Option D was incorrect as "experimental tests of general relativity have confirmed that non-Euclidean space provides a better model for the shape of space".

42. The correct answer is D. Albert Einstein completed a theory of general relativity

This statement can be seen in the last paragraph. Option A is incorrect as whilst George Berkley did complete the essay on Towards a New Theory of Vision it does not state whether this was his most famous work to date.

Option B is incorrect as Immanuel Kant states space is subjective but this is his opinion. Option C is incorrect as four treaties in total are stated not five.

43. The correct answer is B. Greeks knew space as khora

This can be seen in the passage where the "Greeks called khora (i.e. "space")..." Option A is incorrect as physical space is not always conceived in three linear dimensions. Option C is incorrect as the passage does not state when the first evidence of space was found and if it was before the 10th century. Option D is incorrect as there are many theories as to what makes up space entities is only one of them.

44. The correct answer is A. Philosophers have found more evidence about space than mathematicians.

This is as whilst both philosophers and mathematics have studied space there is no evidence to suggest who has found out more. Option B is incorrect as Gottfried Leibniz was a natural philosopher. Option C is incorrect as the passage clearly states "In mathematics, "spaces" are examined with different numbers of dimensions and with different underlying structures". Option D is incorrect as Immanuel Kant was a metaphysician.

45. The correct answer is C. Retroviruses are a type of virus that has single-stranded RNA genomes

The first paragraph states that retroviruses are viruses which have a single-stranded RNA genome.

46. The correct answer is B. ssRNA is converted into dsDNA by reverse transcriptase and combined into the host genome by integrase

Retroviruses contain ssRNA which enters the host cell. Reverse transcriptase converts this copy into dsDNA and integrase integrates this copy into the host genome. (Paragraph 1)

47. The correct answer is D. Retroviruses only use the host cell enzymes

Retroviruses have their own enzymes therefore d is the false statement. The first paragraph states '...integrated into the host cell genome by a viral integrase enzyme."

48. The correct answer is B. By encoding proteins involved in regulating cell growth, infection results in unrestrained cell division

Retroviruses can contain oncogenes, which encode proteins involved in cell growth. This results in uncontrolled cell division associated with tumour growth. (See the last paragraph)

49. The correct answer is A. There are more than 10,000 different languages

This is correct as the passage states that there is an estimate of between 6,000 and 7,000 different languages. Whilst it is an estimate and not definitely the correct amount A is still false as you infer there is more than 10,000 different languages. Option B is incorrect as language is a complex system of communication. Option C is incorrect as in the last paragraph how language has changed through evolution is discussed. Option D is incorrect as the statement "human language relies entirely on social convention and learning" is stated in the passage.

50. The correct answer is B. Language originated when early hominins started gradually changing their primate communication systems.

This is the correct option as this statement can be found in paragraph 3. Option A is incorrect as the passage states that animals can communicate aswell. Option C is incorrect as oral and sign languages contain aphonological system not all forms of language. Option D is incorrect as social grooming and entertainment are ways of how language is used socially but nowhere in the text does it states that humans communicate between each other more.

51. The correct answer is C. A group of languages that descend from a common ancestor is known as a barrier family.

This option is incorrect as a group of languages that descend from a common ancestor is known as a language family not a barrier family. Option A is incorrect as "the scientific study of language is called linguistics" Option B is incorrect as "language is processed in" the "Broca's and Wernicke's areas" of the brain. Option D is incorrect as linguists see the structures of language as having evolved to serve specific communicative and social functions.

52. The correct answer is B. Children generally speak fluently when they are approximately two years old

The passage states that children generally speak fluently when they are approximately three years old. Option A is incorrect as natural language can be converted into secondary media. Option C is incorrect as language does have uses in group identity and social stratification. Option D is incorrect as this passage is stated in the first line of paragraph one.

53. Cyprus cannot be without a President or acting President for more than 45 days. - True

"If there is a vacancy in the office of President, the vacancy is filled by a by-election taking place within a period not exceeding 45 days"

54. A thirty-four-year-old woman cannot run for President in Cyprus. - True

The passage states that a candidate has to be over 35 years old

55. There is no Vice President in Cyprus – Can't tell

The post of Vice President is not discussed in the passage.

56. In Cyprus the presidential term is 6 years - False

A term lasts 5 years.

57. The correct answer is D. Dough is always made by combining all the ingredients at the same time

As paragraph 2 states that a 'pre-ferment' can be used which means some of the flour and yeast is combined and left to ferment overnight.

58. The correct answer is C. The process of making a 'pre-ferment' of yeast and flour

The 'starter method' is the method of mixing yeast, flour and water together the night before. The full explanation of the method is in the 2nd paragraph.

59. The correct answer is A. It makes the bread rise higher

The second paragraph states that the bread will have a better texture using pre-ferment but says nothing about making the bread rise higher. Pre-ferment is used as it is a compromise between the use of baker's year and the complexity of a longer fermentation and it was used to save on baker's yeast as it was originally expensive.

60. The correct answer is D. The longer the rising time of the dough, the less flavour is produced in the bread

The first paragraph states that 'a longer rising time results in more flavour' therefore the last statement is false.

61. The monks were given pensions when the abbey fell in 1538. – Can't tell

It is stated that no records survive about the fall of the Abbey so no information about pensions for monks can be known.

62. Revesby Abbey had domestic buildings arranged around three cloisters - False

The passage states that there were two cloisters

63. At one time the Abbey had an income of £287 - True

"In 1535 the abbey had an income of £287 (placing it among the middle ranks of its order)"

64. The stone monastery was constructed in the twelfth century - True

"Over the latter part of the twelfth century a stone monastery was constructed on the site."

65. The correct answer is A. Prevent an accident

Opening paragraph explicitly states that the aim is to reduce the severity of an accident, which is different than preventing it. The impact assessment refers to a reduction of fatalities and serious injuries (option B). The method of the automated response describes how the system takes action upon detection of imminent collision (option C). A study researching the impact of different systems of the number of insurance claims is also described (option D).

66. The correct answer is A. Many accidents are caused by driver error

This assumption can be reasonably drawn based on the text. If many accidents can be avoided simply by altering a driver to something they have previously not noticed, or by the car autonomously taking control of the vehicle, then the conclusion is natural and reasonable. Option B is not a reasonable assumption as relative accident rates are neither mentioned nor alluded to. The fact that commercial vehicles will be subject to the new rules first is not necessarily because they are involved in more accidents but more likely because they are easier to regulate. There is nothing in the text mentioning the role of the automotive industry.

67. The correct answer is C. Lane departure systems

The study results show that these were not helpful, and possibly are unhelpful, are described. Warning the driver is mentioned as a method these systems use but its helpfulness is not assessed. This is also true of an autonomous action by the car. The usefulness of adaptive headlights is described.

68. The correct answer is D. The Insurance Institute for Highway Safety is a non-profit organisation

All new vehicle types sold in Europe from November 2015 will have Advanced Emergency Braking Systems (option A) however many vehicle sales are likely to be of existing type vehicles or second hand. There is no information about the study in the US being ongoing or otherwise (option B). It's hoped deaths will reduced by around 5,000 per annum after the introduction of this system in the EU but it cannot be assumed that this is the total number of deaths currently (option C).

69. Orcas can be found in the Pacific Ocean - True

The passage states that the Orca is found in all the world's oceans.

70. Despite their name - killer whales do not actually kill people. - False

The passage discusses reports of captive killer whales killing their handlers.

71. The number of killer whales worldwide is in decline. – Can't tell

Worldwide numbers are not mentioned in the passage. Local populations may be threatened but worldwide numbers are not discussed.

72. There are six distinct killer whale types. - False

The passage states that there are up to five distinct killer whale types.

73. The correct answer is C. Patients are usually infected by an oral route

The first paragraph states that patients are usually infected by accidentally ingesting the spores, therefore infected through an oral route.

74. The correct answer is D. CDI only affects patients in healthcare settings

Although patients in healthcare settings such as hospitals and nursing homes are at a higher risk of contracting CDI, there is an increase of community-acquired CDI as stated in paragraph 2.

75. The correct answer is D. CDAD only affects patients on antibiotics

Although CDAD is most commonly associated with patients on or having recently completed a course of antibiotics, CDAD can also be associated with other types of medications such as Proton Pump Inhibitors. See paragraph 3 for further details.

76. The correct answer is D. Basic cleaning of all surfaces when a patient is identified as having CDI.

Basic cleaning of all surfaces will not help reduce the rate of infection of CDI as it states in the first paragraph that basic cleaning will not remove all the spores from the environment. Thorough specialist cleans must be made of areas when patients are identified as having CDI.

77. The Emperor Penguin is the only animal that breeds during the Antarctic Winter – Can't tell

They are the only penguin species that breeds during the Antarctic winter but there may be other animal species that breed during the Antarctic Winter.

78. Emperor Penguins only eat fish and crustaceans. - False

The diet of an Emperor Penguin can also include cephalopods, such as squid.

79. Emperor Penguins can dive to 1,755m. - False

The text states that they can dive up to 535m or 1,755 ft.

80. Emperor Penguins have solid bones. - True

The passage states that "It has several adaptations ...... solid bones to reduce barotraumas".

81. The correct answer is B. Ownership of shares may be documented by issuance of a stock certificate.

This can be seen in the second paragraph where "Ownership of shares may be documented by issuance of a stock certificate". Option A is incorrect as Berkshire-Hathaway Class "B" shares sell under stock ticker BRK.B, not OODHA. Option C is incorrect as preferred stock differs from common stock in that it typically does not carry voting rights but is legally entitled to receive a certain level of dividend payments before any dividends can be issued to other shareholders. Option D is incorrect as there are two types of stock; preferred and common stock.

82. The correct answer is D. Stocks represent a fraction of ownership in a business

This is as shares represent a fraction of ownership in a business not stocks. Option A is incorrect the passage states that "As a unit of ownership, common stock typically carries voting rights that can be exercised in corporate decisions". Option B is incorrect as nothing about the control of stocks is stated in the passage. Option C is incorrect as the statement is correct and can be found in the passage.

83. The correct answer is C. All shares of stock may be issued without associated par value.

This is incorrect as in some jurisdictions shares of stock may be issued without associated par value but not all. Option A is incorrect as the time of business formation the total stock of a corporation is partitioned into shares. Option B is incorrect as "a stock certificate is a legal document that specifies the amount of shares owned by the shareholder" as stated in the passage. Option D is incorrect as the statement is stated in the passage.

84. The correct answer is A. As a unit of ownership, common stock typically carries voting rights that can be exercised in corporate decisions.

This statement can be found in the passage so the statement is true. Option B is incorrect as additional shares may subsequently be authorized by the existing shareholders and issued by the company not just the company. Option C is incorrect as the passage does not discuss what the orion DHC is. Option D is incorrect as the passage does not state what is the most important type of decision in stocks.

85. The correct answer is C. The Butler reforms made secondary education free

The Butler reforms are referred to in the text. Option A is incorrect as the text refers to English and Welsh children, not all British children (i.e. there is no mention of Scotland). Option B is incorrect as uniforms are reported to have reflected the trends of the age between 1870 and 1950. Summer and winter uniforms (option D) are described as being 'sometimes' required.

86. The correct answer is C. School uniform should be broadly similar for both genders.

There is no indication within the text that the genders should wear the same uniform. Nor that this is encouraged practice. All of the other options are mentioned in the text.

87. The correct answer is C. It changed according to season

Whilst this is factual it is not cited as a benefit of school uniform, unlike the other options which are all specifically referred to.

88. The correct answer is A. Blue was selected because it was the cheapest dye

Blue is described as being the cheapest available dye. It is possible other dye colours were cheaper but couldn't be sourced at the time. The fact that the current government is supportive of school uniform and that there is a requirement for it to be affordable is cited in the fourth paragraph. Christ's Hospital is mentioned in the first paragraph.

89.The correct answer is B. 95-99% of DNA from gorillas is the same DNA as humans.

This can be seen in paragraph one which states that "The DNA of gorillas is highly similar to that of a human, from 95-99% depending on what is counted." Option A is incorrect as over 100,000 western lowland gorillas are thought to exist in the wild. Option C is incorrect as there are two types of gorilla species. Option D is incorrect as there are more western lowland gorillas than eastern lowland gorillas.

90. The correct answer is D. Mountain gorillas cannot survive in zoos.

The final paragraph states that no mountain gorillas live in zoos but no reason is given for this. Option A is incorrect as the passage describes the varied elevation and terrain gorillas in Africa live in. Option B is incorrect as the gorilla is described as being the closest relative to humans after the bonobo and chimpanzee. Option C is incorrect as "The separate species and subspecies developed from a single type of gorilla during the Ice Age, when their forest habitats shrank and became isolated from each other"

91. The correct answer is C. Over 95% of living gorillas are western lowland gorillas

The total number of gorillas, based on this text, is >108,624 of which >104,000 are western lowland.

Option A is not definitely true - the range the gorillas inhabit is described as being between 7,200 ft and 14,100ft - not the maximum height of the range. Option B is not true as a gorilla diet is described as predominately herbivorous, not entirely. Option D is incorrect as the 1.6% difference only applies to a comparison of corresponding gene sequences, whilst a difference in the number of gene copies is cited.

92. The correct answer is D. Appearance features are key in distinguishing between species and subspecies of gorilla

Of the features used to distinguish classification of gorilla listed most are related to appearance - size, hair colour and length, facial width. Option A is incorrect as the function of the trinomen is not mentioned. Option B is incorrect as event cited as happening 7 million years ago was divergence of the Hominidae. Option C is incorrect as the list of species and subspecies in the text is described as being agreed upon by most, not all, scientists.

93. The correct answer is B. Competitive surfing always requires a board

This statement can be inferred from the passage as all the forms of surfing mentioned as being 'sport', or which appear to be organised, require boards. Option A is incorrect as " The Guinness Book of World Records recognised a 23.8m wave ride". Option C is incorrect as tow-in surfing is often but not always associated with big wave surfing. Option D is incorrect as surfing waves can also be found in rivers and lakes.

94. The correct answer is D. Waves are required for surfing-related sports

This is as waves are not required for surfing related sports such as paddle boarding and sea kayaking. This option can definitely be shown to be false using the text. Option A is incorrect as the passage says that surfing without a board is very common and although it doesn't explicitly say it is the 'most common' option D is a better answer for the question. Option B is incorrect as three types of standing up surfing are described and the option does not say 'only three'. Option C is incorrect as the native people of the pacific surfed but we cannot know if they were the first or not.

95. The correct answer is B. With the use of U-drive boats, wake surfing has emerged

This is as V- drive boats were used not U-boats. Option A is incorrect as surfing is a surface water sport. Option C is incorrect as body surfing involves using your body and not a board. Option D is incorrect as "The main differences between different standing up surfing styles are the board design and length, the riding style, and the kind of wave that is ridden".

96. The correct answer is D. Surfers can utilize man-made waves

This is correct as the statement can be found in the passage. Option A is incorrect as the motorized water vehicle pulls the surfer into the wave front not away from it. Option B is incorrect as we only know that Garret McNamara surfed the wave in Portugal, not his nationality. Option C is incorrect as the modern day definition of surfing refers to a surfer riding a wave standing up not sitting down.

97. Jiaozi is the Chinese word for banknotes – Can't tell

Jiaozi was the world's first paper-printed currency, which was an innovation of the Chinese Song Dynasty. However, a translation for the word Jiaozi is not provided and nor is the language defined.

98. Cannons were invented by the Song Dynasty – Can't tell

Although the Song Dynasty utilised new weapons such as cannons, it does not necessarily follow that they invented them.

99. Zhang Heng was a Song Dynasty engineer - False

Zhang Heng lived and died 78-139 CE before the Song Dynasty (960-1279 CE).

100. The Dutch introduced windmills to China in the thirteenth century – Can't tell

Although windmills were introduced to China in the thirteenth century, it is not specified where the windmills were introduced from.

100 Decision Making Questions (answers begin on page 139)

20/21

1. The summer was mostly sunny with above average temperatures for the season. Some areas of the country reported water shortages and there was a blanket ban on the use of hosepipes. Farmers' responses depended on the crops they were growing as some thrived in warm dry conditions whereas other crops failed because of the heat and low rainfall.

Select the words 'Yes' or 'No' if the conclusion does or doesn't follow

It did not rain at all this summer	Yes / No
There was a hosepipe ban in areas where water shortages were reported	Yes / No
Some arable crops don't require as much rainfall as others	Yes / No
It was hotter than average every day of the summer	Yes / No
This season benefitted some people	Yes / No

2. The school report was very good. Thomas was achieving his targets in most subjects and the teachers reported that his effort level was either good or excellent in all classes. His progress was, on average, on target. With just two exceptions he was predicted to get top grades in all his subjects.

Select the words 'Yes' or 'No' if the conclusion does or doesn't follow

Thomas put the maximum amount of effort into all his classes	Yes / No
Thomas was making steady progress in all his subjects	Yes / No
Thomas was not meeting targets in some subjects	Yes / No
Thomas is likely to get top grades in several subjects	Yes / No
Thomas had high targets	Yes / No

3. The Lake District ironically does not have many lakes! The bodies of water which some people may erroneously call a lake are called 'Waters' or 'Meres' if they're relatively large and 'Tarns' if they're smaller. There is just one – Bassenthwaite Lake – which is traditionally called 'a lake'. Most of the bodies of water in the district are glacial in origin but there are also a few man-made reservoirs.

Select the words 'Yes' or 'No' if the conclusion does or doesn't follow

The Lake District has been shaped by glaciers	Yes / No
Man-made reservoirs in the district provide water to the population	Yes / No
Mere means lake in another language or dialect	Yes / No
A tarn is smaller than a 'water'	Yes / No
The bodies of water are sometimes misnamed by people	Yes / No

4. Many children who are not motivated by the enjoyment of doing homework are motivated by the high grade they hope to earn because of doing a quality job. Thus, the grade is an incentive, motivating the child to do homework with care and in a timely manner. For children who are not motivated by grades, parents will need to look for other rewards to help them get through their nightly homework and chores.

Select the words 'Yes' or 'No' if the conclusion does or doesn't follow

Some children enjoy doing homework	Yes / No
Many children are motivated by earning a good grade	Yes / No
It is parent's responsibility to help their child get their homework done	Yes / No
Doing homework with care will result in a high grade	Yes / No
Rewards are more effective than punishments	Yes / No

5. Four children all compete in their school sports day – competing for different teams.

The children are: Daniel, Zachary, Amy and Reuben.

The teams are: Red, Yellow, Green and Blue

- The red team came two places behind Zachary's team
- Reuben wasn't in the third-place green team
- Daniel finished one place above Amy

Which of the following MUST be true?

A. Reuben played in the yellow team
B. The blue team was second
C. Amy played in the red team
D. Daniel finished in second place

6. Four siblings – Rachel, Hannah, Grace and Frances – have their birthdays on the 1st, 2nd, 3rd and 4th of different months – January, April, July and October.

- Nobody has a birthday on New Year's Day (1st January)
- Grace's birthday is the last of the year, but not the 1st.
- Someone (not Hannah) celebrates on 4th April
- Frances has her birthday on 1st day of the month

Which of the following MUST be true?

A. Rachel celebrates her birthday in April
B. Hannah has her birthday on 2nd of the month
C. Frances celebrates earlier in the year than Rachel
D. The first birthday of the year is 2nd January

7. Read this information about fruit

- A banana has more calories than a pear
- A pear has more calories than an apple
- Two satsumas are equal in calories to an apple
- Six grapes are equal in calories to one satsuma
- A quarter of a melon has the same calories as a banana and a satsuma combined
- A whole pineapple has the same calories as a whole melon

Which of the following statements is true?

A. A pineapple is equal in calories to four quarters of a melon, 4 bananas and 4 satsumas
B. 16 grapes are the same in calories value to a pear
C. A banana is equal in calories value to three satsumas
D. 24 grapes have fewer calories than two pears

8. This map shows a village green and the buildings around it. The green has a duck pond. The buildings are the pub, the church, the school, the shop and the café.

- The café, which is next door to the church (not around a corner), has a direct view of the pond.
- The pub is in building 1
- The church is next door to the shop (not around a corner)

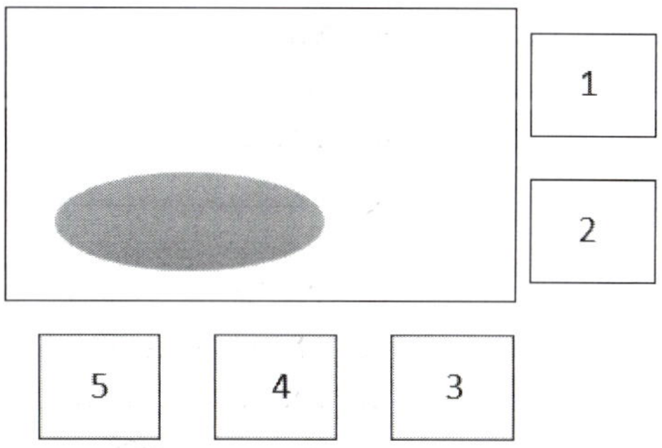

Which buildings occupy buildings 2 and 3?

A. Café and church
B. Church and shop
C. Shop and pub
D. School and shop

9. Encouraging people to spend their holidays in the UK would benefit the UK tourist industry and ensure that people enjoy the many sightseeing and entertainment opportunities the UK has.

Select the strongest argument

A. Yes – holidaying in the UK is cheaper and will enable more families to have holidays
B. Yes – this will ensure that people are knowledgeable about their own country
C. No – people should have choice as to where they spend their holiday
D. No – giving the UK tourist industry an unfair advantage isn't good business practice

10. This is a plan of a zoo. The zoo keeps:

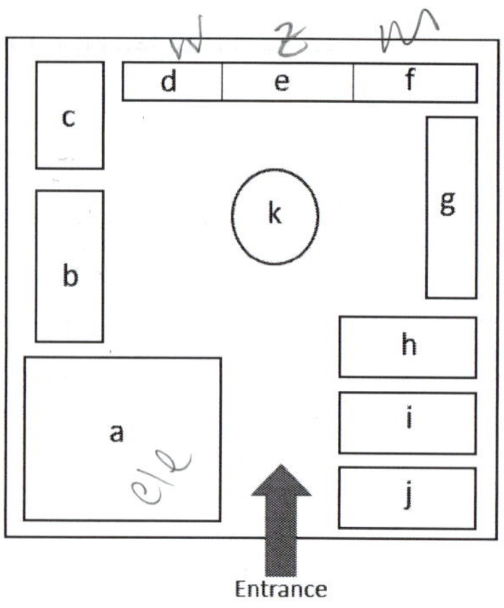

- Birds (in an aviary)
- Elephants
- Fish (in an aquarium)
- Giraffes
- Lions
- Monkeys
- Penguins (in an outdoor pond)
- Snakes (in a reptile house)
- Tigers
- Warthogs
- Zebras

- The elephants live in the largest enclosure
- Sections h, i and j are standalone buildings – an aquarium, an aviary and a reptile pond
- The tigers and lions are next to each other but in totally separate, single enclosures
- The giraffes are could see the lions and tigers, but the penguins are in the way!
- The zebras live between the warthogs and the monkeys

Which animals live in enclosures b, e and h?

A. Elephants, zebras and birds
B. Tigers, warthogs and snakes
C. Lions, zebras and birds
D. Tigers, zebras and penguins

11. Some animals have reached an 'evolutionary dead end' and only survive thanks to the efforts of conservationists. These animals should be allowed to go extinct as extinction is a natural, and desirable, part of evolution.

Select the strongest argument:

A. Yes – humanity interfering in the continuance of a species is as detrimental as contributing to its decline
B. Yes – conservation funding would be better spent elsewhere
C. No – humanity is now part of evolution and should be allowed to protect any species as we see fit
D. No – many of the dying species are of great cultural and educational value

12. There was a lot of upset caused when a resident of a picturesque village in the Cotswolds bought a yellow car. Local people, keen to maintain the ancient beauty of the village, pointed out that the man in question would not be allowed to paint his house, or even the windows and doors of his house, bright yellow as the village is designated a conservation area. However – the owner of the car said that no such rules applied to a vehicle. The debate continues over whether the letter of the law, or the presumed underlying principle, should be applied.
Should the man be allowed to keep his yellow car?

Select the strongest argument

A. Yes – underlying principles can't be applied as they're subjective and unknown
B. Yes – a yellow car can't detract significantly from the appearance of a whole village
C. No – the underlying principle of the rules are to protect the picturesque nature of the village
D. No – the rules should be updated and applied retrospectively

13. When taken globally – the consumption of tea is greater than the consumption of coffee. There are, however, some countries which vastly prefer coffee over tea. Both drinks have costs and benefits on environmental, social, health and economic grounds. Both products are known for being exploitative of the primary workforce which has led to an emergence of 'Fair Trade' versions of the products which enables western consumers to pay a little more but know that their beverage has not contributed to the ongoing exploitation of poor workers.

It is more important to buy fair trade tea than fair trade coffee as tea is the more widely drunk beverage.

Select the strongest argument

A. Yes – as more tea is drunk, more is produced so more people are exploited in this production
B. Yes – tea is a cheaper drink generally which means the exploitation levels are higher per cup
C. No – all products should be exclusively fair trade to ensure the end of worker exploitation
D. No – if rich nations drink more coffee, only drinking fair trade tea will have a limited impact

14. Select the conclusion which can be drawn from the graph

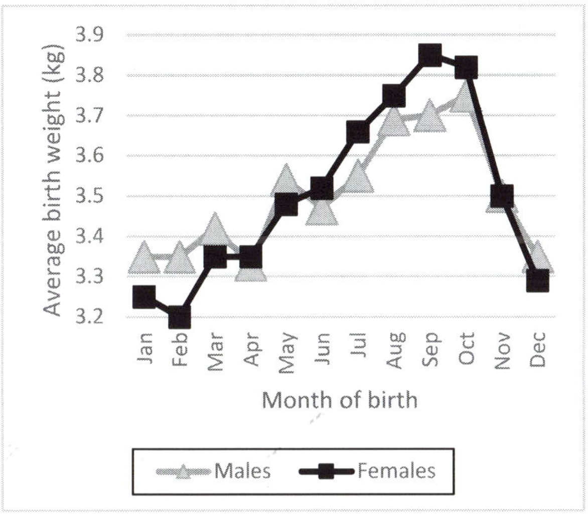

A. Being pregnant throughout the summer leads to bigger babies being born
B. The smallest babies of both genders are born in February
C. Girls vary in average birth rate more than boys
D. The average baby is 3.5kg

15. IQ tests have long been discredited as a general score of intelligence when applied to people from very different national, cultural and economic circumstances. A poor farmer from Sub-Saharan Africa or a Tibetan shepherd is unlikely to excel in an IQ test – but it doesn't mean they lack intelligence. It indicates that the test itself is biased towards people who have received a formal western-style education. The test can be quite useful in differentiating ability within specific population groups though.

UK school children should have their IQs tested to determine their potential.

Select the strongest argument

A. Yes – the IQ test may give teachers a general idea of the child's abilities
B. Yes – UK school children are a population group so internal IQ comparison is valid
C. No – UK school children may differ greatly in their ethnicity, religion and social class
D. No – the IQ test is discredited and shouldn't be used

16. Some African countries have started to routinely dye the tusks of elephants' bright pink as this makes the ivory in their tusks worthless to poachers and stops the poachers killing the elephants. There has been some concern that this approach makes the elephants more vulnerable to predators as bright pink is very noticeable in the African bush. Whilst the approach has had some success there are people who claim that changing the elephant to make it less attractive to the poacher is a back to front way of trying to address the problem of illegal animal poaching and that poachers should continue to be caught and punished to deter future poachers.

Should the practice of dying elephant tusks pink continue?

A. Yes – catching and punishing poachers hasn't stopped the practice so far
B. Yes – anything which protects the continued existence of elephants is justified
C. No – elephants will be killed just as much by predators as poachers if they can't hide
D. No – a market may emerge for pink ivory

17. Music "could face extinction" as a subject in secondary schools in England, researchers have warned. They say music is being squeezed because of pressure on pupils to take subjects included in the EBacc which is a determinant in the school's league table position. Almost two thirds of 650 state school teachers, surveyed by Sussex University researchers, said the EBacc meant fewer students were taking GCSE music. Ministers say the EBacc helps ensure children receive a rigorous education.
The English Baccalaureate or EBacc was brought in by the coalition government in 2010 for pupils achieving GCSE grade C or higher in English, maths, the sciences, a language and geography or history. The percentages of pupils entering and achieving the EBacc are among several measures used by government to determine a school's performance.

Select the words 'Yes' or 'No' if the conclusion does or doesn't follow

Music is not an EBacc subject	Yes / No
The promotion of the EBacc has led to a general decrease in the number of Arts subjects being studied to GCSE	Yes / No
Teachers agree that the promotion of EBacc is to blame for the decrease in uptake of Music	Yes / No
The EBacc is a rigorous education	Yes / No
A school's performance is mainly judged by the percentage of pupils achieving the EBacc	Yes / No

18. Professional athletes should not be allowed to endorse commercial products while they are still competing.

Select the strongest argument

A. Yes – any endorsement by a professional athlete implies that the product advertised contributed to their athletic success
B. Yes – saving all advertising work until after their competitive career is over gives them something to do after they've left the sport
C. No – the public benefit from knowing which products have helped athletes in their health, prowess and general success
D. No – athletes need to make a living and if endorsing products doesn't detract from their performance then it's fine

19. The Venn Diagram represents the menu of a restaurant.

Leah and Caleb visit the restaurant, Leah is Vegan, Caleb is Vegetarian. Which of the following is true of their options?

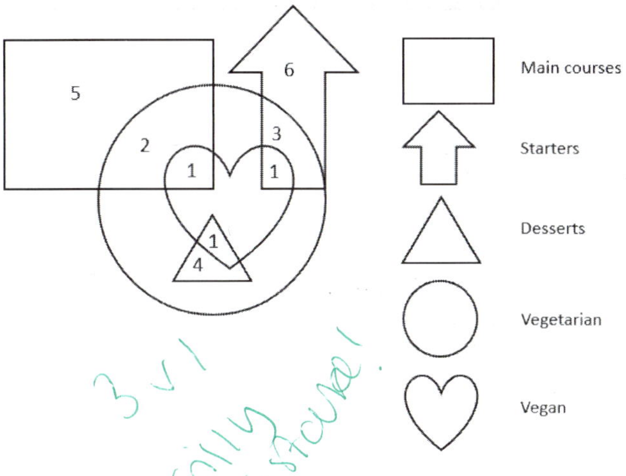

A. If they opt to share a starter or a dessert, they will only have two options

B. Caleb has three times as many main course options as Leah

C. If Leah wants a three-course meal she will only be able to make a choice on one course

D. Leah has only a third of the number of choices as Caleb for the starter.

20. The Venn Diagram represents a school and the extracurricular activities which the children are engaged with. There are 100 girls and 100 boys in the school.

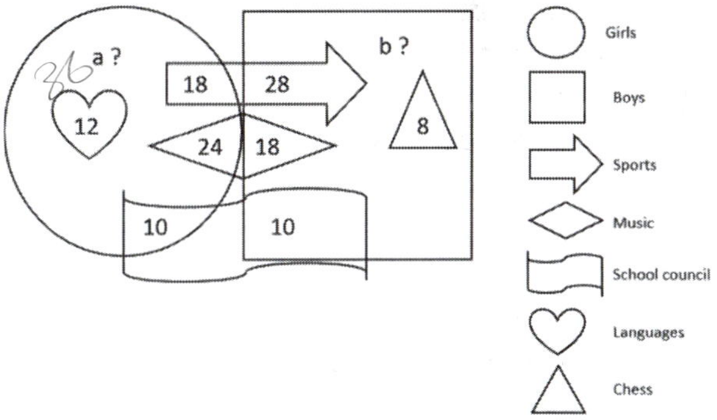

Which of the following is true?

A. 36% of students are not involved in any extracurricular activities

B. There is a school requirement to have equal representation of boys and girls on the school council

C. 42 children are in the school orchestra

D. 12% of the students are learning an extra-curricular language

21. Four colleagues each arrive at work bringing something for the team to share! Anna, Cheyenne, Rabia and Touba arrived carrying tea bags, cake, fruit and flowers. Who arrived with what in which order?

- The fruit arrived last – not with Cheyenne or Anna
- Rabia arrived before Cheyenne
- Touba arrived immediately after Anna (who had the teabags)
- The flowers arrived immediately before Cheyenne

Which of the following MUST be true?

A. Touba brought the cake
B. Anna arrived second
C. The flowers arrived first
D. Cheyenne arrived third

22. A political party interviewed 500 people to ascertain what their local concerns were. The interviews were unstructured, and the Venn Diagram shows the subjects raised and by how many residents.

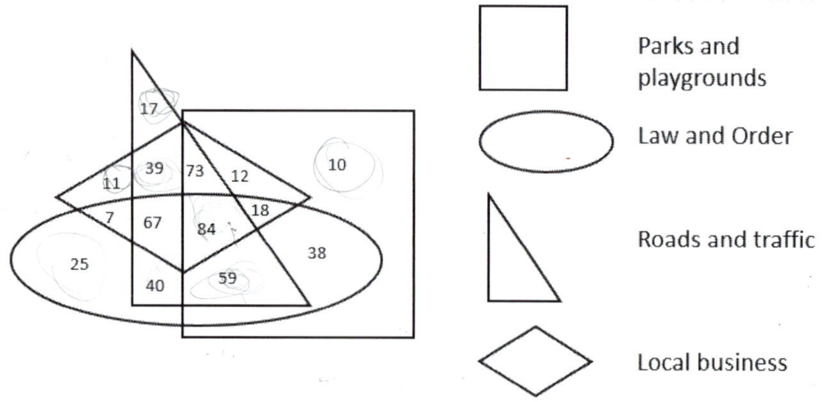

Which of the statements is true?

A. 84% of the residents were concerned about all the subjects mentioned
B. Around 1 in 8 residents only mentioned one subject
C. Less than 1% of people were just concerned for Law and Order and Local Business
D. Parks and Playgrounds were of most concern to the whole group

23. Which combination elicited the most responses?

A. Parks and Playgrounds and Law and Order
B. Law and Order and Roads and Traffic
C. Roads and Traffic and Local Business
D. Parks and Playgrounds and Roads and Traffic

24. Some zeps are zips.
No zips are zops.
Some zops are zups. No zops are zeps.
Some zups are zaps.
Which Venn Diagram represents this best?

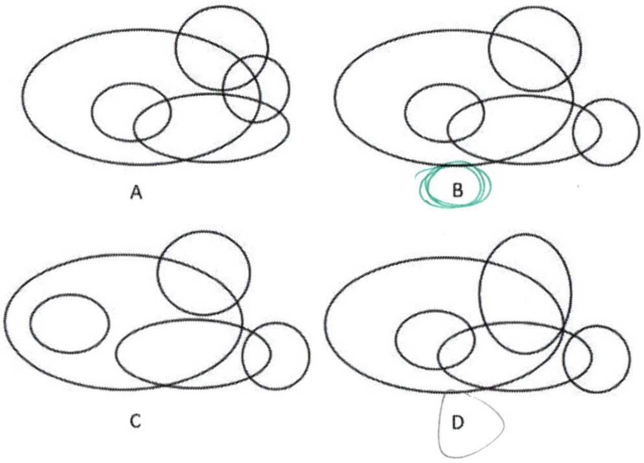

25. 'Extreme' online shopping offers many benefits to their customers including Next Day Delivery, a 25% discount on your first order and 5% cashback on all your orders in the first year!

Which of the Venn Diagram segments would 'Extreme' online shopping be place in?

a b c d e

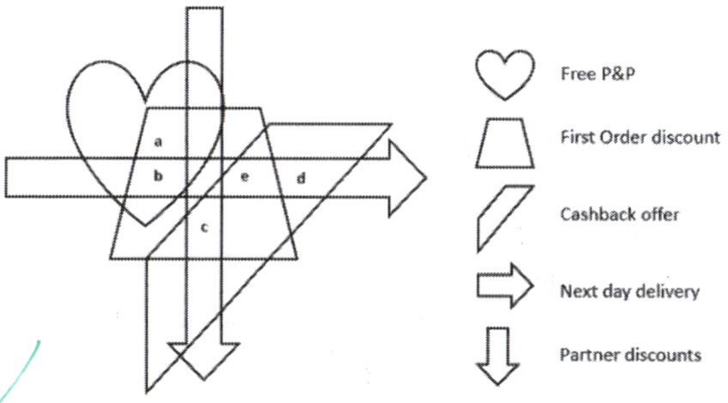

26. Three people are playing darts. They calculate the likelihood of each of them winning is:

Tom	20%
Andre	30%
Ethan	50%

Tom thinks that if they play three games of darts there is a better than 50% chance he will win at least once. Is he right?

A. Yes – he has three chances to win and his chance of winning is 1 in 5. 3 is more than half of 5.
B. Yes – his chance of not winning once is 80% but his chance of not winning at all is only 48.8%
C. No – he would need to play five times to be correct
D. No – his chance of not winning once is 80% but his chance of not winning at all is 51.2%

27. A football team have analysed 10 years of results and come up with this information about the circumstances that affect the likelihood of them winning.

Home match +8%
Away match -7%
Won the last match +12%
80%+ capacity crowd +5%
3 or more absent teammates -10%

The team are now playing at a neutral ground in a Cup Match. They won their last match but have 3 team members out with illness. (Assume a 50% chance of victory as a base).
What is the chance of victory?

A. 43%
B. 45%
C. 50%
D. 55%
E. 57%

28. Gerald has two ponds in his garden. Pond 1 has eight red fish and two yellow fish. Pond 2 has four red fish and six yellow fish.
Gerald takes out two fish; one from Pond 1 and one from Pond 2.
He is more likely to get two red fish than to get a yellow fish from Pond 1 followed by a red fish from Pond 2.

A. Yes, yellow fish from Pond 1 are the least likely single occurrence
B. Yes, two red fish are the most likely combination
C. No, there are more combinations that give a one yellow and one red fish
D. No, a red fish from Pond 1 is the most likely single occurrence

29. Jamila has a drawer full of mixed socks. She has animal decorated socks and flower decorated socks. There are eight identical animal socks and six identical flower socks.
She randomly removes a sock, puts it back, shakes the drawer, and then randomly takes a second sock. She believes she is more likely than not to pick two socks of the same type. Is she correct?

A. Yes, the probability of choosing two of the same is 24/49
B. Yes, the probability of choosing two of the same is 25/49
C. No, the probability of choosing two the same is 24/49
D. No, this would only be true if there were 8 flower socks

30. All Jads are Jids. Some Jids are Jods. No Juds are Jeds. All Jeds are Jads.
Select the words 'Yes' or 'No' if the conclusion does or doesn't follow

All Jeds are Jids — Yes / No
Some Jods are Jads — Yes / No
Some Jeds are Jods — Yes / No
A Jod could be a Jad — Yes / No
No Juds are Jids — Yes / No

31. Physical, climatic, and biological factors can contribute to endemism. The orange-breasted sunbird is exclusively found in the fynbos vegetation zone of southwestern South Africa. The glacier bear is found only in limited places in Southeast Alaska. Political factors can play a part if a species is protected, or actively hunted, in one jurisdiction but not another

Select the words 'Yes' or 'No' if the conclusion does or doesn't follow

A protected species is likely to enjoy better outcomes than a non-protected one — Yes / No
Multiple factors play an equal part in endemism — Yes / No
The orange breasted sunbird cannot be found in Europe — Yes / No
Political factors play a part in endemism only over international borders — Yes / No
Where humanity impacts the environment, it may also impact endemism — Yes / No

32. A risk factor is any attribute, characteristic or exposure of an individual that increases the likelihood of developing a disease or injury. Some examples of the more important risk factors are being underweight, unsafe sex, high blood pressure, tobacco and alcohol consumption, and unsafe water, sanitation and hygiene.

Select the words 'Yes' or 'No' if the conclusion does or doesn't follow

Exposure to risk factors is largely in the control of any individual — Yes / No
People with multiple risk factors are more likely than not to develop the disease — Yes / No
Risk factors apply to individuals rather than populations — Yes / No
Some risk factors have a bigger impact than others — Yes / No
Obesity is a risk factor — Yes / No

33. The family hosted a barbecue over the weekend. They served meat and vegetarian sausages, beef burgers, vegetable kebabs and chicken drumsticks. Some of their guests were vegetarian but most were not. Some of the non-vegetarians enjoyed some of the vegetarian food. There was also a selection of drinks, salads and a cake for dessert.

Select the words 'Yes' or 'No' if the conclusion does or doesn't follow

There was more than one drink option available	Yes / No
Some non-vegetarians enjoyed the vegetable kebabs	Yes / No
There was only one dessert option	Yes / No
The barbecue happened on a Saturday or Sunday	Yes / No
The barbecue happened at the family's home	Yes / No

34. Jenny, Kevin, Steve and Helen travelled by boat, car, plane and train to engage in a beach holiday, a city break, a shopping trip and a walking holiday.

- The beach holiday is a plane trip away
- Steve and Kevin don't like going on boats so wouldn't travel on holiday on one
- Jenny went shopping
- The man who went walking travelled by car
- The train travelled to the city break

Which of the following must be true?

A. Helen went to the beach
B. Jenny travelled by boat
C. Steve went on the walking holiday
D. Kevin went on the city break

35. Four cars (a red, blue, black and silver one) were each brought to a garage for some repairs. The cars were brought in on Monday, Tuesday, Wednesday and Thursday. They needed new tyres, new brake pads, a new exhaust and new light bulbs.

- The first car of the week needed to have new tyres
- The brake pads were fitted two days after the blue car had its exhaust replaced
- The red car was fixed one day before the silver car

Which of the following is true?

A. The brake pads were fixed on Wednesday
B. The red car needed new bulbs
C. The black car was fixed on Tuesday
D. The exhaust was fixed after the red car

36. Eight people (four women and four men) are sitting around a table. They are:

Women	**Men**
Paula	Brian
Kay	Tim
Claire	Andy
Sylvia	Ross

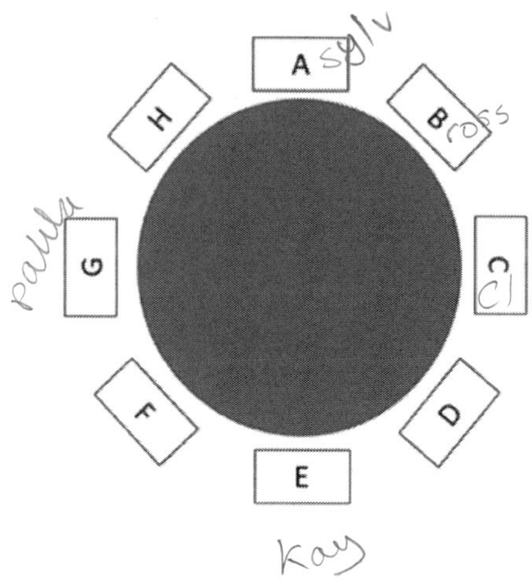

- They are sitting alternating between men and women.
- Only one person (a woman) has a seat letter which corresponds to her initial
- Brian and Andy are separated by Paula – neither of them is sitting beside Claire.
- Sylvia is sitting beside Ross (who is in seat B)

Where are Tim and Kay seated?

A. Seats B and A
B. Seats D and E
C. Seats F and G
D. Seats H and A

37. This shows the parking spaces outside an office building. The cars parked are owned by Carole, Sheila, Caroline, Jan and Betty.

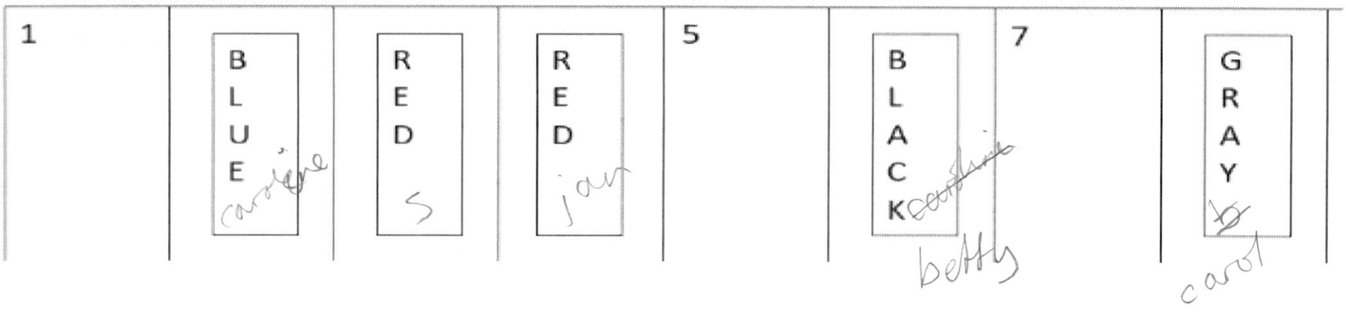

- Sheila is parked between two cars, next to Jan but not next to Betty
- Caroline does not drive the black car, nor is she parked in space 8.
- Carole is parked adjacent to a single empty space, her car isn't red.

Which of the following statements must be true?

A. Caroline drives a blue car
B. Jan drives a red car
C. Betty is parked in space 6
D. The blue car is in space 3

38. Drinking two litres of water a day is not medically necessary or even desirable if you have a balanced diet with plenty of fresh fruit and vegetables.

Select the strongest argument below

A. Yes – fruit and vegetables have a high enough water content to keep you hydrated
B. Yes – drinking too much water can be dangerous
C. No – there is no harm in drinking a lot of water
D. No – modern fruit and vegetables dry out in storage and on shelves

39. Shopping centres with car parks should strictly monitor their 'disabled' and 'parent and child' car parking spaces to stop people who aren't in need occupying spaces.

Select the strongest argument below

A. Yes – the spaces are allocated for a reason and not enforcing them disregards that reason
B. Yes – it is commercially sensible to cater for all customers including parents and the disabled
C. No – the additional costs of this service would simply be passed to the customer
D. No – most people respect these spaces and wouldn't use them anyway

40. 'Brain Training' apps and games are worth trying as even if they don't always produce empirical improvement in cognitive function, they can't do any harm and they are fun!

Select the strongest argument below

A. Yes – anything which exercises cognitive skill sets is worthwhile
B. Yes – brain training exercises are a more useful than other screen time activities
C. No – it's a pointless exercise if there is no hard data suggesting it is useful
D. No – people spend too much time honing 'hard' skills at the expense of soft skills

41. Parents should be allowed to take their children on holiday in school term time, with the consent of the head teacher.

Select the strongest argument below

A. Yes – family time is just as important as schooling
B. Yes – but only if the head teacher thinks the children can afford the time
C. No – parents should value the education of their children over that of entertainment
D. No – parents who can't afford holidays out of term time should stay at home

42. Which of the following statements is a logical conclusion to draw.

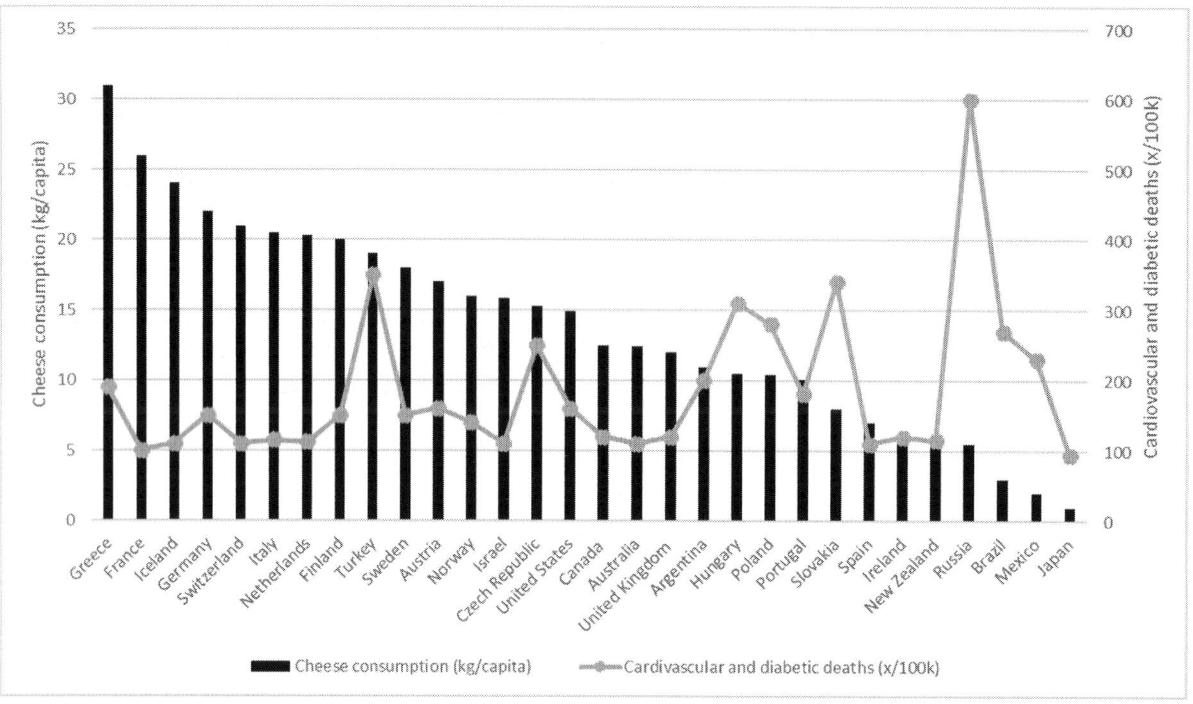

A. High cheese consumption is associated with more cardiovascular deaths
B. The global median cheese consumption rate is around 15kg per capita
C. There is no general, discernible trend shown on this chart
D. Some national and ethnic groups are more prone to cardiovascular disease than others

43. It is better to continually revise throughout an academic year than to cram for hours for a month just before your exams.

Select the strongest argument below

A. Yes – you will retain information much better if you are slow and steady in your approach
B. Yes – you will have really organised revision notes to work from
C. No – your revision efforts will detract from your ongoing coursework
D. No – you can't revise for an exam until you have covered all the curriculum

44. There is overwhelming evidence showing that starting school later is best, and the practice in many countries, such as Sweden and Finland. These countries have better academic achievement and child well-being, despite children not starting school until age 7.

The fear is that the English system – which was introduced in 1870 to get women back into work, rather than because of any educational benefit to children – is now causing profound damage. A similar story applies in the rest of the UK, and there is pressure for greater formality in preschools in other countries, such as the US.

The English school system should, therefore, be changed so that children start at aged 7 in order to protect them from profound harm.

Select the strongest argument below

A. Yes – the wellbeing of children should be of greater import than any other consideration
B. Yes – any system which hasn't been updated for over a century needs an overhaul
C. No – the system should be changed only if benefits for one group aren't at the expense of other groups
D. No – changing the level of formality in pre-school settings will protect children without such a radical change

45. There was a compulsory and an additional reading list for the course. There were nine required texts but over a hundred additional texts. The average length of book was 218 pages. One student has worked out that he can read 500 pages per week. He has twenty weeks in which he can do his reading.

Select the words 'Yes' or 'No' if the conclusion does or doesn't follow

The student will have time to read all his compulsory texts	Yes / No
It would take the student more than double his available time to read the whole list	Yes / No
There are at least 110 books on the total list	Yes / No
The course is in a literary subject	Yes / No
There are under 2000 pages of compulsory reading	Yes / No

46. People who rely on satnav could be at risk of losing their ability to navigate, an expert has warned.

Writing in the journal Nature, former president of the Royal Institute of Navigation Roger McKinlay argues that our reliance on GPS technology is misplaced and could be eroding our innate way-finding abilities. "If we do not cherish them, our natural navigation abilities will deteriorate as we rely ever more on smart devices," he wrote.

McKinlay believes huge investment will be needed before navigation systems will be good enough to allow technologies such as autonomous vehicles to take off. In the meantime, he argues, we need better research into systems for navigation while children should be encouraged to learn how to find their way around by more traditional means.

Schools should teach navigation and map reading as life skills.

Select the strongest argument below

A. Yes – relying on technology, which can fail, puts you in a dangerous position
B. Yes – navigation and map reading are useful spatial and logic skills
C. No – as technology advances essential 'life skills' inevitably change such as fire making
D. No – if navigation skills are 'natural' or 'innate' there is no need to teach them

47. This Venn diagram shows the various attractions available at several theme parks in the UK.

Assuming each theme park featuring a rollercoaster actually has three rollercoasters then how many rollercoasters are there in these theme parks in total?

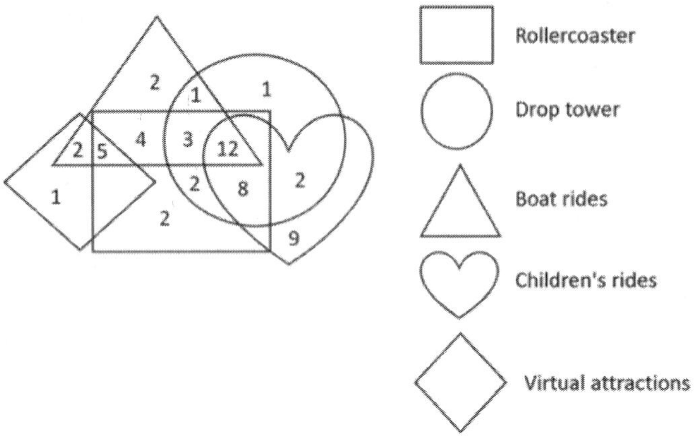

A. 36
B. 54
C. 102
D. 108
E. 162

48. The four largest theme parks by visitor number feature four out of five of these attractions. Which one do they all lack?

A. Rollercoasters
B. A drop tower
C. Boat rides
D. Children's rides
E. Virtual attractions
F.

49. Five couples each had their first child last year. Men: Andrew, Christopher, Geoff, Geraint, Martin. Women: Brenda, Claire, Nancy, Samantha, Sylvia. Babies: two daughters and three sons. Birth months: January, March, July, September and November

- Brenda and Samantha both had daughters. Neither of them had their baby is November
- Martin and his wife had their baby boy in January, two months before Andrew became a father
- Nancy gave birth in November. Two months after Samantha.
- Geoff and Sylvia are married and celebrated the arrival of their firstborn in July.

Which of the following must be true?

A. Andrew had a new baby daughter
B. Geraint had a baby with Samantha
C. Christopher had his baby in November
D. Christopher had his baby before Samantha

50. Which of the four scenarios is represented by this Venn Diagram?

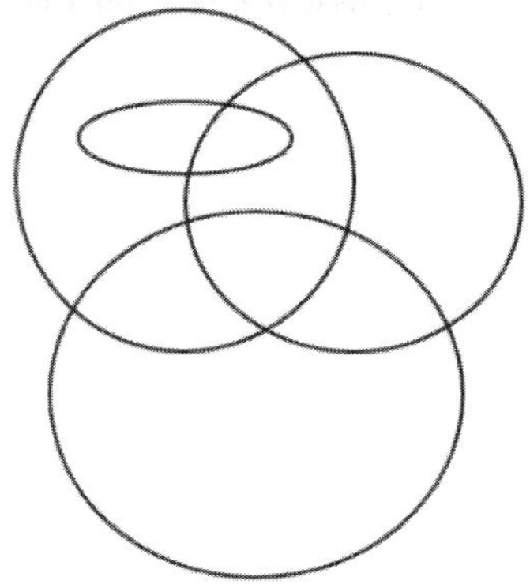

A. The flower displays all had a mixture of colours. Red, purple and pink were combined as was red and white and purple and blue. Only a few displays had fewer than three colours and all of the displays had a great deal of foliage.

B. A group shared their weekend activities. Many had watched TV; some watched TV and played sports; some watched TV, played sports and did housework. Some people watched TV and did housework. Some people saw family but all of those had either played sports or done housework as well.

C. When planning meals for the week the cook decided to make chicken, tomatoes and cheese her key ingredients and planned to make her meals using primarily these ingredients. She later sees that she also has some bacon but decides that this ingredient doesn't mix well with either cheese or tomatoes so only plans to use it in conjunction with chicken.

D. There were many dogs in the park. Some of the dogs had long fur, some were playing with a ball and some were on a lead. None of the dogs on a lead were playing with a ball. Only the dogs on a lead were wearing a collar.

51. A short haul travel company have identified the four key priorities different customers have asked for in their mini-breaks. They have classified their locations using the below Venn Diagram.

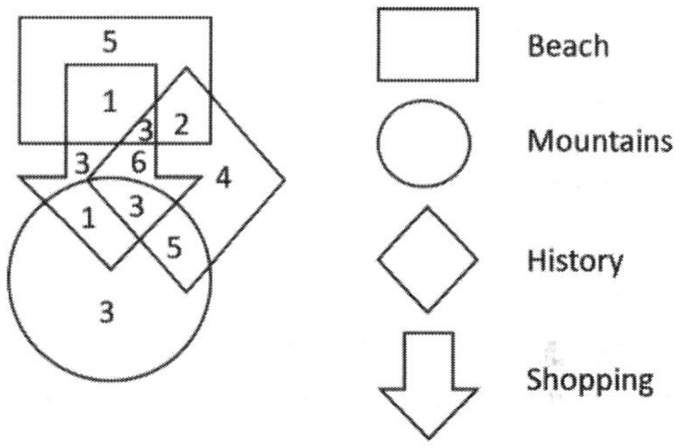

Which combination of attractions can't be enjoyed simultaneously?

A. Beach and mountains
B. Mountains and history
C. History and shopping
D. Beach and shopping

52. A family want to enjoy the beach and some history on their holiday. How many options do they have?

A. 2
B. 3
C. 5
D. 6

53. A record company has compiled the below Venn Diagram about its music groups. A group is defined as three or more artists. Most are only vocalists but there are some musicians (who play instruments in the group) as well. 'Success' is defined as a certain number of record sales.

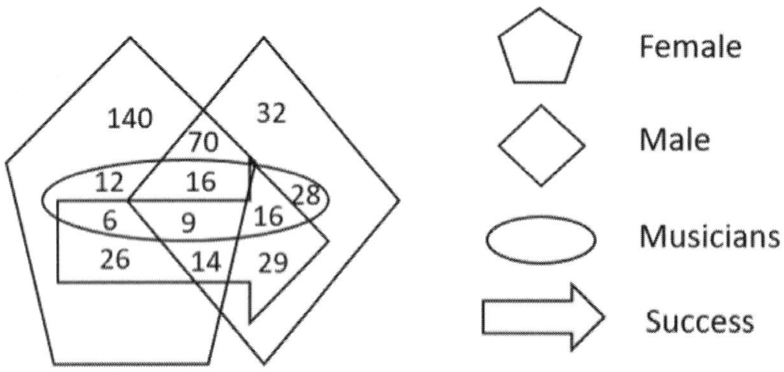

As a proportion the total number of mixed gender groups – how many achieve success?

A. 13%
B. 20%
C. 21%
D. 25%
E. 32%

54. Debbie and John have 4 children. They eat dinner together every night. Debbie burns the dinner three times a fortnight. When Debbie cooks 5 out of the 6 family members are satisfied with the nutritional quality of the meal. John burns the dinner once a week. When John cooks only 1 member of the family is dissatisfied with the nutritional quality of the meal.

Considering only the likelihood of burning and the satisfaction of the family members John should cook dinner.

A. Yes, the family are more satisfied with the meals that John cooks
B. Yes, satisfaction is equal, and Debbie is more likely to burn the dinner
C. No, the family are more satisfied by a meal cooked by Debbie
D. No, both have the same level of satisfaction and Debbie burns the dinner less often

55. You have a bag full of scrabble tiles. There are two of each of the five vowels and one each of all 21 of the other letters (consonants).

If you pick three random letters in turn without replacement you have a 1 in 26,970 probability of choosing the word cat?

A. Yes, there is one fewer tile at each subsequent pick and 31 x 30 x 29 = 26,970
B. No, it is 4 in 26,970 as there are 2 tiles for each vowel
C. No, it is twice as likely as this because there are two tiles for each vowel
D. No, there is less chance than this as there are a total of 31 tiles in the bag

56. Sam is using a random number generator to choose his pizza today. There are two types of base, deep pan or thin & crispy. There are five different toppings and three types of cheese. He will choose a base with 1 topping and 1 cheese. There is one possible combination that Sam hates, how likely is it that this combination will be picked.

A. There are 30 possible combinations which gives a 3% chance of picking the hated combination
B. There are 15 combinations so there is a 1 in 15 chance that any specific combination is picked
C. Each choice is independent so there is a 1% chance of choosing a single combination
D. There is a 1% chance of choosing that combination as 0.5+0.2+0.3 = 1

57. There are 30 students in a class. 18 are studying Art. 17 are studying Music. Kathleen is chosen at random. There is a 2 in 5 chance that Kathleen does not study Art?

A. Yes, there are 12 out of 30 students that do not study Art
B. No, there are 18 + 5 students who study Art, the probability is 23/30 that Kathleen does not
C. No, 18+17 = 35 so there is a 1 in 6 chance that Kathleen does not study Art
D. No, 18+17 = 35 so there is a 1 in 7 chance that Kathleen does not study Art

58. All flips have flops. Some flips have flops which have flups. Some flips have fleps and some have flaps. No flips have fleps AND flaps.

Select the words 'Yes' or 'No' if the conclusion does or doesn't follow

All flips have flups	Yes / No
Flips could have flups and flaps	Yes / No
Some flips don't have flops	Yes / No
All flips have either fleps or flaps	Yes / No
Not all flips have flups	Yes / No

59. There was a sale at the clothes shop. 80% of their stock was offered at a reduced price, with half of that being reduced by 50% or more. The shop was keen to sell off winter stock so most of the biggest reductions were on winter coats and knitwear.

Select the words 'Yes' or 'No' if the conclusion does or doesn't follow

20% of the shop's stock was being sold at full price	Yes / No
40% of sales during this period were from half price (or less) products	Yes / No
Half of the clothes in the shop were being sold at half price or less	Yes / No
Knitwear was being sold at less than half price	Yes / No
This sale took place during the spring time	Yes / No

60. Recent news reports have suggested that people who drink five cups of coffee per day reduce their risk of Liver Cancer by half. A lower reduction can be achieved with smaller amounts of coffee. Decaffeinated coffee also offers some protection but to a lesser extent.

Select the words 'Yes' or 'No' if the conclusion does or doesn't follow

1 cup of coffee per day could reduce the risk of Liver Cancer by 10%	Yes / No
Many more tea drinkers will get Liver Cancer than coffee drinkers	Yes / No
It's possible the caffeine has some protective effect	Yes / No
The exact mechanism of this reported impact is not definitely known	Yes / No
This research could lead to thousands of lives being saved per year	Yes / No

61. A sixth form advertise the following:

- ***95% of previous students achieved B B B or better in their A-levels***
- ***75% students got to their first-choice university, everyone else got their insurance place or secured a university space through clearing***
- ***40% students went to a Russell Group University (top tier universities)***
- ***15% students go to Oxford or Cambridge (ultra-top tier universities)***

Select the words 'Yes' or 'No' if the conclusion does or doesn't follow

5% of students did not achieve well in their A-levels and needed to use clearing

to get a university place — Yes / No

All the students went to university — Yes / No

Students routinely take 3 A levels — Yes / No

25% of students use clearing to get a university place — Yes / No

At least 20% of students select a non-Russell group / Oxbridge university as their first choice — Yes / No

62. The three tallest children in the class of 30 are all boys but the average height of the girls is taller than the average height of the boys. There are equal numbers of girls and boys. Their teacher has noted that some of the children have grown over 5cm in the last year.

Select the words 'Yes' or 'No' if the conclusion does or doesn't follow

The shortest child in the class is a boy — Yes / No

Both boys and girls could have grown 5cm in the last year — Yes / No

There are 15 girls in the class — Yes / No

Girls are typically taller than boys as children — Yes / No

5cm is significant growth for a child in one year — Yes / No

63. Five people had just submitted application forms for a new driving license. The five people – Aiden, Brodie, Lily, Melanie and Peter – were an architect, an engineer, a doctor, a lawyer and a politician. Their birthdays were on April 4, June 27, July 8, October 26 and December 6.

- Brodie was born in October, later in the year than Lily the architect.
- The politician (not Aiden or Melanie) was born on December 6
- Of Melanie and the person born on July 8 – one is the Lawyer and the other the Doctor
- The doctor and Lily have the closest birthdays

Which of the following must be true?

A. The engineer had their birthday before the doctor
B. Aiden is a doctor
C. Lily has her birthday before the Lawyer
D. Brodie is a Politician

64. Zippo's Fun Park has four rollercoasters! They were installed three years apart and have four different top speeds! The rollercoasters are called 'Zippo's Train Ride', 'Space Rocket', 'The Excitement Factor' and 'Firework Fury'. They were installed in 2003, 2006, 2009 and 2012. Their top speeds are 30mph, 50mph, 70 mph and 80mph.

- The first rollercoaster to be installed in the park is not the fastest one or Firework Fury
- Space rocket is the latest addition to the park, it doesn't go as fast as the one installed three years earlier
- Visitors in 2006 were excited to ride the new 70mph rollercoaster

Which of the following must be true?

A. Zippo's Train Ride is the slowest in the park
B. The earliest rollercoaster in the park in the slowest
C. Firework Fury has a top speed of 70mph
D. The Excitement Factor is the fastest rollercoaster in the park

65. Four people were relocating from their home city for various reasons. One is retiring, one has a new job, one is moving to be closer to their family and the other is moving to study. The places they are moving to are London, Cardiff, Edinburgh and Liverpool.

Can you deduce why and where to Shanna, Amna, Vy and Alex were moving?

- It is not Shanna who has a place at the University of Liverpool to continue her studies
- Amna is excited about her new job.
- Alex is moving to London, the person who is retiring is going to Cardiff

Which of the following is true?

A. Alex is moving to be closer to her family
B. Vy is going to work in Liverpool
C. Amna isn't moving to Edinburgh
D. Shanna is going to study in Cardiff

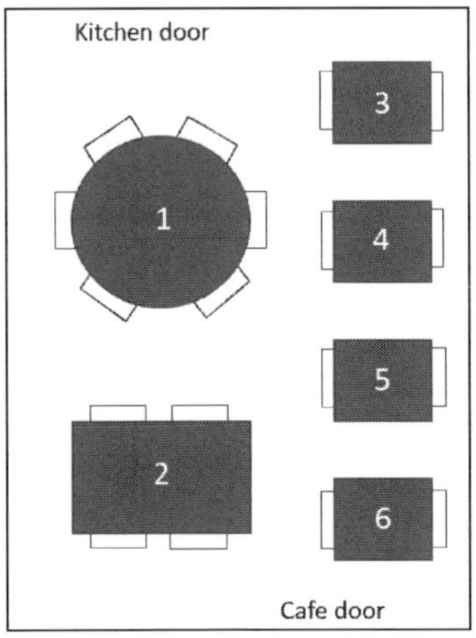

66. There are two parties of four people seated in this café. There is also a couple sitting on an even numbered table. A single diner is sitting on the table closest to the café door. When Mike and Heather go into the café for a meal, which two tables are available for them?

A. 1 and 2
B. 2 and 3
C. 3 and 5
D. 4 and 6

67. A café is compiling a list of their best-selling item on different days of the week. They analyse their sales for Monday, Wednesday, Friday and Sunday. The four days each reveal a different best-selling foodstuff (items 1, 3, 6 and 7) and drinks (items 1, 3, 4 and 6).

Breakfast menu:	Drinks:
1. Toast and marmalade	1. Tea
2. Beans on toast	2. Americano
3. Sausage sandwich	3. Latte
4. Egg and bacon	4. Cappuccino
5. Croissant	5. Espresso
6. Pain au Chocolat	6. Hot chocolate
7. Full English Breakfast	7. Orange Juice
8. Full Vegetarian Breakfast	8. Fruit smoothie

- Obviously – most people need to begin their week with a strong cup of tea!
- It seems that a combination of hot chocolate and toast and marmalade is very popular
- The full breakfast is most enjoyed on a Sunday (presumably when people have a little more time) but a couple of days before that people enjoy a Pain au Chocolat with a Latte

Which of the following is true?

A. On Monday people enjoy Tea and a Full Breakfast
B. On Wednesday people enjoy Hot chocolate and Toast and marmalade
C. On Thursday people enjoy Latte and Pain au Chocolat
D. On Sunday people enjoy Tea and a Full breakfast

68. Public transport should be heavily subsidised in order to tackle traffic congestion

Select the strongest argument from the options below:

A. Yes – many people find that driving is quicker than a bus or train so happily pay the extra cost
B. Yes – one bus can carry as many people as 40 cars but take up far less space on the road
C. No – it's not the cost of public transport which stops people using it but the fact it is less convenient
D. No – subsidising any venture artificially manipulates the market and prevents problems self-correcting

69. Older people who are under-occupying large houses should be given an incentive to downsize. This would ease the house crisis which is causing many young families to live in crowded conditions.

Select the strongest argument from the options below:

A. Yes – it is not fair that some people live alone in very large houses whilst large families are crammed into small homes.
B. Yes – if the incentive were fair and there was no compulsion involved then this could help a lot of people
C. No – older people are attached to their homes by sentiment and memory and shouldn't have to move
D. No – young families living in close proximity promotes close family relationships and need not be discouraged

70. University tuition fees should vary according to how much direct contact time (lectures, tutorials, seminars etc) the course entails. A philosophy degree (which may only require 6 hours of lectures per week) costs the same as an engineering degree (where there are 30 hours of lectures / direct contact per week)

Select the strongest argument from the options below:

A. Yes – everything else you buy is priced according to its value rather than being a standard amount
B. Yes – people who do higher contact courses such as medicine or engineering are likely to earn more in the long run so can pay back a bigger debt
C. No – an effective way to ensure that high contact courses can be made affordable to everyone is for lower contact courses to subsidise them
D. No – all higher education is subsidised and paying an equal amount shows that different disciplines are equally valued by society

71. End of life decisions regarding medical care should be made by doctors, who are able to assess the situation with a scientific and objective eye.

Select the strongest argument from the options below:

A. Yes - family members cannot make these decisions due to their lack of medical knowledge and grief
B. Yes - only a doctor knows if a patient is likely to be in pain, or has a chance of recovery
C. No – a consensus should always be sought between medics and family members
D. No – doctors should do everything they can to save someone even if it seems pointless

72. All of our hotel rooms have en-suite facilities with most of those having both a bath and shower. We have three rooms with four poster beds and all of the rooms at the front of the hotel enjoy stunning views of the lake. There are two rooms on the ground floor which are suitable for people with mobility issues. We also have one family room which can sleep a family of four.

Select the words 'Yes' or 'No' if the conclusion does or doesn't follow

Pete and Lizzie would like a room with a four-poster bed and a lake view.

Can this hotel definitely accommodate this? Yes / No

Mr and Mrs King have two children. Would the family room have en-suite facilities? Yes / No

Mrs Ashdown uses a wheelchair. Would the room she can use definitely

have a lake view? Yes / No

More than half of the rooms in the hotel have a lake view Yes / No

The hotel has at least two storeys Yes / No

73. A cosmetics company is launching a new line of hand creams. All of the hand creams are suitable for sensitive skin. Three of the new range have flower fragrances. One contains beeswax. All except one are quick absorb and the other is a heavy 'night hand cream' intended to give 'dry hands an intensive overnight burst of moisture'.

Select the words 'Yes' or 'No' if the conclusion does or doesn't follow

Half of the new hand creams have a flower fragrance Yes / No

The beeswax hand cream doesn't have a flower fragrance Yes / No

The night hand cream is suitable for sensitive skin Yes / No

There are at least three varieties Yes / No

The beeswax hand cream is quick absorb Yes / No

74. A travel agent is comparing the cost of holidays to various European destinations

	Spain	Italy	Greece
Flights – per person	£250	£400	£550
Accommodation – per unit of up to six people	£500	£600	£200
Typical meal out – per person	£8	£7	£5
Typical attraction cost – per person	£10	£11	£8

Select the words 'Yes' or 'No' if the conclusion does or doesn't follow

For a family of four the additional flight costs make a holiday to Greece, in local accommodation, less economical than either of the other destinations Yes / No

A couple on holiday in Greece go out for two meals every day and visit one attraction every day. After fourteen days they recoup the extra money spent on an airfare to Greece rather than Italy. Yes / No

The cheap flights to Spain make the biggest difference to the overall holiday cost Yes / No

If a family could drive to the destination for the cost of one airfare, then a Greek holiday would be the most economical Yes / No

The cost of meals out or attractions makes up less than 10% of the total value of a holiday Yes / No

75.

International Tourist Arrivals and Receipts in Sub-Saharan Africa, 2010

Region	Total tourist arrivals	Total long hauls	Receipts (US$, million)	Average contribution to GDP (%)
Southern Africa	10,626,127	2,509,893	8,599	3.4
East Africa	11,905,651	3,944,858	6,332	5.5
West Africa	4,419,061	1,748,555	2,676	2.0
Central Africa	1,075,408	654,168	631	1.7
Total	**28,026,247**	**8,857,474**	**18,238**	**2.6**

Select the words 'Yes' or 'No' if the conclusion does or doesn't follow

Southern African nations collectively have a larger economy than the other regions Yes / No

Southern and East Africa had similar numbers of non long-haul tourist arrivals. (within 250,000) Yes / No

Tourism in Africa is worth less than 20 billion US dollars. Yes / No

Central Africa had the highest proportion of long-haul arrivals Yes / No

If more long-haul flights flew into Central Africa, their tourist industry would grow Yes / No

76. A mother leaves four equal length lists of chores for her two sons and two daughters to do while she is at work. Half of the chores she asked her daughters to do are done. The whole list of kitchen related chores is completed but only half of the jobs she wanted done in the living room are done. One of her sons does not do any of his chores but the other completes his list and does some of the chores on his sister's list as well.

Select the words 'Yes' or 'No' if the conclusion does or doesn't follow

The two daughters did some of their chores Yes / No

There was more than one job in more than one room on the lists Yes / No

The kitchen was tidier than the lounge when the mother got home Yes / No

Only one child completed their list of jobs Yes / No

Three of the four children did something from their list Yes / No

77. One city has three football teams. They all play in the same league with 17 other teams. Between the three of them the blues won the most matches this season, but the reds scored the most goals. The team that plays in white beat both of their local rivals in all league matches – the reds and the blues, home and away. None of the teams won any trophies.

Select the words 'Yes' or 'No' if the conclusion does or doesn't follow

The blue team finished highest of the three in the league table	Yes / No
The blue team lost at least twice	Yes / No
The white team had more than four wins during the season	Yes / No
The red team failed to score against the white team	Yes / No
The blue team won the league	Yes / No

78. Gregory is growing pea plants, he notices that plants with green pods have a 1 in 3 chance of having yellow seeds, the remainder have green seeds. Half of plants grown from green seeds have purple flowers and half have white flowers. Plants grown from yellow seeds have white flowers.

He has 4 plants grown from green seeds and 2 plants grown from yellow seeds that have been mixed up.

He gives two plants at random to his grandmothers. The probability that they both produce purple flowers is one third

A. Yes, because only two of the plants from green seeds will give purple flowers
B. Yes, because there is a 1 in 3 chance of having yellow seeds which give purple flowers
C. No, because one third is the probability of having yellow seeds from a green pod
D. No, it is much lower than one third as most of the plants produce white flowers

79. A bag contains 4 green beads and 2 red beads. A bead is taken from the bag and then replaced before drawing another bead. The probability of drawing 2 red beads is half that of drawing one red and then a one green bead.

A. Yes, because the green beads are twice as common as the red ones
B. Yes, because the probability of drawing two green beads is 3/9
C. No, because green is the most common colour bead
D. No, because the chance of drawing two red beads is 1/9

80. The Venn Diagram shows the colours used in the uniforms of all the primary schools in locality. Most schools have one colour which is combined with black, white or grey, but a few have more than one colour in their tie

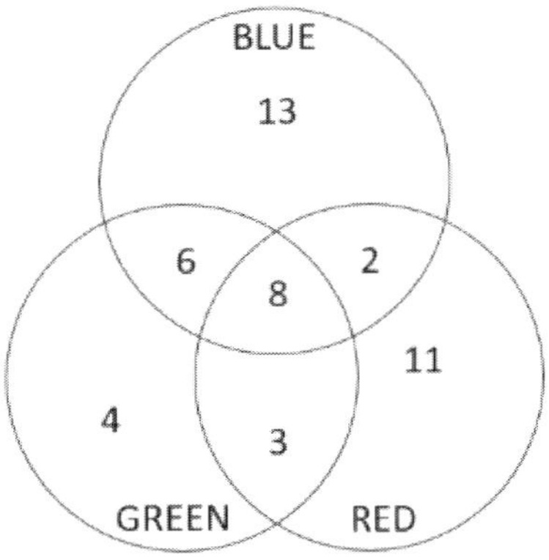

How many schools have two colours in their uniform?

A. 6
B. 9
C. 11
D. 19

81. Based on the diagram, which of the following statements are true?

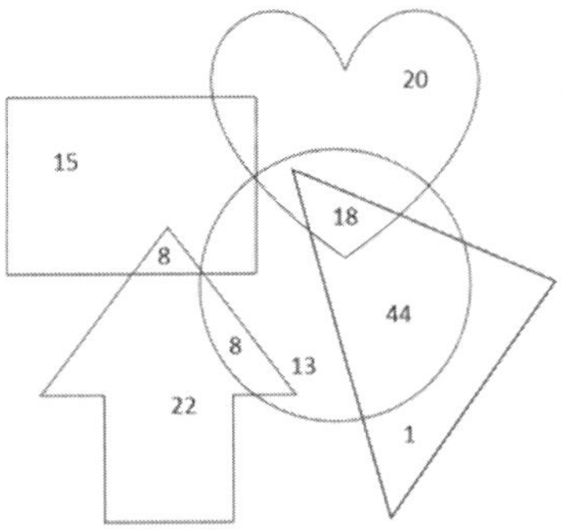

The rectangle represents commuters who cycle
The arrow represents commuters who drive
The triangle represents commuters who walk
The circle represents commuters who catch the train
The heart represents commuters who catch the bus

A. More commuters cycle and drive than commuters who only catch the train
B. The number of commuters who walk, catch the bus and catch the train are equal to the number who cycle to work
C. The number of commuters who catch the bus is the same as the number of commuters who drive
D. The are 30 more commuters who catch the train and walk than there are commuters who only cycle to work

82. On a housing estate in Cardiff, the homes have different features.

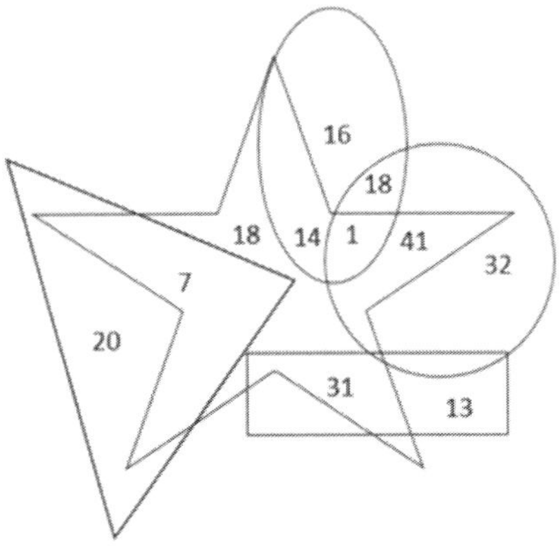

The oval represents home which have a patio

The triangle represents homes which have a driveway

The circle represents homes which have a garage

The rectangle represents homes which have a porch

The star represents homes which have a garden

Based on the diagram, which of the following statements are false?

A. Houses that have a garden and a patio are less common than the houses that have a patio and a garage
B. The number of houses that have a porch and a garden are more than the houses that have driveways
C. There are 26 less houses that have a garden and a driveway than houses that only have a garage
D. Houses that have a garden, patio and a garage are the least common

83. There is a summer scheme with 100 children. There are 60 boys and 40 girls. Half of the children are taking part in the Sports day. 30% of them are taking part in the Theatre production.

Which diagram represents this data set?

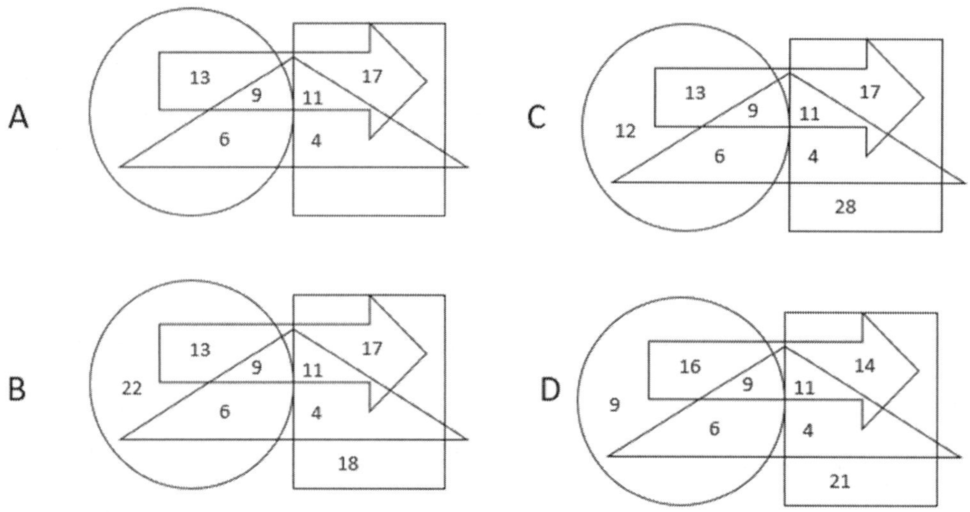

A. A
B. B
C. C
D. D

84. A survey of a village school with a large pupil population shows that a child who lives more than 6 miles from the school has a probability of 1 of being driven to school. A child who lives within 400 yards of the school has a probability of 0 of being driven to school. Of the rest 10%, are driven to school, 10% take the bus, 5% ride a bicycle and the rest walk to school. 4 children who live 1 mile from school are chosen at random. The most likely outcome is that all but one of them walk to school.

A. Yes, because at least a quarter of children do not walk to school
B. Yes, because 65% of children walk to school which is most of them
C. No, because 65% of children walk to school which is most of them
D. No, because a probability of 0 means this is an impossible event

85. Jenny is booking a package holiday and is choosing between two tour operators. Johnsons Tours has a delayed flight rate of 2% and makes last minute room alterations for 2 in 25 customers. Jacksons Tours flights arrive on time 98% of the time and are able to guarantee the same room as booked for 45 out of 50 customers.

Considering only the likelihood of a delayed flight or a room alteration should Jenny book with Jacksons Tours?

A. Yes, because at Johnsons Tours are more likely to make a room alteration
B. Yes, because at Johnsons Tours are more likely to have a flight delay
C. No, because at Johnsons Tours are less likely to make a room alteration
D. No, because at Jacksons Tours are less likely to have a flight delay

86. An African elephant weighs more than an Asian elephant. A giraffe and a hippopotamus weigh about the same. A rhinoceros weighs more than a crocodile but less than a giraffe.

Select the words 'Yes' or 'No' and drop them to the appropriate places if the conclusion does or doesn't follow

An Asian elephant weighs more than a giraffe	Yes / No
A hippopotamus weighs more than a crocodile	Yes / No
A crocodile is the smallest animal described here	Yes / No
A rhinoceros weighs less than a giraffe	Yes / No
An African elephant is the largest animal described here	Yes / No

87. The largest land mammal in the world is the African Elephant. Other mega-fauna (large mammals) include the Asian Elephant, the Hippopotamus and the Giraffe. Mega-fauna as usually defined as being over 1000Kg (1 metric ton) but this causes problems as the weight range for some creatures (such as the rhinoceros and crocodile) crosses this threshold leading to a discussion over whether they class as mega-fauna or not.

Select the words 'Yes' or 'No' and drop them to the appropriate places if the conclusion does or doesn't follow

African elephants usually weight more than 1 metric ton	Yes / No
As adult crocodile may weigh less than 1 metric ton yet still be mega-fauna	Yes / No
A full-grown giraffe is typically heavier than a full-grown rhinoceros	Yes / No
There are some definitions of mega-fauna which don't include the 1000kg weight limit	Yes / No
There are sea mammals which are bigger than land mammals	Yes / No

88. Matthew was the oldest child in the group of five. He was born immediately before Elliot. Chris was the second youngest. Oli was right in the middle. James was also in the group.

Select the words 'Yes' or 'No' and drop them to the appropriate places if the conclusion does or doesn't follow

There were five boys in this group	Yes / No
James was the last born	Yes / No
Elliot is older than Oli	Yes / No
Chris is older than Oli	Yes / No
Matthew was the firstborn of the group	Yes / No

89. As many as 2,529 products have shrunk in size over the past five years, but are being sold for the same price, official figures show.

The Office for National Statistics (ONS) said it was not just chocolate bars that have been subject to so-called "shrinkflation".

It said toilet rolls, coffee and fruit juice were also being sold in smaller packet sizes.

At the same time 614 products had got larger between 2012 and 2017.

Most of the items getting smaller were food products.

Select the words 'Yes' or 'No' and drop them to the appropriate places if the conclusion does or doesn't follow

Some non-food products are being sold in smaller sizes for the same price	Yes / No
Chocolate bars have been the subject of Shrinkflation	Yes / No
All product package sizes are shrinking	Yes / No
This data is gained from the observation of consumers	Yes / No
The ONS primarily concerns itself with retail data such as this	Yes / No

90. Their study suggests there's now a one in three chance of monthly rainfall records being broken in England and Wales in winter.
The estimate reflects natural variability plus changes in the UK climate as a result of global warming.
But a supercomputer was needed to understand the scale of increased risk.

Select the words 'Yes' or 'No' and drop them to the appropriate places if the conclusion does or doesn't follow

There was extensive flooding in 2014 in the UK	Yes / No
Monthly rainfall records for England and Wales are likely to be broken 4 times a year	Yes / No
Experienced meteorologists are calculating the risks	Yes / No
Global warming is the main cause of the downpours	Yes / No
There is a natural variability to the UK climate	Yes / No

91. Dr Daniels saw four children in surgery this morning. None of them were particularly ill so each was presented with a different coloured lollipop and told it would make them feel better! Hurrah for placebos! Can you work out which child (Isabelle, Amelia, Benjamin and Matthew) had which imagined ailment (hurty foot, aching fingers, sore hair or bumpy freckles) and which coloured lollipop cured them of their ills (red, orange, green or purple).

- Dr Daniels assured his patient that red lollipops were medicine for aching fingers
- Benjamin was cured by a green lollipop – but not for sore hair
- Isabelle's bumpy freckles were cured by her lollipop which was not purple

Which of the following must be true?

A. Amelia had a purple lollipop
B. Matthew had sore hair
C. Isabelle was cured by a red lollipop
D. The aching fingers were cured by a red lollipop

92. Four classes each did an assembly on a famous composer. Which class (years 2, 3, 4 and 5) did their assembly on which day (Monday, Tuesday, Thursday and Friday) about which composer (Handel, JS Bach, Mozart and Beethoven).

- Year 5 went first, three days before the Handel presentation.
- The youngest year group (year 2) presented of Mozart – the child genius – three days after the school had learned about Beethoven from year 4

Which of the following must be true?

A. The Handel presentation was the day after the Beethoven presentation
B. Year 3 presented their composer on Wednesday
C. The first composer to be presented was JS Bach
D. Year 5 presented Handel

93. Four cats have four different fur colours and four different servants.

The cats are: Tiddles, Fluffy, Whiskers and Obadiah
Their fur colours are: Black, Tabby, Ginger, White
Feline servants: Miss Price, Mr Fudding, Sir Timpson and the Dibble family

- Sir Timpson gave his cat the regal name Obadiah
- The Dibble family own the ginger cat
- Fluffy is a white, long haired cat
- Mr Fudding is the willing servant of Whiskers, who is not a black cat!

Which of the following is true?

A. The black cat is Tiddles
B. Miss Price owns the tabby cat
C. Whiskers is a ginger cat
D. Sir Timpson owns the black cat

94. Susan has knitted a blanket using four colours of yarn (red, blue, green and yellow) made up of 16 squares as shown. There are four squares of each colour.

- **The corner squares (A, D, M and P) feature two red and two yellow squares**
- **There are two diagonal lines of symmetry**
- **B is green and C is blue**

A	B	C	D
E	F	G	H
I	J	K	L
M	N	O	P

Which of the following statements must be true?

A. G and J are red
B. F and K are the same colour
C. There is a vertical line of symmetry
D. D and M are yellow

95. Four friends take it in turns to cook dinner each month. They each choose a different cuisine and take charge for one night.

The friends are Brandy, Wanda, Floyd and Noel. The cuisines they cooked are TexMex, Indian, Italian and Moroccan. They meet for dinner February, April, June and August.

- The group really enjoy Moroccan food in February (it wasn't cooked by Floyd)
- Brandy cooked for the group in a month beginning with the letter A
- The final meal on this table was an Italian feast, enjoyed 2 months after Wanda cooked

Which of the following must be true?

A. Noel cooked Moroccan food
B. Brandy cooked in April
C. Wanda cooked TexMex food
D. They didn't have Italian food in August

96. There should be a wide variety of media in terms of culture, information and ideas. People should be able to choose from a wide range of alternatives according to their different needs, points of view, beliefs and tastes. For this to be achieved there needs to be diversity of ownership and real opportunities for access to all main voices and interests in society.

With this statement in mind – Is it important for government regulation to act against potential monopolies within society?

Select the strongest argument

A. Yes – government needs to ensure that there is balance and equality in the media
B. Yes – if one entity controls too much of the media they could have undue influence over the populace
C. No – if government interferes with media then they could clamp down on negative coverage
D. No – A wide range of media will naturally happen in a free, democratic society

97. A major obesity programme introduced into more than 50 primary schools in the West Midlands has failed to have any significant effect on children's weight. Children were given a year of extra physical activity sessions, a healthy eating programme and cookery workshops with their parents. Families were invited to activity events, including sessions run by Aston Villa football club.

But at the end of 30 months, there was no difference in obesity between those children who took part and those who did not.

Do schools have a role in tackling the childhood obesity epidemic?

A. Yes – they should still play a part in conjunction with wider action by other agencies
B. Yes – this programme has not been successful but other programmes will work better
C. No – the failure of this programme shows that the issue cannot be easily or quickly solved
D. No – schools should concern themselves with academic education and not tackling lots of social ills

98. Capital punishment is often supported by populations of nations where it is used but rarely in populations where it was stopped many years ago.

Support for capital punishment wanes when people are not regularly exposed to it.

Select the strongest argument from the options below:

A. Yes – people who have not grown up with state execution find it barbaric and unusual
B. Yes – people are far more squeamish now and the history of public execution horrifies most people
C. No – no-one is regularly exposed to executions so exposure can't be a factor in support
D. No – there are many variations between populations and causal links are hard to establish

99. Is censorship, the changing or the suppression or prohibition of speech or writing that is subversive of the common good, a necessary part of modern society?

Select the strongest argument from the options below:

A. Yes – the common good is the highest principle at stake here
B. Yes – modern society cannot withstand subversion without causing damage to the people
C. No – some censorship may be desirable but it's not necessary
D. No – without knowing who defines 'subversive' and 'common good' a conclusion cannot be drawn

100. The exact mechanism of climate change, which is the cause of the increased regularity of severe weather, and how humans contribute to it are uncertain. Therefore, all efforts to arrest the process are speculative. It is not known if climate change can be halted or slowed but an increase in severe weather events of all kinds will certainly cause harm to populations, infrastructures, economies and society.

Efforts should be made to tackle climate change even if we are uncertain that they will work.

Select the strongest argument from the options below:

A. Yes – uncertain and speculative do not mean there is no chance of success and the harm of doing nothing is unacceptable
B. Yes – it is better to try something which turns out to be ineffective than to do nothing
C. No – money and effort would be better spent trying to protect people from these weather events
D. No – we cannot win the battle with climate change and must adapt to a new normal

100 Decision Making Question Answers

1.It did not rain at all this summer **No**
The rainfall is described as 'low', not none.
There was a hosepipe ban in areas where water shortages were reported **Yes**
The hosepipe ban was a blanket ban, but it did apply in these areas
Some arable crops don't require as much rainfall as others **Yes**
The farmer's responses show that different crops respond differently to weather
It was hotter than average every day of the summer **No**
It was hotter than average for the season – not every single day
This season benefitted some people **Yes**
Some farmers found their crops 'thrived'

2. Thomas put the maximum amount of effort into all his classes **No**
His effort score was 'good' in some classes, rather than excellent
Thomas was making steady progress in all his subjects **No**
His progress was on target – when taken as an average.
Thomas was not meeting targets in some subjects **Yes**
His was achieving his targets in most subjects – not all.
Thomas is likely to get top grades in several subjects **Yes**
There are 'just two' exceptions (indicating that it's a small number) and the rest of his subjects are described as 'all' suggesting there is a larger number.
Thomas had high targets **Yes**
Although this is not explicitly stated, we know he is set to get mostly top grades based on his achieving those targets

3. The Lake District has been shaped by glaciers **Yes**
The 'lakes' in the district are mostly glacial in origin
Man-made reservoirs in the district provide water to the population **No**
There is no mention of the destination of the man-made reservoirs contents, nor their uses
Mere means lake in another language or dialect **No**
There is not enough information in the text to conclude that.
A tarn is smaller than a 'water' **Yes**
This is described in the text
The bodies of water are sometimes misnamed by people **Yes**
The erroneous use of the word 'lake' is described.

4. Some children enjoy doing homework **Yes**
Apparently! Many don't though!
Many children are motivated by earning a good grade **Yes**
This is the group of many who aren't motivated by the enjoyment of doing homework
It is parent's responsibility to help their child get their homework done **Yes**
This text suggests this to be true - parents will need to look for other rewards etc.
Doing homework with care with result in a high grade **No**
It's what they hope to achieve, not a guaranteed outcome
Rewards are more effective than punishments **No**
There is nothing to suggest this in the text.

5. C. Amy played in the red team

We know that the green team placed third. Thus – if the red team was two placed behind Zachary's team it must have come fourth, and Zachary must have been in the second placed team. If Daniel finished one place above Amy, they must have finished in 3rd and 4th places respectively. Amy came fourth, so she must have played in the red team.

6. A. Rachel celebrates her birthday in April

Grace's birthday is in October and must be on 2nd or 3rd of the month as the April birthday is on 4th. April 4th is neither Hannah nor Grace's birthday. It also cannot be Frances' birthday as she celebrates on 1st of her month so April 4th must be Rachel's birthday.

7. D. 24 grapes have fewer calories than two pears

Option A: A pineapple is equal in calorific value to a melon – no need for the extra bananas and satsumas
Option B: We have no specifics on the calorific value of a pear – other than it's more than an apple so we can't know this.
Option C: We have no specific information about the calorific value of a banana – other than it's more than a pear.
Option D: 6 grapes = 1 Satsuma
12 grapes = 2 satsumas = 1 apple
24 grapes = 4 satsumas = 2 apples
An apple has fewer calories than a pear, so 2 apples must have fewer calories than 2 pears.

8. D School and shop

The café must be in building 5, 4 or 2 to have a direct view of the pond, therefore the church must be in building 5, 4, 3 or 1.

The pub is building 1 so the café cannot be in building 2 and must be building 5 or 4 meaning the church must be building 5, 4 or 3.

As the church is also next door to the shop it must be building 4 as that is the only one with two next door neighbours. Therefore, the café must be building 5 and the shop must be building 3.

9. C. No – people should have choice as to where they spend their holiday

This option counters the suggestion that is would be good to 'encourage' people to behave a particular way.
Option A – introduces the idea of price which is not mentioned in the original proposition
Option B – introduces the idea of 'education' which is not warranted by the original proposition
Option D – introduces the idea of 'business practice'. There is no mention of any other tourist industry in the proposition.

10. C. Lions, zebras and birds
Enclosures b and c contain the lions and tigers (we don't know which animal lives in which enclosure)
Enclosure e must contain the zebras – only one animal lives between two others as we know that h, I and j are buildings and a, b and c don't contain warthogs or monkeys. Enclosure h contains either birds, snakes or fish.

11. A. Yes – humanity interfering in the continuance of a species is as detrimental as contributing to its decline
If extinction is both natural and desirable, then humanity should not interfere either way
Option B brings funding into the discussion where it was not previously mentioned
Option C comes across as very arrogant and ignores the desirability of extinction in some circumstances
Option D introduces cultural and educational values into a biological debate
12. A. Yes – underlying principles can't be applied as they're subjective and unknown
The underlying principle is described as 'presumed' in the text and is not a codified and properly expressed 'thing'
Option B – this assumes the impact of a yellow car is not that bad, despite it causing a lot of upset
Option C – the underlying principle is only presumed and can't be confidently asserted as here
Option D – this introduces the notion of changing the 'rules' which is a step further than the question asks.

13. D. No – if rich nations drink more coffee, only drinking fair trade tea will have a limited impact
This is the only argument which considers the fact that some countries vastly prefer coffee over tea making any drive to drinking fair trade tea (rather than coffee) a pointless exercise.
Option A is full of assumptions. More tea may be drunk and produced but it doesn't necessarily mean there is more exploitation. It's possible that the exploitation of tea producers is only minor compared to horrific injustice meted out to coffee producers
Option B introduces the issue of cost which is not necessarily proportionate to the exploitation
Option C broadens the argument from tea and coffee to 'all products' and makes a wild claim that 'fair trade' can end all worker exploitation

14. C. Girls vary in average birth rate more than boys
This can be seen as girls occupy both the lowest and highest points of the graph.
Option A is very Northern Hemisphere centric
Option B is incorrect as boys are equally small in February and April
Option D is incorrect as the graph does not tell us how many babies are born in each month

15. B. Yes – UK school children are a population group so internal IQ comparison is valid
The IQ test is called 'quite useful' within a specific population group – of which UKCAT school children are one.
Option A is vague and talks of a 'general idea' which wouldn't be very useful at all
Option C lists ways in which UK school children may vary – none of which are specifically mentioned in the text. In themselves they are not good enough reasons to discount the IQ test.
Option D claims the IQ test has been discredited rather than specifically discredited as a global measure.

16. A. Yes – catching and punishing poachers hasn't stopped the practice so far
The current practice (as demonstrated by the words 'continue to be') clearly has not been entirely successful hence the development of a new attempt.
Option B is very broad is its use of the word 'anything'. Anything could include genocide of the entire African population and making the whole continent an elephant sanctuary.
Option C is unwarranted as there has only been 'some concern' that predators may find the elephants easier to spot and nothing to suggest that even if this is the case that predators will kill as many elephants as poachers.
Option D is an assumption

17. Music is not an EBacc subject **Yes**
This is clear from the text
The promotion of the EBacc has led to a general decrease in the number of Arts subjects being studied to GCSE **No**
Only music is discussed here – not Arts subjects in general
Teachers agree that the promotion of EBacc is to blame for the decrease in uptake of Music **No**
Two thirds of teachers say this
The EBacc is a rigorous education **No**
The minister says it helps ensure children receive a rigorous education - not that it is one in itself
A school's performance is mainly judged by the percentage of pupils achieving the EBacc **No**
It's one of several measures

18. D. No – athletes need to make a living and if endorsing products doesn't detract from their performance then it's fine
This is a pragmatic response to a pithy statement.
Option A assumes that all endorsements are intended to communicate a link to an athlete's sporting success which is unwarranted – they could, for example, advertise a car or a brand of shampoo.
Option B assumes that athletes won't have anything to do when the sporting part of their career is over, and also that advertising work will be available to them afterwards.
Option C rewrites advertising as being of public benefit!

19. B. Caleb has three times as many main course options as Leah
Caleb has three options, Leah only has one.
Option A - there is only one vegan option for either starter or dessert
Option C - Leah will only have one option for starter, main and dessert courses
Option D - Leah only has one option for starters whereas Caleb has four (as he can eat vegan food as well as vegetarian food).

20. A. 36% of students are not involved in any extracurricular activities
There are 200 children in the school – 128 of whom are engaged in some extracurricular activity. This amounts to 64%. The answer option is about the percentage of children are not involved in any extracurricular activities – hence 36%.
Option B cannot be known from the data. There may be a requirement but just because there are currently equal numbers does not mean that there is.
Option C cannot be known - having music lessons does not automatically equate to being in the school orchestra
Option D - 12 of the girls are learning a language. This is not the same as 12% of the total student body.

21. C. The flowers arrived first
Touba must have arrived last – with the fruit. The fruit was last but not with Anna or Cheyenne and Rabia arrived before Cheyenne so can't have arrived last.

As Touba arrived immediately after Anna with the teabags – Anna must have arrived third with the tea bags. As Rabia arrived before Cheyenne she must have arrived 1st and Cheyenne arrived 2nd. The flowers arrived immediately before Cheyenne so must have arrived 1st with Rabia.

22. B. Around 1 in 8 residents only mentioned one subject

The total of the survey is 500 and 63 only mentioned one subject - this is close to 1 in 8.
Option A - 84 individual residents mentioned everything - not 84%
Option C - 7 cited just these two concerns. This is slightly more than 1%
Option D - 294 people mentioned parks and playgrounds. This compares to 338 mentioning Law and Order, 379 mentioning roads and traffic and 311 mentioning Local Business

23. B. Law and Order and Roads and Traffic

40 people spoke about this combination.
The other options were as follows:
A. Parks and Playgrounds and Law and Order 38
C. Roads and Traffic and Local Business 39
D. Parks and Playgrounds and Roads and Traffic 0

24. The correct answer is B.

The large oval represents zeps.
The small fully enclosed circle is zaps.
The upper circle is zips.
The long small oval is zups.
The small circle, not intersecting with the largest one, is zops.

25. E

26. D. No – his chance of not winning once is 80% but his chance of not winning at all is 51.2%

Playing fourth time would make winning at least once more likely than not.
With three games the probability that he will not win at all = 0.8 x 0.8 x 0.8 = 0.512 which is equal to 51.2%.
The chances of his winning at least once is 100% - 51.2% = 48.8%.

27. B. 45%

The base starting point is 50% - 7% for being away (neutral is still away for the team)
– 10% for the absent team members
+ 12% for the last match victory = 45%

28. A. Yes, yellow fish from Pond 1 are the least likely single occurrence

The most likely combination is a red fish from Pond 1 and a yellow fish from Pond 2. The least likely combination is a yellow fish from Pond 1 and red fish from Pond 2.
Although there are more combinations that give one red fish and one yellow - the question asks for fish from a specific pond at each step.

29. B. Yes, the probability of choosing two the same is 25/49

The two events are independent as the first sock was replaced before another was selected.
Probability of choosing two the same = (4/7 x 4/7) + (3/7 x 3/7) = (16/49) + (9/49) = 25/49 = 51.02%
Probability of choosing two different = (4/7 x 3/7) + (4/7 x 3/7) = (12/49) + (12/49) = 24/49 = 48.98%

30. All Jeds are Jids ***Yes***
Some Jods are Jads ***No***
Some Jeds are Jods ***No***
A Jod could be a Jad ***Yes***
No Juds are Jids ***No***

31. A protected species is likely to enjoy better outcomes than a non-protected one **No**
The only statement is that 'political factors can play a part' – not necessarily one which will lead to better outcomes
Multiple factors play an equal part in endemism **No**
The text only states that all three do play a part. Not that they have equal importance or impact.
The orange breasted sunbird cannot be found in Europe **Yes**
The bird can exclusively be found in southwestern South Africa
Political factors play a part in endemism only over international borders **No**
The text uses the term jurisdiction, which is a wider definition than international borders
Where humanity impacts the environment, it may also impact endemism **Yes**
If humanity can change the physical, climatic or biological factors it will change the endemism too

32. Exposure to risk factors is largely in the control of any individual **No**
Whilst some of the factors listed are in the control of an individual, it is clearly not an exhaustive list.
People with multiple risk factors are more likely than not to develop the disease **No**
There is no statistics associated. The risk could increase from 1% to 2% and the disease still be very unlikely.
Risk factors apply to individuals rather than populations **Yes**
Whilst it might seem counter intuitive seeing as the list of risk factors includes society wide issues, the test does only ascribe risk factors to individuals.
Some risk factors have a bigger impact than others **Yes**
Some risk factors are described as 'more important'.
Obesity is a risk factor **No**
Obesity is not listed

33. There was more than one drink option available **Yes**
Some non-vegetarians enjoyed the vegetable kebabs **No**
We only know that non-vegetarians enjoyed some of the vegetarian food – it's possible this was just the vegetarian sausages and salads
There was only one dessert option **Yes**
Given that every other menu item is detailed, and the dessert is described as 'a cake' this is a logical conclusion
The barbecue happened on a Saturday or Sunday **Yes**
The event is described as happening over the weekend.
The barbecue happened at the family's home **No**
The family hosted the event but not necessarily at their home

34. B. Jenny travelled by boat

This puzzle can't be completed.

The beach trip goes with the plane. The walking trip goes with the car and can't be taken by Helen as a man went on this trip. The city break goes with the train so, the shopping trip – which Jenny did – must be by boat.

35. B. The red car needed new bulbs

The Monday job was new tyres so the Tuesday job must have been the blue car and its exhaust as two days after that – Thursday (the last day in the puzzle) must have been the brake pads. Hence option A and C are incorrect. The red car was fixed one day before the silver car and as we know the blue car was fixed on

Tuesday. That then means the red car got fixed on Wednesday and the silver car on Thursday. Bulbs is the only fix which hasn't been assigned so it must apply to the red car.

36. B. Seats D and E

Claire is sitting in seat C. Brian and Andy must be in Seats F and H with Paula in seat G. Ross is in Seat B and Sylvia in Seat A. The only 'male' seat not assigned in D so Tim must be sitting there.

37. C. Betty is parked in space 6

Sheila must be parking in space 3, Jan in either space 2 or 4. Betty is not in space 2 or 4. Caroline is not in space 6 or 7 so she must be in space 2 or 4 along with Jan. Space 6 and 8 must be occupied by Carole and Betty. Carole is adjacent to one empty space so must be in space 8.

38. A. Yes – fruit and vegetables have a high enough water content to keep you hydrated

Option B the idea that too much water could be dangerous is a far reach from 'or even desirable'.
Option C doesn't address the proposition as there is no suggestion of harm.
Option D introduces a whole new subject with no basis.

39. A. Yes – the spaces are allocated for a reason and not enforcing them disregards that reason

This is the only argument which directly responds to the argument of stopping people who aren't supposed to use these spaces using them. Option B adds in a commercial consideration which might be true but doesn't directly answer the original statement. Option C also adds in the element of cost without warrant. Option D assumes that the original argument isn't valid.

40. A. Yes – anything which exercises cognitive skill sets is worthwhile

The proposition says that these exercises don't 'always' produce empirical improvement which shows that sometimes they do. Thus – it is a worthwhile endeavour.

Option B assumes other screen activities is less worthwhile which is unfounded given that we don't know what the 'other screen activities' are.

Option C takes doesn't always produce empirical improvement and converts it to the much more damning 'no hard data'.

Option D introduces the notion of hard and soft skills and assumes that Brain Training only concentrates on the former.

41. B. Yes – but only if the head teacher thinks the children can afford the time

This argument puts the power in the hands of the head teacher.

Option A is vague as there may be reasons to take children out of school other than 'family time'. Also – there is a false equivalency about family time and schooling.

Option C is somewhat judgemental. It is possible to value education and still wish to take children out of school for various reasons – not limited to 'entertainment'.

Option D is also very harsh and judgemental.

42. C. There is no general, discernible trend shown on this chart

The red line goes up and down as the cheese consumption data decreases. Even if there was a clear link it is important to remember that correlation does not equal causation, so the word 'associated' in option A is problematic. Option B is incorrect as we have no data about the population sizes of the countries shown in the graph so don't know if any particularly large or small populations have skewed the data. Option D is illogical as we only have information about one dietary factor and nationality.

43. D. No – you can't revise for an exam until you have covered all the curriculum

The word 'revise' means that this option makes a lot of sense. Option A makes assumptions about how effective your memory is. Option B only seems to suggest that continual revising is writing revision notes. Option C assumes you cannot adequately do coursework whilst also revising.

44. D. No – changing the level of formality in pre-school settings will protect children without such a radical change

Option A offers a simplistic statement but not a solution. Option B suggests the age of a system is the key problem. Option C is vaguer than option D.

45. The student will have time to read all his compulsory texts **No**
The average length of book is an average taken from over 100 texts. It is possible that the nine compulsory texts are all much longer than average.
It would take the student more than double his available time to read the whole list **Yes**
The minimum number of books on the list is 110 (over 100 additional and 9 compulsory). The average 218 pages per book, at a rate of 500 pages per week, would result in a read time of over 47 weeks.
There are at least 110 books on the total list **Yes**
There are 'over 100' additional texts and 9 compulsories
The course is in a literary subject **No**
There are many courses which require extensive reading
There are under 2000 pages of compulsory reading **No**
The average quoted is for the whole list. It may not apply to the compulsory list.

46. C. No – as technology advances essential 'life skills' inevitably change such as fire making
Option C is the best as it does not directly challenge any of the elements of the proposition or contain an unwarranted assumption. Option A may be true but means we are put in danger every time we climb aboard a plane, into a car or even use an elevator. Option B assumes that navigation and map reading are necessary for spatial awareness and that spatial awareness is a key skill which must be learned. Option D is also based on an assumption that navigation skills are innate which contradicts the premise that such skills should also be taught

47. D. 108

There are 36 parks with rollercoasters. 36 x 3 = 108

48. E. Virtual attractions

No park with virtual attractions has three other types of attraction

49. A. Andrew had a new baby daughter

The whole puzzle cannot be completed.

Martin had his baby in January and Andrew in March. Samantha had her baby girl in September and Nancy had her baby in November. Geoff and Sylvia had their baby in July. The other girl was born to Brenda who must have given birth in March as Martin - the January father – had a boy. Therefore, Andrew must have had a daughter with Brenda.

50. B. A group shared their weekend activities. Many had watched TV; some watched TV and played sports; some watched TV, played sports and did housework. Some people watched TV and did housework. Some people saw family but all of those had either played sports or done housework as well.

The lowest circle represents watching TV
The two larger circles represent playing sports or doing housework
The small circle represents seeing family

51. A. Beach and mountains

52. C. 5

53. C. 21%

There are 109 mixed gender groups (70+16+9+14)
Of these 23 achieve success (9 + 14)
23 / 109 (X100) = 21.2

54. B. Yes, satisfaction is equal, and Debbie is more likely to burn the dinner
John burns the dinner once a week which is equivalent to twice a fortnight - less often than Debbie.

55. C. No, it is twice as likely as this because there are two tiles for each vowel
There is a 1/31 probability of choosing the letter c, a 1/15 (or 2/30) probability of choosing the vowel a, and a 1/29 probability of choosing the letter t. This is equal to a probability of 1 / (31*15*29) which is 1 in 13,485 or 2 in 26,970. This is twice as likely as 1 in 26,970.

56. A. There are 30 possible combinations which gives a 3% chance of picking the hated combination.

2 bases types x 5 toppings = 10
10 x 3 cheese types = 30 different possible combinations.
B is incorrect as there are 30 combinations not 15
C is incorrect as although each choice is independent there is a greater than 1% chance of choosing a single combination
D is incorrect as decimal probabilities are not added together to calculate the probability of one combination

57. A. Yes, there are 12 out of 30 students that do not study Art

18 + 17 = 35. There are 30 students in the class so there must be 5 that study both Art and Music. There are 12 students that study only Music, 13 students that study only Art and 5 that study both.

For Kathleen to be part of the group that do not study Art she must be one of the 12 that study only Music.

58. All flips have flups **No**
Flips could have flups and flaps **Yes**
Some flips don't have flops **No**
All flips have either fleps or flaps **No**
Not all flips have flups **Yes**

59. 20% of the shop's stock was being sold at full price **Yes**
Only 80% of stock was in the sale
40% of sales during this period were from half price (or less) products **No**
We don't have information about sales
Half of the clothes in the shop were being sold at half price or less **No**
Half of 80% is only 40%
Knitwear was being sold at less than half price **Yes**
The biggest reductions (50% or more) was mostly winter coats and knitwear
This sale took place during the spring time **No**
This is an assumption which can't be concluded definitively.

60. 1 cup of coffee per day could reduce the risk of Liver Cancer by 10% **No**
There is nothing to suggest the relationship is linear
Many more tea drinkers will get Liver Cancer than coffee drinkers **No**
The exact incidence of Liver Cancer is not referred to, nor any potential protective value of tea
It's possible the caffeine has some protective effect **Yes**
The lesser protective value of decaffeinated coffee makes this a logical conclusion
The exact mechanism of this reported impact is not definitely known **Yes**
The word 'suggested' shows us that the report writers have found a correlation but not necessarily any causation
This research could lead to thousands of lives being saved per year **No**
There are no incidence levels. Nothing to warrant to suggestion of thousands. Also – nothing to suggest that Liver Cancer is a big killer.

61. 5% of students did not achieve well in their A-levels and needed to use clearing to get a university place **No**
All the students went to university **Yes**
Students routinely take 3 A levels **No**
25% of students use clearing to get a university place **No**
At least 20% of students select a non-Russell group / Oxbridge university at their first choice. **Yes**

62. The shortest child in the class is a boy **No**

We don't have enough information to conclude or assume this
Both boys and girls could have grown 5cm in the last year **Yes**
There are 15 girls in the class **Yes**
Girls are typically taller than boys as children **No**
This is not a global sample and no specific conclusion can be drawn
5cm is significant growth for a child in one year **No**
Just because the teacher has noted it does not mean it is significant

63. B. Aiden is a doctor

April 4	Melanie	Lawyer
June 27	Lily	Architect
July 8	Aiden	Doctor
October 26	Brodie	Engineer
December 6	Peter	Politician

64. C. Firework Fury has a top speed of 70mph

2003	Unknown	Unknown
2006	Firework Fury	70mph
2009	Unknown	80mph
2012	Space Rocket	Unknown

65. A. Alex is moving to be closer to her family.

Shanna	Retiring	Cardiff
Amna	Job	Edinburgh
Vy	Study	Liverpool
Alex	Family	London

66. C. 3 and 5

The two parties of four must be sitting on tables 1 and 2. As the table closest to the café door (table 6) and the other even numbered table are occupied the correct answer is option C.

67. B. On Wednesday people enjoy hot chocolate and toast and marmalade.

Monday	Tea	Sausage sandwich
Wednesday	Hot chocolate	Toast & Marmalade
Friday	Latte	Pain au chocolat
Sunday	Cappuccino	Full breakfast

68. B. Yes – one bus can carry as many people as 40 cars but take up far less space on the road

Option B is the only argument which addresses the way that public transport can ease congestion as the original proposition states. Option A suggests that driving is quicker assuming that congestion is not really a problem. Option C introduces the idea of convenience and makes an assumption about people's motivations. Option D is more ideological and general and doesn't directly address the subject at hand.

69. B. Yes – if the incentive were fair and there was no compulsion involved then this could help a lot of people.

This stresses the need for a fair incentive and no compulsion whilst acknowledging it could help many people. Option A is rather emotive. Option C suggests that older people may 'have to move' which is not argued by the proposition at all. Option D suggests that overcrowding has some positive benefits which is based on assumption.

70. C. No – an effective way to ensure that high contact courses can be made affordable to everyone is for lower contact courses to subsidise them

Option A is based on a generalisation (and assumption) that things generally are priced by value. Option B makes a generalisation that high contact courses lead to high earnings. Option D assumes that all disciplines are equally valued by society.

71. C. No – a consensus should always be sought between medics and family members

The strongest argument is option C as it is the only one which attempts to meet the requirements of all parties. Option A assumes the ignorance of family members which is something of an assumption. Option B also assumes that only those specific medically trained people have any insight into the situation. Option D assumes that doctors don't already do this.

72. Pete and Lizzie would like a room with a four-poster bed and a lake view. Can this hotel accommodate this?
No
We don't know if any of the four poster bedrooms are at the front of the hotel.
Mr and Mrs King have two children. Would the family room have en-suite facilities? **Yes**
All of the rooms have en-suite facilities so this must include the family room suitable for four people.
Mrs Ashdown uses a wheelchair. Would the room she can use definitely have a lake view? **No**
We don't know if either of the downstairs rooms are at the front.
More than half of the rooms in the hotel have a lake view? **No**
We don't know how many rooms are at the front of the hotel.
The hotel has at least two storeys **Yes**
As there is a ground floor with two rooms and many other rooms there must be at least two floors.

73. Half of the new hand creams have a flower fragrance **No**
We don't know how many there are
The beeswax hand cream doesn't have a flower fragrance **No**
It might do
The night hand cream is suitable for sensitive skin **Yes**

They all are
There are at least three varieties **Yes**
The beeswax hand cream is quick absorb **No**
Not necessarily

74. For a family of four the additional flight costs make a holiday to Greece, in local accommodation, less economical than either of the other destinations **Yes**
A Greek Holiday would cost £2,400 (4 x flights + accommodation) whereas a Spanish holiday would cost £1,500 and an Italian one would cost £2,200
A couple on holiday in Greece go out for two meals every day and visit one attraction every day. After fourteen days they recoup the extra money spent on an airfare to Greece rather than Italy. **No**
The couple save £7 each per day (two meal savings of £2 and one attraction saving of £3 each) which is £14 per day in total. Over fourteen days they'll save £196 which won't cover the extra spent on both airfares.
The cheap flights to Spain make the biggest difference to the overall holiday cost **Yes**
The flights are costed per person. All other expenses won't add up to recoup this cost if anyone goes elsewhere
If a family could drive to the destination for the cost of one airfare then a Greek holiday would be the most economical **Yes**
The accommodation is best value in Greece and the saving on other costs would recoup the extra on travel as well.
The cost of meals our or attractions makes up less than 10% of the total value of a holiday **No**
This is not a valid conclusion as meals out / attractions may be daily costs which are priced per person. We don't have enough information to draw a conclusion.

75. Southern African nations collectively have a larger economy than the other regions **Yes**
South African nations got the highest number of 'receipts' (income) from tourism but their GDP was less affected. We can conclude therefore than the economy outside of tourism must be larger.
Southern and East Africa had similar numbers of non long-haul tourist arrivals. (within 250,000) **Yes**
Southern Africa had 8.12million non long-haul tourist arrivals. East Africa had 7.96 million.
Tourism in Africa is worth less than 20 billion US dollars. **No**
This table only pertains to Sub-Saharan Africa – not the continent as a whole
Central Africa had the highest proportion of long-haul arrivals **Yes**
If more long-haul flights flew into Central Africa their tourist industry would grow **No**

76. The two daughters did some of their chores **No**
We know that half of the chores allocated to the daughters were completed but we also know that one of the sons did jobs from the daughter's list as well.
There was more than one job in more than one room on the lists **Yes**
There are chores (plural) described for the kitchen and 'jobs' (plural) described for the lounge
The kitchen was tidier than the lounge when the mother got home **No**
We don't know the nature of the chores or the state of the rooms before
Only one child completed their list of jobs **Yes**
One son completed his chores. We know that neither of the daughters did as only half of their work was completed and at least some of these jobs were done by the son who completed his own list.
Three of the four children did something **No**
We only know for certain that one of the children did any jobs at all.

77. The blue team finished highest in the league table **No**
The blue team lost at least twice **Yes**
The white team had more than four wins during the season **No**
The red team failed to score against the white team **No**
The blue team won the league **No**

78. D. No, it is much lower than one third as most of the plants produce white flowers
A is incorrect as there is a total of 6 plants, 2 of which will produce purple flowers. (2/6*1/5)
B is incorrect as yellow seeds do not produce purple flowers
C is incorrect as although one third is the probability of having yellow seeds from a green pod this scenario does not involve the colour of the pod
D is correct.

79. A. Yes, because the green beads are twice as common as the red ones
A is correct as to calculate the probability of the two options you multiply the probability of each event. As green beads are twice as common as red ones the probability of drawing two red balls (1/9) is half that of drawing one of each (2/9).
B is incorrect as the probability of drawing two green beads is not relevant. It is also 4/9 not 3/9
C is incorrect as being the most common colour bead is not the relevant fact, it is the fact that it is exactly twice as common as red.
D is incorrect at the probability of drawing two red being 1/9 does not prevent the probability of drawing one of each being 2/9 which it is.
1 green, 1 red = 4/6 x 2/6 = 8/36 = 2/9

80. C. 11

81. C. The number of commuters who catch the bus is the same as the number of commuters who drive
A. More commuters cycle and drive than commuters who only catch the train. - False
B. The number of commuters who walk, catch the bus and catch the train are equal to the number who cycle to work. – False
C. The number of commuters who catch the bus is the same as the number of commuters who drive. – True
D. The are 30 more commuters who catch the train and walk than there are commuters who only cycle to work. – False

82. C. There are 26 less houses that have a garden and a driveway than houses that only have a garage
A. Houses that have a garden and a patio (14) are less common than the houses that have a patio and a garage (18). True
B. The number of houses that have a porch and a garden (31) are more than the houses that have driveways (27). True
C. There are 26 less houses that have a garden and a driveway (7) than houses that only have a garage (32). False, there are 25 less.
D. Houses that have a garden, patio and a garage are the least common. True

83. C
Venn diagram A does not account for the children on the scheme who are not taking part in either activity detailed. Venn diagram B does not account for the fact there are more boys on the scheme that girls. Venn diagram D has ten too few boys.

84. C. No. because 65% of children walk to school which is most of them
A is incorrect as the most likely outcome is that they all walk to school
B is incorrect as the most likely outcome is that they all walk to school
C is correct as the most likely outcome is that they all walk to school
D is incorrect as the probability of 0 does not apply to this group of children

85. C. No. because at Johnsons Tours are less likely to make a room alteration
Both tour operators have the same likelihood of a delayed flight and Johnsons Tours make room alterations for 2 in 25 (or 4 in 50) customers and Jacksons Tours make room alterations for 5 in 50 customers. Johnsons Tours is least likely to make a room alteration.

86. An Asian elephant weighs more than a giraffe **No**
There is no comparison between the elephants and the other animals
A hippopotamus weighs more than a crocodile **Yes**
A hippopotamus weighs about the same as a giraffe which weighs more than a rhinoceros which weighs more than a crocodile
A crocodile is the smallest animal described here **No**
We have no information about how elephants fit into the size order
A rhinoceros weighs less than a giraffe **Yes**
This is explicitly stated
An African elephant is the largest animal described here **No**
There is no comparison between the elephants and the other animals.

87. African elephants usually weight more than 1 metric ton **Yes**
As adult crocodile may weigh less than 1 metric ton yet still be mega-fauna **No**
There is a discussion and no conclusion can be drawn
A full-grown giraffe is typically heavier than a full grown rhinoceros **Yes**
Giraffes apparently are always included in mega-fauna as a species whereas there is some discussion regarding the rhino
There are some definitions of mega-fauna which don't include the 1000kg weight limit **Yes**
The 'usually defined' shows us that some variation is present in the definition.
There are sea mammals which are bigger than land mammals No
There is no information about sea mammals. The fact of the African elephant being the largest land mammals does not mean that there are other mammals from elsewhere which are larger.

88. There were five boys in this group **No**
There is no mention of the sex of the children. The names are not all obviously gender specific
James was the last born **Yes**
Elliot is older than Oli **Yes**
Chris is older than Oli **No**
Matthew was the firstborn of the group **Yes**

89. Some non-food products are being sold in smaller sizes for the same price **Yes**
There is mention of toilet roll and only 'most' products getting smaller were food products.
Chocolate bars have been the subject of Shrinkflation **Yes**
It's not only chocolate bars, but they are included
All product package sizes are shrinking **No**
614 products got larger in the time frame
This data is gained from the observation of consumers **No**
The data is gathered by ONS
The ONS primarily concerns itself with retail data such as this **No**
The ONS may have many other concerns other than retail data

90. There was extensive flooding in 2014 in the UK **No**
Monthly rainfall records for England and Wales are likely to be broken 4 times a year **No**
It just pertains to winter
Experienced meteorologists are calculating the risks **No**
A super computer is
Global warming is the main cause of the downpours **No**
It is a cause, maybe not the main one
There is a natural variability to the UK climate **Yes**

91. D. The aching fingers were cured by a red lollipop

Unknown	Aching fingers	Red
Benjamin	Hurty foot	Green
Isabelle	Bumpy freckles	Orange
Unknown	Sore hair	Purple

92. C. The first composer to be presented was JS Bach

Monday	Year 5	Bach
Tuesday	Year 4	Beethoven
Thursday	Year 3	Handel
Friday	Year 2	Mozart

93. D. Sir Timpson owns the black cat

Obadiah	Black	Sir Timpson
Tiddles	Ginger	Dibble family
Fluffy	White	Miss Price
Whiskers	Tabby	Mr Fudding

94. B. F and K are the same colour

Given the diagonal lines of symmetry then F and K must be the same colour but we don't know which colour that is. We don't know from the clues that G and J are red (although they are on the diagram), likewise we can't know that D and M are yellow. There cannot be a vertical line of symmetry if B is green and C is blue.

95. A. Noel cooked Moroccan food

February	Noel	Moroccan
April	Brandy	Indian
June	Wanda	TexMex
August	Floyd	Italian

96. B. Yes – if one entity controls too much of the media they could have undue influence over the populace

This option directly addresses monopoly (lack of diversity of ownership) which is the proposition being discussed.

Option A overreaches the role of government in asking them to ensure balance and equality. Whilst diverse ownership may achieve this the government is only being asked to ensure diverse ownership. Option C doesn't really address the proposition as there is no suggestion that the government is being invited to take editorial control. This option may be making a broader point, but it doesn't address the proposition specifically. Option D is based on an assumption which can neither be supported not refuted by the proposition or accompanying quote.

97. A. Yes – they should still play a part in conjunction with wider action by other agencies

This argument is not especially strong but it is stronger than the others on offer.

Option B confidently suggests that other programmes will work better which is not warranted from any of the information given. Option C assumes that because this one programme failed then the problem itself is complex and difficult (we may use our existing knowledge to conclude the same thing but this section is about recognising when we bring our own assumptions to an analysis). Option D moves from childhood obesity – a social ill – to suggesting schools shouldn't tackle lots of social ills. It also creates a assumed definition of 'academic education' which does not include health matters.

98. D. No – there are many variations between populations and causal links are hard to establish.

We are given very little information and this argument is quite correct – there is not enough to establish a causal link. Option A and B makes assumptions about what people are feeling and that their objection to capital punishment is largely emotional. Option C makes a bold assumption about people's motivations and the interpretation of the word 'exposed'.

99. D. No – without knowing who defines 'subversive' and 'common good' a conclusion cannot be drawn

Option A confidently asserts the highest principle without justification. Option B similarly fails to question what subversion means and goes further in asserting that it will certainly be damaging. Option C is vague whereas option D is far more specific.

100. A. Yes – uncertain and speculative do not mean there is no chance of success and the harm of doing nothing is unacceptable.

Option B is quite fatalistic and doesn't recognise the nuance between uncertain and ineffective. Option C only suggests protection of people and not the other areas which severe weather is said to harm. Option D makes big assumptions about climate change which cannot be justified with the text given.

100 Quantitative Reasoning Questions (answers begin on page 175)

The following table shows the results of students taking language exams last semester.

Grade	Percentage of Students
A*	4%
A	16%
B	30%
C	27%
D	22%
F	1%

Total number of students per year = 230

1. How many students received a grade C? Give the answer to the nearest whole number

A. 27
B. 9
C. 54
D. 62
E. 26

2. If all students who attained a grade below C must re-sit their exams, how many pupils (to the nearest whole number) will this be?

A. 52
B. 23
C. 53
D. 46.9
E. 52.9

3. The exam board decided to drop the mark required for an A* grade to 89%. This meant that two of the A-grade students now have an A* grade instead. What percentage of students will now have an A*? Give the answer to the nearest whole number.

A. 6%
B. 5%
C. 11%
D. 4%
E. 14%

4. If the number of students achieving a B grade the following year increased by 35%, how many students will gain a B grade if the total number of students remains 230. Give the answer to the nearest whole number.

A. 150
B. 93
C. 65
D. 69
E. 93.2

1.364

The following table shows the local petrol prices during July.

Petrol Station	Price (in pence)
Supermarket	1.30
Shore Garage	1.33
PB Garage	1.31
Pump House	1.33
Motorway Services	1.45

5. What is the difference between the average petrol price and motorway petrol price?

A. 0.12
B. 0.11
C. 0.15
D. 0.10
E. 0.14

6. There are 420 staff members in an insurance firm. 41% are in customer services, 25% are in management, 12% are in sales, 8% are in accounting and 14% in Human Resources

How many staff members are employed in the accounting department?

A. 30
B. 50
C. 34
D. 51
E. 3360

7. The following table shows the number of fish sold at a pet store on a Saturday.

Item	Number Sold	Price of each fish
Tetras	29	£2.75
Goldfish	20	£4.50
Catfish	17	£5.00
Platy	15	£2.50
Guppy	25	£3.00

Did the Goldfish, Catfish or Tetras earn the most income?

A. Goldfish
B. Tetras
C. Catfish
D. Tetras and Catfish
E. Can't tell

8. The table shows the number of cars parked in a long stay car park.

Colour	Number
Silver	51
Red	64
Black	75
Blue	35

What percentage are black?

A. 24%
B. 16%
C. 33%
D. 23%
E. 28%

9. What percentage of winter sales was made up of the deck and patio chairs? Give the answer to one decimal place.

The following table shows the winter sales in a chair factory.

Product	Sales (thousands)
Dining Room Chairs	38.4
Deck Chairs	4.1
Patio Chairs	20.6
Desk Chairs	73.2
Folding Chairs	51.6

A. 13.2%
B. 25%
C. 13%
D. 13.1%
E. 24.7%

10. How many desk chairs and folding chairs were sold?

A. 124,800
B. 125
C. 124.8
D. 66.4
E. 124,000

11. In the summer the only change was that the number of patio chairs sold tripled. What percentage of total sales in the summer was made up by patio chairs? Round the answer to one decimal place.

A. 61.8%
B. 32.8%
C. 26.9%
D. 32.9%
E. 27.0%

12. During the following winter the sales of dining room chairs increased by 3.7 %. How many dining room chairs were sold to the nearest whole number?

A. 40,000
B. 45,352
C. 40
D. 39,821
E. 42,100

13. How many pounds sterling would you get if you exchange 300 Euros. Round the answer to 1 decimal place.

The following table shows currency exchange rates.

Currency	Exchange Rate (to £1)
Euro	0.73
U.S Dollar	1.87
Indian Rupees	40.01
Japanese Yen	143.19
Hong Kong Dollar	11.92

A. £410.95
B. £219.00
C. £410.96
D. £411.00
E. £219.52

14. If someone were to exchange 37 Rupees and 42 US Dollars, how much money would they receive in Pounds Sterling?

1480·37

0·92·5

A. £23.38
B. £1975.00
C. £42.25
D. £152.47
E. £23.37

15. If 153 U.S. Dollars was exchanged for £47 in the following week, what is the new exchange rate? Give the answer to 2 decimal places.

A. 0.30
B. 0.31
C. 3.25
D. 0.33
E. 3.26

16. One customer is going on holiday and has £150 to spend. They need to get 30 Euros and change the remaining money into Rupees. How many Rupees will they have?

A. 2.72
B. 5,125.28
C. 3.20
D. 4,801.20
E. 4,357.09

The following table shows the annual simple interest rate for various bank accounts.

Account	Annual Rate
Super Saver	0.6%
Golden Saver	1.1%
Standard Saver	0.4%
Reserve Account	0.2%
Current Account	0.1%

17. If £1358.00 was put into the Super Saver account, how much extra money would the saver have after one year?

A. £8.15
B. 81.48
C. £8.14
D. £1366.14
E. £1366.15

18. If a saver was to have £7650.00 in the Current Account for one year and then move their full balance into a Standard Saver account for a further year, how much money would they have at the end of the two years?

A. £7688.28
B. £7688.25
C. £7491.02
D. £11,781.00
E. £7611.91

19. A saver deposits a lump sum at the beginning of the year. After payment of interest over a full year in the Super Saver account, the saver has £439.67. What was the original amount put into the account?

A. £437.03
B. £414.78
C. £437.05
D. £263.80
E. £263.81

20. How much would a saver have after keeping £51,438.43 in the Reserve Account for 2 years?

A. £51,644.18
B. £51,644.39
C. £51,644.38
D. £53,516.54
E. £53,516.53

The following table shows the distribution of staff at the IT Consultancies Company.

Department	Number of Staff
Customer Services	41%
Accounting	8%
Sales	12%
Management	25%
Human Resources	14%

Total number of staff = 160

21. How many staff members are employed in the Sales department? Give the answer to the nearest whole number

A. 13
B. 160
C. 19
D. 13.3
E. 19.2

22. How many people are employed in the Accounting and Human Resources departments? Give your answer to the nearest whole number.

A. 29
B. 28.6
C. 28
D. 35
E. 34

23. If one member of staff moves from the Sales department to Customer Services department, what percentage of the company does the Customer Services department now make? Give your answer to the nearest whole number.

A. 41%
B. 40%
C. 42%
D. 41.3%
E. 43%

24. To reduce costs the IT Consultancies Company decide to make two of the Management staff redundant. What percentage of the company will the Management department now make up? Give your answer to one decimal place.

A. 24.1%
B. 23.7%
C. 23.8%
D. 24.8%
E. 24.0%

25. The following table shows the items sold at a market stall on a Saturday

Did the Bananas, Oranges or Carrots earn the most income?

Item	Number Sold	Price of each Item
Orange	21	12p
Apple	44	21p
Banana	18	56p
Pear	21	67p
Carrot	34	12p
Potato	29	87p
Parsnip	43	99p

A. Bananas
B. Oranges
C. Carrots
D. Bananas and Carrots
E. Can't tell

26. What fraction of the total sales (units) was made up by the Oranges?

A. 21/200
B. 1/10
C. 3/60
D. 21/205
E. 7/60

27. If the Parsnips had been sold at an 80% discount, what would the new price be?

A. 79p
B. 19p
C. 5p
D. 4p
E. 20p

28. In the following week the unit sales of Potatoes increased by 60%. What revenue did they bring in that week?

A. £139.20
B. £40.02
C. £40.37
D. £52.20
E. £46.00

Monday sales for Coffee House's most popular beverages.

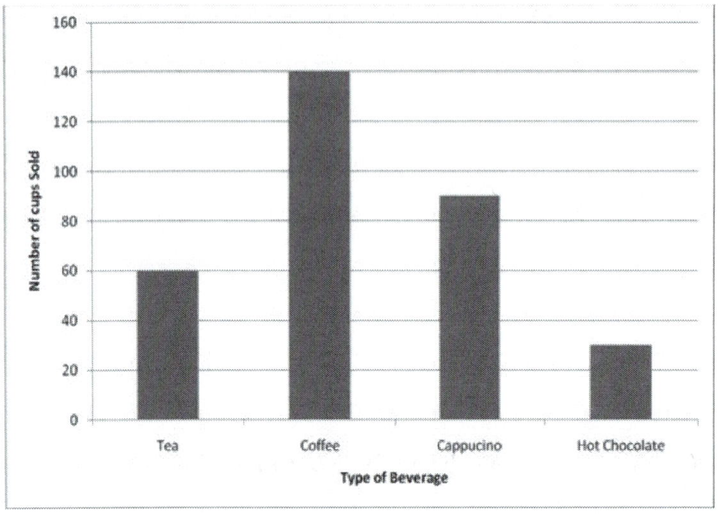

Cost per cup: Tea = £1.00, Coffee = £2.50, Cappacino = £3.25, Hot Chocolate = £2.70

29. How much revenue did the Cappuccino bring in?

A. £3.35
B. £260.00
C. £325
D. £292.50
E. £27.69

30. What percentage of units sold are cups of tea?

A. 60%
B. 53.3%
C. 18.75%
D. 15.87%
E. 10.58%

31. The next day Hot Chocolate sales saw an increase of 27%. How many more cups of Hot Chocolate were sold? Give your answer to the nearest whole number.

A. 8.1
B. 38
C. 38.1
D. 8
E. 1

32. On average, how much was paid for each cup sold on Monday? Give the answer to two decimal places.

A. £2.45
B. £2.36
C. £2.37
D. £2.44
E. £2.25

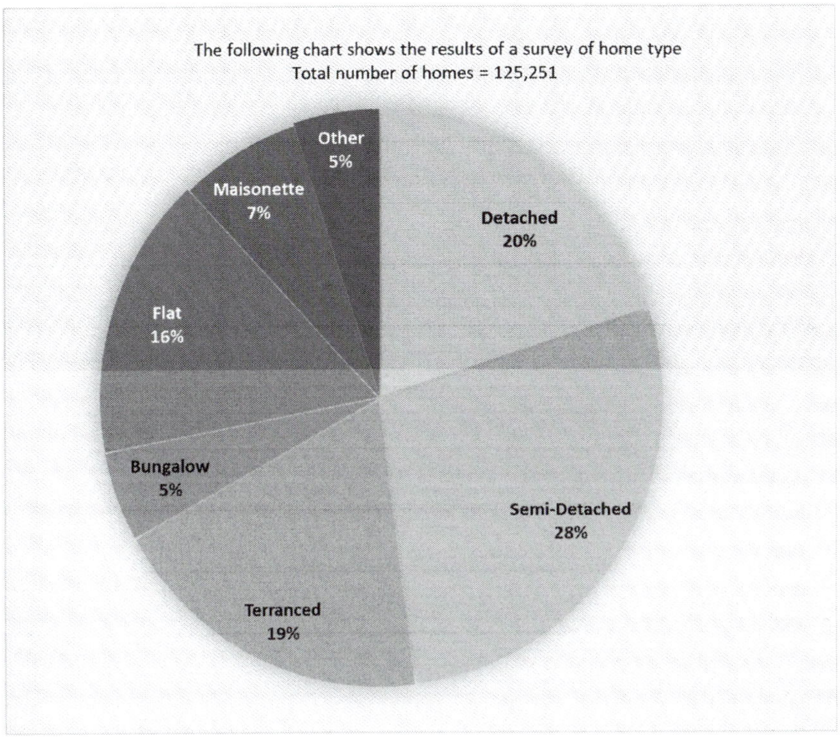

33. How many homes are terraced properties? Give the answer to the nearest whole number.

A. 6592
B. 6590
C. 25,050
D. 23,798
E. 212,525

34. The average number of people living in a flat is three. How many people in total live in the flats? Give the answer to the nearest whole number.

A. 20,040
B. 6,680
C. 60,120
D. 7,828
E. 23,485

35. What fraction of homes are of either the Detached or Bungalow type?

A. 2/7
B. 1/4
C. 20/5
D. 1/3
E. 2/5

36. If 30% of the homes which fall under the 'others' category are canal boats, how many homes are canal boats?

A. 37,575
B. 1,879
C. 837
D. 25,050
E. 213

The table shows the number of balls used in a game

Colour	Number
Red	49
Blue	147
Green	98
Yellow	49

37. What fraction of the balls are blue?

A. 3/7
B. 49/21
C. ¼
D. 7/21
E. 2/7

38. What percentage of the balls are yellow?

A. 14%
B. 49%
C. 25%
D. 7/21
E. 21%

39. What is the ratio of red balls to green balls?

A. 1:4
B. 1:7
C. 1:2
D. 1:3
E. 1:14

40. Later in the game 42 purple 'bonus' balls were added. What percentage of the total balls were bonus balls? Round the answer to two decimal places.

A. 10.90
B. 10.91
C. 12.24
D. 8.16
E. 8.17

Ingredients to make 6 scones

Ingredients	Liquid
200g flour	300 ml milk
25g sugar	
50g fruit	
30g margarine	
2 tsp bicarbonate of soda	

41.. What percentage of the not liquid ingredients is the sugar? There is 2.7g of bicarbonate of soda in a teaspoon. Round the answer to 1 decimal place.

A. 8.1%
B. 8.2%
C. 8.0%
D. 12.4%
E. 12.42%

42. If 1 gram (g) is equal to 0.035 ounces (oz.): How many ounces of margarine are in the scone the answer to two decimal places.

A. 1.05 oz
B. 857.14 oz
C. 10.50 oz
D. 0.12 oz
E. 1.1 oz

43.If you wanted to make 15 scones, how many grams of flour would be required?

A. 600
B. 3,000
C. 500
D. 400
E. 700

44. Using the recipe for 6 scones, a Baker used sultanas for 54% of the fruit and raisins for the rest. What was the weight of the raisins used?

A. 27g
B. 23 g
C. 25g
D. 24g
E. 28g

45. If the typical breaking distance of a car travelling at 40mph increases by 70% compared to its typical breaking distance at 30mph, what would the longest typical breaking distance be of these cars travelling at 40mph?

Information for consumers about different cars

	Cost to buy	Average fuel consumption (mpg)	Typical braking distance at 30mph (metres)	Top Speed (mph)
Car A	£15,400	44.8	11.2	130
Car B	£12,000	38.2	13.1	105
Car C	£17,000	54.1	9.6	120
Car D	£13,000	32.5	14.5	110
Car E	£14,000	34.9	13.1	100

A. 22.27m
B. 10.15m
C. 19.04m
D. 24.65m
E. 27.55m

46. If Car A is travelling at 60% of its top speed and is 3 miles ahead of Car D which is travelling in the same direction, how long would it take Car D to draw level with Car A if Car D is travelling at 72% of its top speed?

A. 2 hours 30 minutes
B. 2 hours 15 minutes
C. 3 hours 30 minutes
D. 3 hours
E. 2 hours 45 minutes

47. If a litre of fuel costs £1.32 and there are 4.546 litres in a gallon, how far on average would Car B be able to travel with £30 worth of fuel?

A. 157 miles
B. 174.5 miles
C. 191 miles
D. 221.5 miles
E. 195.5 miles

48. Someone travels an average of 15000 miles a year, assuming fuel costs £1.32 per litre and there are 4.546 litres in a gallon, which car would be the cheapest for them to buy and run over the first five years considering cost and fuel usage?

A. Car A
B. Car B
C. Car C
D. Car D
E. Car E

Road distances travelled by a vehicle to a number of towns

Town	Miles
Townville	37.41
Weston	4.79
Tulip Town	78.28
Popular	123.76
Grampton	48.49

49. If it takes four hours to get to Tulip Town, at what average speed would the vehicle be travelling? Give the answer in miles per hour (mph)

A. 313
B. 23
C. 78
D. 20
E. 40

50. How long would it take to get to Townville if the vehicle was travelling at an average speed of 70 mph. Round the answer to the nearest whole minute.

A. 30 mins
B. 53 mins
C. 32 mins
D. 26 mins
E. 37 mins

51. The vehicle travels half way to Popular at an average speed of 50 mph and stops for a 15-minute break. It travels the remainder of the journey at 70 mph. How long did the journey take? Give the answer to the nearest whole minute.

A. 127 mins
B. 131 mins
C. 187 mins
D. 142 mins
E. 172 mins

52. The vehicle travels for 1 hour at 30 mph. It then travels on the motorway at an average speed of 70 mph for 3.5 hours. What was the total distance travelled?

A. 275 miles
B. 100 miles
C. 225 miles
D. 50 miles
E. 250 miles

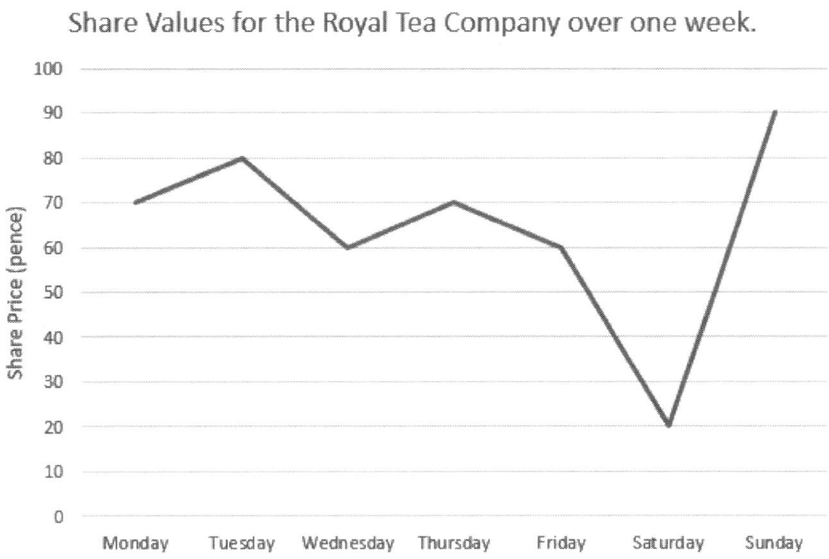

53. What was the biggest daily drop in share price during the week?

A. 60p
B. 20p
C. 70p
D. 40p
E. 50p

54. What was the overall percentage change in share price over the week? Give the answer to the nearest whole number

A. 20% increase
B. 28% increase
C. 29% increase
D. 129% increase
E. 70% increase

55. If 50 shares were purchased on Tuesday and sold on Friday, how much money would have been made or lost? Give the answer in pounds (£).

A. Lost £50
B. Gained £10
C. Lost £20
D. Lost £10
E. Gained £20

56. In the following week the average share price increased by 2%. What was the average share price that following week? Round the answer to 1 decimal place.

A. 65.6p
B. 74.1p
C. 65.5p
D. 61.2p
E. 66.3p

The ages of Green Bowls Club Members

Member Ages
69
84
58
62
49
63
58
61
17
62
73
64

57. What is the average (mean) age of club members? Round the answer to the nearest whole number.

A. 60
B. 62
C. 61
D. 67
E. 68

58. What is the range of ages at the bowls club?

A. 67
B. 61
C. 60
D. 60.8
E. 68

59. The club would like to decrease the mean age of members by 20%. What would the new mean age be? Give the target mean age to the nearest whole number.

A. 41
B. 54
C. 76
D. 67
E. 48

60. The following month the club recruited additional members with the following ages: 23, 58, 24 & 18. What percentage decrease was seen in the average (mean) age?

A. 87%
B. 8%
C. 9%
D. 14%
E. 12%

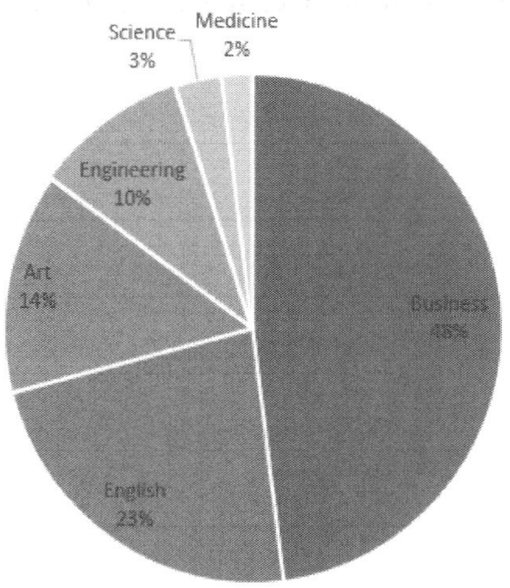

Degrees chosen by school leavers

61. How many school leavers chose to study an Art degree? Round the answer to the nearest whole number.

A. 24
B. 48
C. 47
D. 85
E. 23

Total number of school leavers choosing to study a degree = 340

62. How many more students chose to study Business than those who chose English as a degree?

A. 163
B. 85
C. 78
D. 25
E. 62

63. 10 % of the students who chose to study Business will be doing the degree entitled "Business and Management". How many students will this be?

A. 34
B. 48
C. 17
D. 35
E. 16

64. The remaining 40 students leaving school that year decided to go straight into a job. What percentage of school leavers was this? Round the answer to 2 decimal places.

A. 10.53
B. 11.70
C. 10.5
D. 11.76
E. 11.8

Produce from the allotment

Produce	Number
Cabbage	2
Carrots	32
Potatoes	12
Tomatoes	68
Rhubarb	4
Turnips	7
Runner beans	77

65. What percentage of the produce was made up of tomatoes? Give the answer to the nearest whole number.

A. 68%
B. 32%
C. 36%
D. 34%
E. 33%

66. The gardener decided to sell 60 % of his runner beans at the market for 5p per whole unit. How much money did he make? Give the answer in pounds (£).

A. £0.56
B. £3.85
C. £2.30
D. £3.00
E. £2.43

67. The gardener wants to sell some of his carrots and make at least £8. If he sells each carrot for 87p, how many whole carrots would he have to sell?

A. 8
B. 10
C. 8.7
D. 9
E. 7

68. The next day the gardener decides to sell all his potatoes at 70p. He then buys 12 strawberries for 30p each and 6 eggs for 23p each. How much money will he have left? Give the answer in pounds (£).

A. £3.60
B. £3.42
C. £3.00
D. £0.17
E. £4.98

8.4
− 3.6
− 1.38

Densities of liquid samples

Liquid	Density (kg/m³)
Sample 1	100.03
Sample 2	87.11
Sample 3	146.09
Sample 4	89.44

Density in a kilograms per cubic metre

69. What is the average density of the liquid samples?

A. 58.98
B. 422.67
C. 105.67
D. 100.03
E. 105.66

70. How much would 7 cubic metres of Sample 4 weigh?

A. 626.08 kg
B. 0.08 kg
C. 630.00 kg
D. 12.78 kg
E. 12.77 kg

71. Density used to be measured in ounces/gallon. 1 kilogram per cubic metre is equal to 0.16 ounces/gallon, what is the density of Sample 2 in ounces per gallon?

A. 544.44
B. 87.11
C. 86.95
D. 16.00
E. 13.94

72. If 1 cubic metre is equal to 1000 litres, how many litres of Sample 3 would weigh 5kg?

A. 0.03
B. 29.22
C. 29,218
D. 730.45
E. 34.23

Book Type	Percentage Book Sales
Romance	46%
Crime	7%
Autobiography	11%
Science Fiction	3%
Children's	32%
Dictionary	1%

Total number of books sold = 65

73. How many Crime books were sold? Give the answer to the nearest whole number.

A. 9
B. 7
C. 6
D. 8
E. 5

74. If all of the Romance and Science Fiction books sold were donated by a local library, how many books would be donated in total? Give the answer to the nearest whole book.

A. 49
B. 32
C. 16
D. 31
E. 31.85

75. If 50 % of the Children's books sold were Fantasy books, how many Science Fiction and Fantasy books were sold in total? Give answer the nearest whole number.

A. 34
B. 12
C. 16
D. 53
E. 19

76. If the number of Crime books sold the following week increased by 45%, give the number of Crime books sold if the total number of book sales remains at 65. Round to the nearest whole book.

A. 7
B. 5
C. 29
D. 33.8
E. 34

During some rocket trials, a team of engineers were recording the performance of the engine. They measured a thrust force of 1.1 Newtown and were expecting a chamber pressure of 130 psi (pounds per square inch). However, the pressure inside a chamber was 140 psi.

77. If 1 bar is equal to 14.504 psi, what was the measured pressure inside the rocket chamber in bars? Round the answer to one decimal place.

A. 10
B. 8.9
C. 2030.6
D. 1885.52
E. 9.7

78. If the area inside the chamber is 6.5 inches squared, how many pounds of force were exerted over the entire chamber area?

A. 21.5 pounds
B. 0.05 pounds
C. 910 pounds
D. 845 pounds
E. 140 pounds

79. During later trials the engineers were able to improve the rocket performance so that it was now providing a thrust force of 1.3 N. If 1 N = 0.225 lbf (pound-force), what was the increase in performance in pound-force? Round the answer to 2 decimal places

A. 0.29 lbf
B. 0.05 lbf
C. 0.89 lbf
D. 0.04 lbf
E. 5.78 lbf

80. During later trials the chamber pressure had also increased to 150 psi. If 1 bar is equal to 14.504 psi what was the increase in chamber pressure in bar?

Round the answer to 1 decimal place.

A. 10.3 bar
B. 0.7 bar
C. 145.0 bar
D. 9.6 bar
E. 1.0 bar

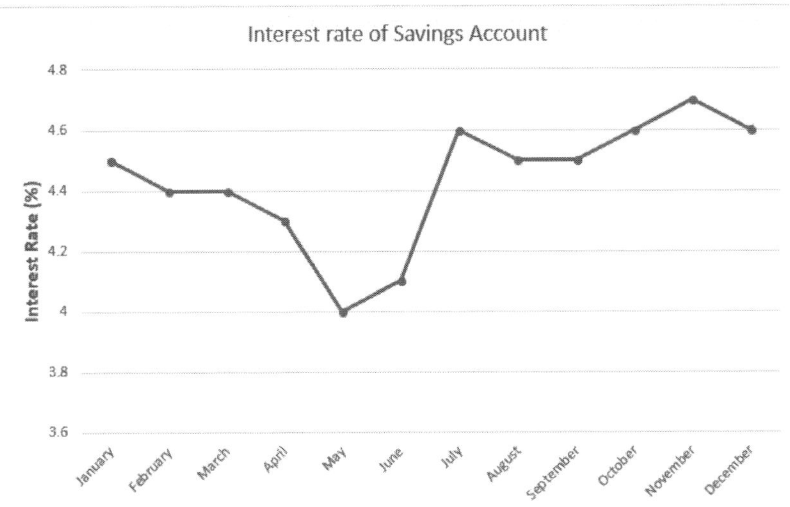

81. For what fraction of the year was the interest rate more than 4.4%?

A. 7/12
B. 3/4
C. 9/12
D. 1/6
E. 1/12

82. Between what months was the biggest fall in interest rate?

A. June and July
B. April and May
C. January and February
D. May and July
E. March and May

83. If the total money in the account in August was £140,000; how much money would have been paid in interest during August?

A. £31,111
B. £6,300
C. £133,971
D. £525
E. £63,000

84. If £13,482 was put into the savings account at the beginning of the year, at the end of which month should the money be withdrawn for the most profit to be made?

A. July
B. May
C. November
D. January
E. December

Cost of sending mail	
Letter Price	L = 0.3a x 0.2b
Parcel Price	P = 0.2a x 0.2b x 0.9c
Where a = width, b = length and c= depth in centimetres (cm) and the prices are in pence (p)	

85. What would be the price of sending a letter which had a width of 10 cm and length of 15 cm?

A. 9p
B. 6p
C. 6.5p
D. 35p
E. 7p

86. How much would it cost to send a package that had width of 10 cm, a length of 12 cm and a volume of 3,600 cm^3?

A. 5184p
B. 31p
C. 15,552p
D. 156p
E. 130p

87. The postal office decided to increase the price of sending letters by adding a 5p charge to those which have lengths over 50 cm. What formula would be the most appropriate to use for letters with lengths over 50 cm?

A. L + 5 = 0.3a x 0.2b
B. L = 0.3a x 0.2b + 5
C. L = 0.3a x (0.2b + 5)
D. L = 0.3a x (0.2b x 5)
E. L = (0.3a + 5) x 0.2b

88. If the price of a parcel was £5, and it had a length of 13 cm and a width of 5 cm, what was the depth of the parcel to the nearest cm?

A. 192cm
B. 213.7cm
C. 1170cm
D. 556cm
E. 214cm

89. A group of students were devising a game to help them learn about probability. They put the following items into a bag.

- **3 green balls**
- **2 blue balls**
- **5 red cars**
- **2 green cars**
- **2 yellow cars**

What is the probability that the first object picked out of the bag is a yellow car?

A. 1/5
B. 2/15
C. 2/5
D. 1/7
E. 2/7

90. If the first object selected was the yellow car, what is the probability that the second object selected is green? Give the answer to three decimal places.

A. 0.385
B. 0.357
C. 0.400
D. 2.600
E. 0.154

91. All of the objects were returned to the bag. The students then decided to add three red balls to the bag. What is the probability that a red ball will be selected now? Give the answer to three decimal places.

A. 0.167
B. 5.667
C. 0.300
D. 0.214
E. 0.176

92. The students decided to play a new game which involved selecting coloured counters from a jar of 62 counters. They picked out 10 counters and only one of them was blue. They worked out that the probability of the eleventh counter being blue was 13/52. At the beginning of the game, what was the probability that the first counter picked could be blue?

A. 7/31
B. 14/52
C. 13/52
D. 13/62
E. 14/31

93. A presidential election has just been completed in this fictional nation which has exactly one million registered voters. In the past the 'first past the post' system has been used (where the person with the most votes wins) but this has now been replaced by the 'single transferable vote' systems under which votes won by the least successful candidate are re-allocated according to the voters' alternative choice. This process is repeated until a clear winner emerges having more than half of the votes cast. The table shows the first and second votes after the count.

1st choice votes	Abbot 261457			Baines 238766			Carter 210555			Dewar 189445		
2nd choice votes	Baines 98750	Carter 102099	Dewar 60608	Abbot 109744	Carter 109744	Dewar 19278	Abbot 90554	Baines 80554	Dewar 39447	Abbot 57889	Baines 68889	Carter 92667

What majority would have been reported for the winner under the old system?

A. 261457
B. 22691
C. 72012
D. 26%
E. 32468

94. What proportion of the vote was recorded for the loser on the first count? (to the nearest whole number)

A. 19%
B. 21.05%
C. 29%
D. 22%
E. 21%

95. After the reallocation of votes, what proportion did the leader hold?

A. 34%
B. 31%
C. 307655
D. 32%
E. 33%

96. Who was elected?

A. Abbot
B. Baines
C. Carter
D. Dewar
E. Can't tell / none of them

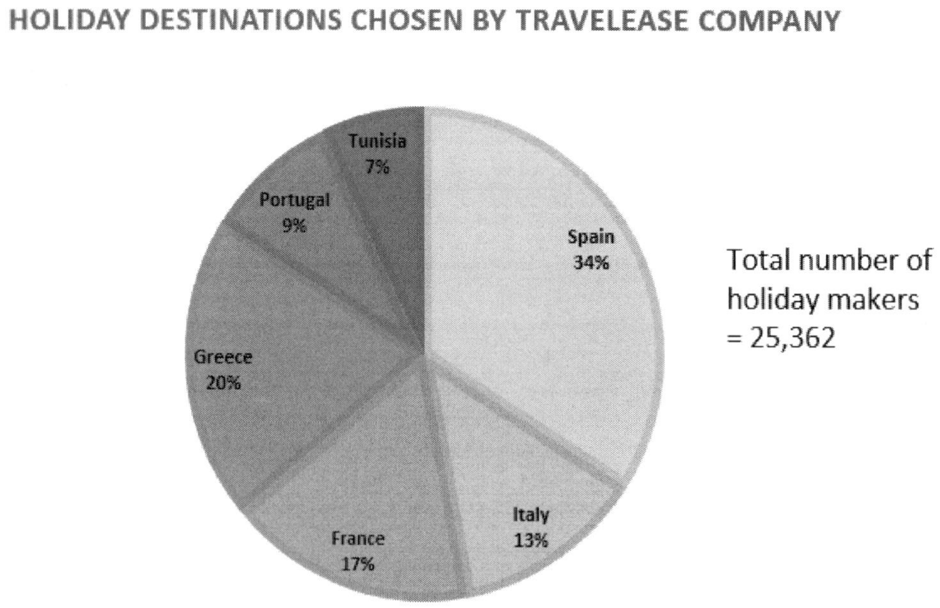

97. How many people decided to travel to Italy?

A. 1362
B. 330
C. 1951
D. 3297
E. 4227

98. How many extra people decided to travel to Spain than Tunisia?

A. 1775
B. 939
C. 6848
D. 8623
E. 746

99. 34 % of the travellers going to Spain will actually be visiting one of the small Balearic Islands. How many people will be travelling to the Balearic Islands?

A. 745
B. 8623
C. 17246
D. 2932
E. 22

100. The same year TravelEase added another country to its list of destinations: Austria. If an additional 163 people travelled to this destination, what percentage of the total TravelEase travellers visited Tunisia? Give your answer to 1 decimal place.

A. 6.9%
B. 7.0%
C. 6.4%
D. 0.6%
E. 7.1%

100 Quantitative Reasoning Question Answers

1. The correct answer is : **D.** 230 x 0.27 = 62.1 = 62 students.

2. The correct answer is : **C**. Grade D + F = 23%; 230 x 0.23 = 52.9 = 53 students (to the nearest whole student)

3. The correct answer is: **B**. Initially 9 students have an A*-grade: 230 x 0.04 = 9.2 = 9, two more students = 11; ((11/230)x100) = 4.78 = 5%

4. The correct answer is: **B**. 230 x 0.30 = 69 students; 69x1.35 = 93.2 = 93 students.

5. The correct answer is: **B**. Average = (1.30 + 1.33 + 1.31 +1.33 + 1.45)/5
Average = 1.34, 1.45-1.34 = 0.11

6. The correct answer is option **C**: 34
420 × 0.08 = 33.6. We round to 34 as there can not be 0.6 of an employee

7. The correct answer is option **A**. Goldfish
The question only asks you to compare three fish. Of these:
Goldfish - 20 x £4.50 = £90
Tetras - 29 x £2.75 = £79.75
Catfish - 17 x £5.00 = £85

8. The correct answer is **C**. 33%
The total number of cars is (51+64+75+35) = 225.

9. The correct answer is: **D.** Total sales = 187.9 (thousand). Deck and patio chair sales = 4.1 + 20.6 = 24.7.
Percentage of sales = (24.7/187.9) × 100 = 13.145 =13.1 to one d.p.

10. The correct answer is: **A.** 73.2 + 51.6 = 124.8 thousand = 124,800

11. The correct answer is: **E.** Tripled sales: 20.6 × 3 = 61.8, New total sales = 229.1. Percentage of sales = (61.8/229.1)×100 = 26.975 = 27.0 to 1 d.p.

12. The correct answer is: **D.** 38.4 (×1000) × 1.037 = 39820.8 = 39, 821

13. The correct answer is: **D**. 300/0.73 = 410.9589 = £410.96, rounding to 1 decimal place gives £411.0

14. The correct answer is: **A**.
37/40.01 = 0.9248
42/1.87 = 22.4599
0.9248 + 22.4599 =£23.3847 or £23.38 to 2 decimal places.

15. The correct answer is: **E**. 153/47 = 3.255 = 3.26

16. The correct answer is: **E.**

30/0.73 = 41.09589 = 41.10.
Remaining money = £150 - 41.10 or 108.90 left to exchange for rupees.
108.90x40.01 = 4,357.089 the closest option is 4,357.09

17. The correct answer is: **A.** 1358.00 × 0.006 = 8.148 = 8.15

18. The correct answer is **A.**
7650 × 1.001 = 7657.65 at the end of year one
7657.65 × 1.004 = 7688.2806 or 7688.28 at the end of year two.
19. The correct answer is **C.** 439.67/1.006 = 437.05

20. The correct answer is **A**. £51644.18
The account is simple interest. 0.2% of £51,438.43 is £102.88
£102.88 × 2 = £205.75
£51,438.43 + £205.75 = £51644.18

21. The correct answer is: **C**. 160 × 0.12 = 19.2 = 19

22. The correct answer is: **D.**
160 × 0.08 = 12.8
160 × 0.14 = 22.4
12.8 + 22.4 = 35.2 or 35 to the nearest whole number

23. The correct answer is: **C.**
160 × 0.41 = 65.6
(66.6/160)x100 = 41.625 or 42% to the nearest whole number

24. The correct answer is: **A.**
Originally: 160 × 0.25 = 40.
Two less members of the management team: 40-2 = 38.
Also two less employees in the whole company: 160-2 = 158.
The new percentage is: (38/158) × 100 = 24.05 = 24.1 (to 1 d.p).

25. The correct answer is**: A.**
Bananas: 18 × 56 = 1008p (£10.08)
Oranges: 21 × 12 = 252 (£2.52)
Carrots: 34 × 12 = 408 (£4.08)

26. The correct answer is: **B.**
Total units sold = 21+44+18+21+34+29+43 = 210
Oranges sold = 21/210 = 1/10

27. The correct answer is: **E**. 99 × 0.2 = 19.8 = 20p

28. The correct answer is: **C.**
New number of units sold = 29 × 1.6 = 46.4potatoes
New Revenue = 46.4 × 87p = 4,036.8p = £40.37

29. The correct answer is: **D**. 90 × 3.25 = £292.50

30. The correct answer is: **C**.
Total sales = 60+140+90+30 = 320
Percentage Tea = (60/320) × 100 = 18.75%

31. The correct answer is: **D**. 30 × 0.27 = 8.1 or 8 to the nearest whole number

32. The correct answer is: **A**.
Total revenue = (60×1.00 + 140×2.50 + 90×3.25 + 30×2.70) = 783.5
Total units = (60+140+90+30) = 320
Average spend = 783.5/(320) = 2.4484 or 2.45 to 2 decimal places.
33. The correct answer is: **D**. 125,251 x 0.19 = 23,797.69 = 23,798 homes.

34. The correct answer is: **C**.
125,251 x 0.16 = 20,040.16 Flats
20,040 × 3 = 60,120 people in Flats

35. The correct answer is: **B**. 20 + 5 % = 25% = 25/100 = 1/4

36. The correct answer is: **B.**
125,251 x 0.05 = 6,262.55 Other homes
6,262.55 x 0.30 = 1878.765 = 1879 canal boats.

37. The correct answer is **A**. 3/7
Blue balls proportion = 147/Total balls
= 147/(49+147+98+49)
= 147/343
= 21/49
= 3/7

38. The correct answer is **A**. 14%
Yellow ball % = (49/343) x 100 = 14.29 or 14% to the nearest whole number.

39. The correct answer is **C** 1:2
49:98 = 7:14 = 1:2
Alternatively, 49:98 = 0.5 which is 1:2 expressed as a ratio

40. The correct answer is **B.** 10.91
Bonus ball % = 42 / (343+42) x 100 = 10.91%

41. The correct answer is **A.** 8.1%
Total weight = 200 + 25 + 50 + 30 + (2 × 2.7) = 310.4
Percentage Sugar = (25/310.4) × 100 = 8.05 = 8.1%

42. The correct answer is **A**. 1.05oz
30 g × 0.035 = 1.05 oz.

43. The correct answer is **C.** 500
(200/6) × 15 = 500

44. The correct answer is **B**. 23g
Raisins would be 100-54% = 46%
Weight of raisins is 46% of 50g = 50 × 0.46 = 23 g

45. The correct answer is **D**. 24.65m
The car with the longest typical breaking distance is Car D, if it was travelling at 40mph it's typical breaking distance would be 170% of the distance shown in the table therefore 14.5 × 1.70 = 24.65

46. The correct answer is **A**. 2 hours 30 minutes
Car A's top speed is 130mph, it is therefore travelling at 130 × 0.6 = 78mph, Car D's top speed is 110mph, it is therefore travelling at 110 × 0.72 = 79.2mph, this means Car D is travelling at 1.2mph faster than Car A. Car D will therefore take 3 miles / 1.2 mph = 2.5 hours to reach Car A

47. The correct answer is **C**. 191 miles
A gallon of fuel costs £1.32 × 4.546 = £6, this means £30 worth of fuel is 30 / 6 = 5 gallons. Car B travels an average of 38.2 miles per gallon, meaning that on 5 gallons of fuel it would travel 5 × 38.2 = 191 miles

48. The correct answer is **B**. Car B
A gallon of fuel costs £1.32 × 4.546 = £6
Car A costs £15,400 + (15000/44.8)x6x5 = £25444.64
Car B costs £12,000 + (15000/38.2)x6x5 = £23780.00
Car C costs £17,000 + (15000/54.1)x6x5 = £25317.93
Car D costs £13,000 + (15000/32.5)x6x5 = £26846.15
Car E costs £14,500 + (15000/34.9)x6x5 = £27393.98
Therefore, the cheapest car to run overall is Car B.

49. The correct answer is **D**. 20
(78.28/4) = 19.57 = 20 mph

50. The correct answer is **C.** 32 mins
37.41/70 = 0.5344 hours; 0.5344 × 60 = 32.066 = 32 mins

51. The correct answer is **D.** 142 mins
61.88/50 = 1.2376 hours travelled at 50mph
1.2376 × 60 = 74.256 minutes
61.88/70 = 0.884 hours travelled at 70mph
0.884 × 60 = 53.04 minutes
74.256 + 53.04 + 15 minutes break = 142.296 mins or 142 mins to the nearest whole minute.

52. The correct answer is **A**. 275 miles
(1×30) + (3.5×70) = 275 miles

53. The correct answer is **D**. 40p
The biggest drop in share price was from Friday to Saturday (60 - 20 = 40 p)

54. The correct answer is **C**. 29% increase
The share price went from 70p on Monday to 90p on Sunday, an increase of 20p
% increase in share price = (20/70) × 100
% increase in share price = 28.5714% or 29% to the nearest whole number

55. The correct answer is **D**. Lost £10
50 × 80p = 4000p paid on Tuesday
50 × 60p = 3000p sold on Friday
The shares were bought for 1000p (£10) more than they were sold for

56. The correct answer is **A**. 65.6p
Average price this week = (70+80+60+70+60+20+90)/7 = 64.2857
Increase of 2% = 64.2857 × 1.02 = 65.571 or 65.6p to 1 decimal place

57. The correct answer is **C**. 61
Mean age = (69+84+58+62+49+63+58+61+17+62+73+64)/12.
Mean age = 720/12 = 60

58. The correct answer is **A**. 67
Range = highest age – lowest age
84 – 17 = 67

59. E. 49
Target mean age = 80% of current mean
Current mean age = (69+84+58+62+49+63+58+61+17+62+73+64)/12
Current mean age = 720/12 = 60
Target mean age = 60 × 0.80 = 48

60. E. 12%
Previous mean = (69+84+58+62+49+63+58+61+17+62+73+64)/12
Previous mean = 720/12 = 60
New Mean = (720 + 23+58+24+18)/(12+4)
New Mean = 843/16 = 52.6875
Decrease = 60 – 52.6875 = 7.3125
% Decrease = (7.3125/60) × 100 = 12.1875 or 12%

61. The correct answer is **B**. 48
340 × 0.14 = 47.6 = 48

62. The correct answer is **B.** 85
340 × 0.48 = 163.2 = 163; 340 × 0.23 = 78.2 = 78; 163-78 = 85

63. The correct answer is **E.** 16
340 × 0.48 = 163.2; 163.2 × 0.10 = 16.32 =16

64. The correct answer is **A.** 10.53
(40/(340+40)) × 100 = 10.52632 = 10.53

65. The correct answer is **D.** 34%
(68/(2+32+12+68+4+7+77) × 100 = (68/202) × 100 = 33.66 = 34%

66. The correct answer is **C**. £2.30
77 × 0.6 = 46.2 (but you can not sell 0.2 of a bean) so 46. 46 × 5 = 230p = £2.30

67. The correct answer is **B.** 10
8.00/0.87 = 9.195 i.e. he would have to sell at least 10 whole carrots to make £8

68. The correct answer is **B.** £3.42
Potatoes sold = 12 × 0.70 = £8.40; Strawberries = 12 × 0.30 = £3.60; Eggs = 6 × 0.23 = £1.38; £8.40 - 3.60 - 1.38 = £3.42

69. The correct answer is **C**. 105.67
(100.03+87.11+146.09+89.44)/4 = 422.67/4 = 105.6675 = 105.67

70. The correct answer is **A**. 626.08 kg
Density = kg/m^3
Density = mass/volume
mass = density × volume

mass = 89.44 × 7
mass = 626.08 kg

71. The correct answer is **E**. 13.94
87.11 × 0.16 = 13.9376 = 13.94

72. The correct answer is **E**. 34.23
Density = kg/m^3 = mass/volume; volume = mass/density = 5/146.09 = 0.0342254 m^3; 0.0342254 × 1000 = 34.23 litres

73. The correct answer is **E**. 5
65 x 0.07 = 4.55 = 5 whole books.

74. The correct answer is **B**. 32
Romance + Sci Fi = 46 + 3 = 49%
65 x 0.49 = 31.85 = 32 books (to the nearest whole book)

75. The correct answer is **B**. 12
Fantasy books: 50% of 32% = 16%; Science Fiction + Fantasy: 3% + 16% of total sales i.e. 0.19 x 65 = 12.35 = 12 books.

76. The correct answer is **A**. 7
65 x 0.07 = 4.55 = 5 books; 5 x1.45 = 7.25 = 7 books.

77. The correct answer is **E**. 9.7
The measured/actual pressure was 140 psi; 140/14.504 = 9.6525 = 9.7 bar

78. The correct answer is **C**. 910 pounds
Chamber pressure was 140 pounds per square inch. 140 pounds per square inch gives a total of 140x6.5 = 910 pounds

79. The correct answer is **B** 0.05lbf
Increase in thrust = 1.3-1.1 = 0.2 N
Increase in pound-force = 0.2 × 0.225 = 0.045 or 0.05 lbf to 2 decimal places

80. The correct answer is **B**. 0.7 bar
Increase in chamber pressure = 150 - 140 = 10 psi
Number of bar = 10/14.504 = 0.689 or 0.7 bar to one decimal place

81. The correct answer is **A**. 7/12
7 months (January and July to December) = 7/12

82. The correct answer is **E**. March and May
The biggest fall was seen between March and May (4.4 to 4%)

83. The correct answer is **D**. £525
140,000 × 0.045 = £6,300. 6300/ 12 = 525

84. The correct answer is **E.** December
The money should be left in the bank account for the entire year, because money will not be lost even when the interest rate falls.

85. The correct answer is **A**. 9p

L = 0.3 (10) × 0.2 (15) = 3 × 3 = 9p

86. The correct answer is **E.** 130p
10 × 12 = 120 cm2; 3600/120 = 30 cm = depth;
P = 0.2 (10) × 0.2 (12) × 0.9 (30)
P = 2 × 2.4 × 27 = 129.6p
P = 130p

87. The correct answer is **A.** L + 5 = 0.3a x 0.2b

88. The correct answer is **E.** 214cm
£5 = 500p; P = 500
500 = 0.2 (5) × 0.2 (13) × 0.9c
500 = 1 × 2.6 ×0.9c
c = 500/ (2.6x0.9)
c = 213.675
c = 214 cm

89. The correct answer is **D**. 1/7
The total number of objects in the bag is 14. There are 2 yellow cars in the bag. Probability = 2/14 = 1/7

90. The correct answer is **A**. 0.385
The total number of objects is 14. When the yellow car is removed the new total is 13. There are 5 green objects. Probability = 5/13 = 0.3846 = 0.385.

91. The correct answer is **E**. 0.176

There are now three more objects in the bag, bringing the total to 17. Probability = 3/17 = 0.176

92. The correct answer is **A**. 7/31
At the beginning of the game there would have been 52+10 = 62 counters and 1 + 13 blue counters = 14. The probability of picking a blue counter at the beginning = 14/62 = 7/31.

93. The correct answer is **B**. 22691
The highest vote is 261457 and the second is 238766. The difference is 27691
261457 - 238766 = 22691

94. The correct answer is **E**. 21%
900223 voted in total, 189445 of those voted for Dewar. (189445/900223) × 100 = 21%

95. The correct answer is **A**. 34%
After Dewar is eliminated his votes are re-allocated to the other contestants according to the voters second choice. The 68889 allocated to Baines bring his total to 307656 which is the highest at this point.
307655/900233 = 34%

96. The correct answer is **E.** Can't tell / none of them
The scenario states that the transfer of votes will go ahead until a candidate has more than 50% of the vote. This does not happen as after the first transfer the highest number of votes is held by Baines at 307655 which is only 34% of the vote.

97. The correct answer is **D**. 3297
25362 × 0.13 = 3297.06 = 3297

98. The correct answer is **C**. 6848
34% - 7% is 27%.

27% of 25362 = 0.27 x 25362
27% = 6847.7
27% = 6848

99. The correct answer is **D**. 2932
Those visiting Spain is 34% of 25362 = 0.34 x 8623.08
Those visiting the Balearic Islands are 34% of 8623.08 = 8623.08 × 0.34
Those visiting the Balearic Islands = 2931.8 or 2932

100. The correct answer is **B**. 7.0%
Originally there were 25362 × 0.07 = 1775.34 travellers to Tunisia. With Austria the total number of travellers is now (25362 + 163) = 25525. New Tunisia percentage = (1775.34/25525)×100 = 6.955 = 7.0 % (1.d.p)

100 Abstract Reasoning Questions **(answers begin on page 196)**

Set A | Set B

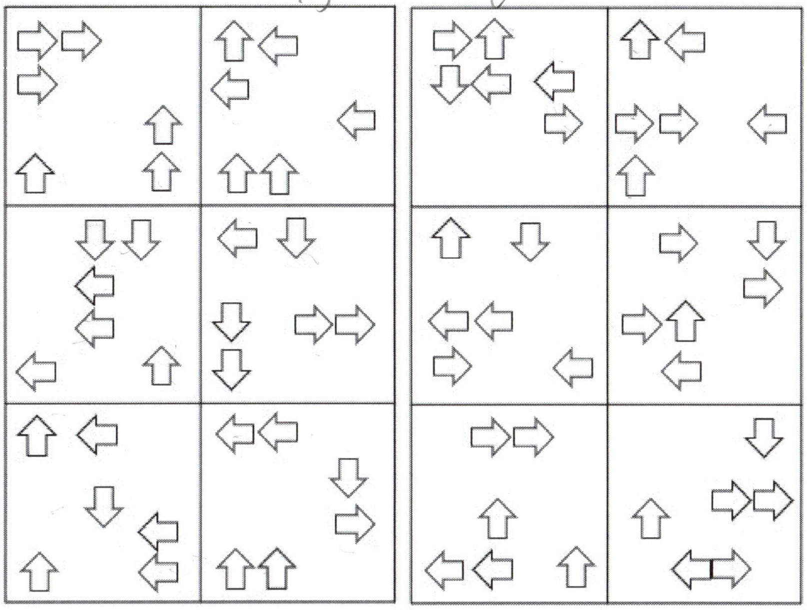

1 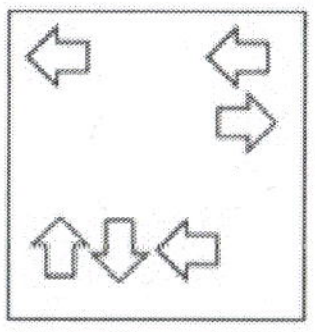
Set A
Set B
Neither

2 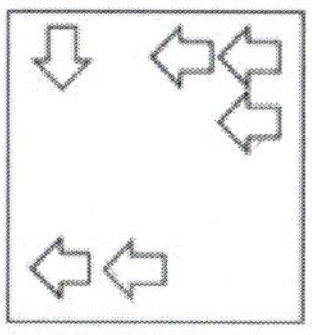
Set A
Set B
Neither

3 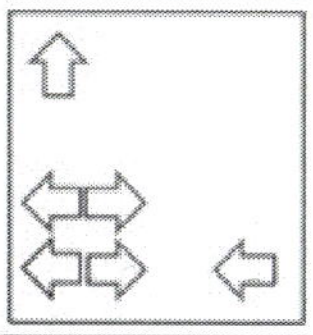
Set A
Set B
Neither

4 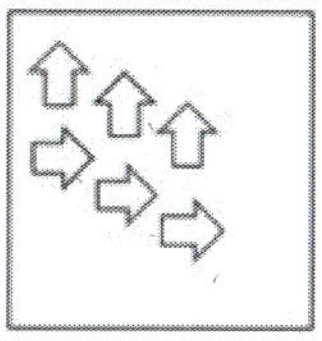
Set A
Set B
Neither

5 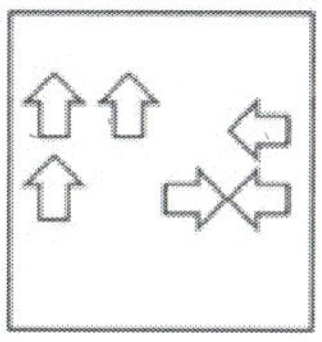
Set A
Set B
Neither

To which of the two sets do the following shapes belong?

Set A | Set B

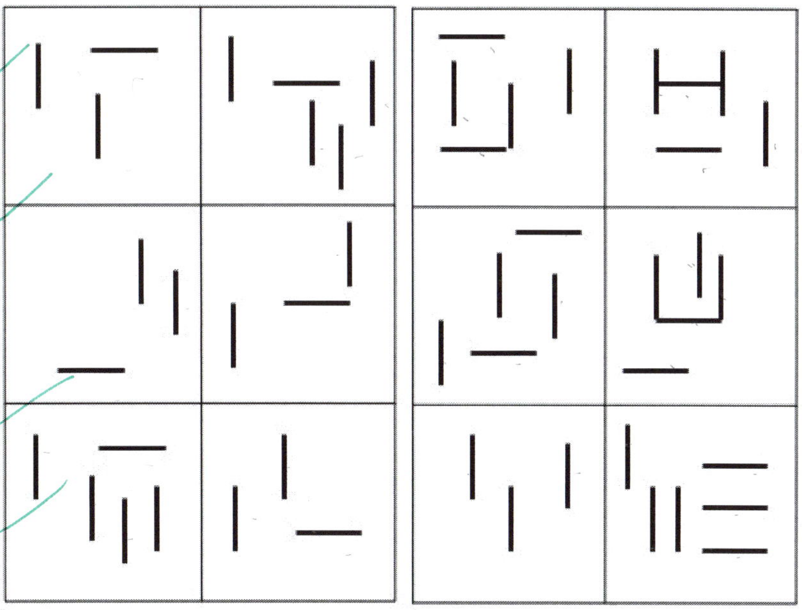

6 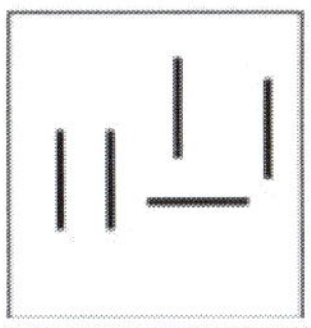
Set A
Set B
Neither

7 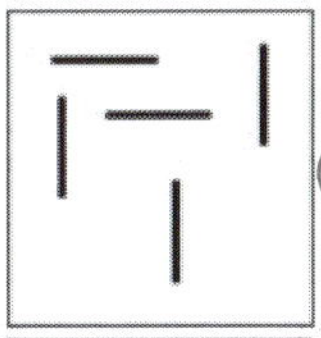
Set A
Set B
Neither

8 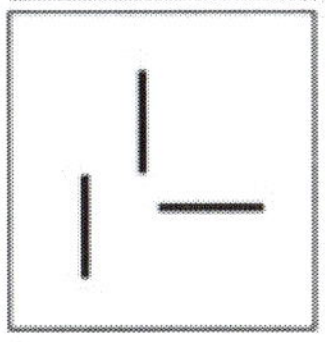
Set A
Set B
Neither

9 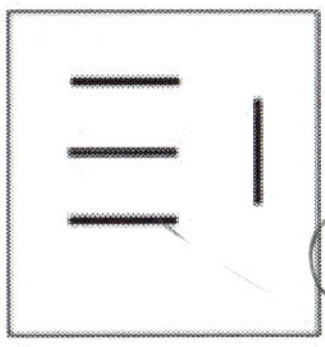
Set A
Set B
Neither

10 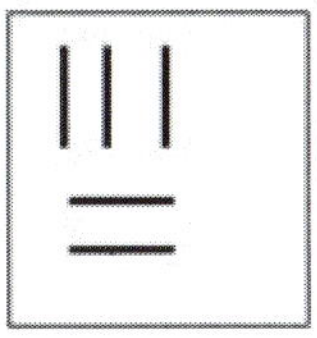
Set A
Set B
Neither

Set A

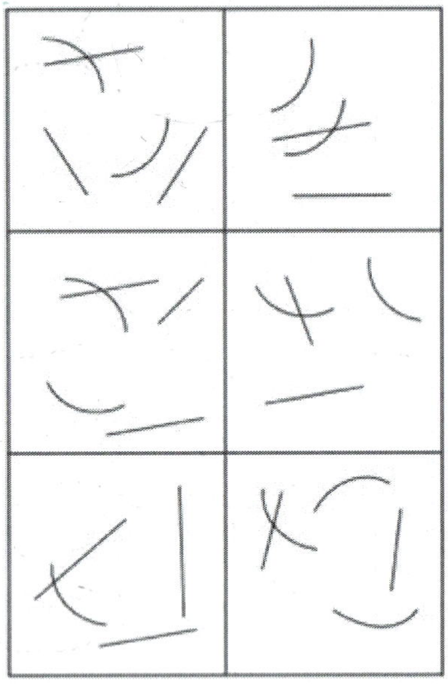

Set B

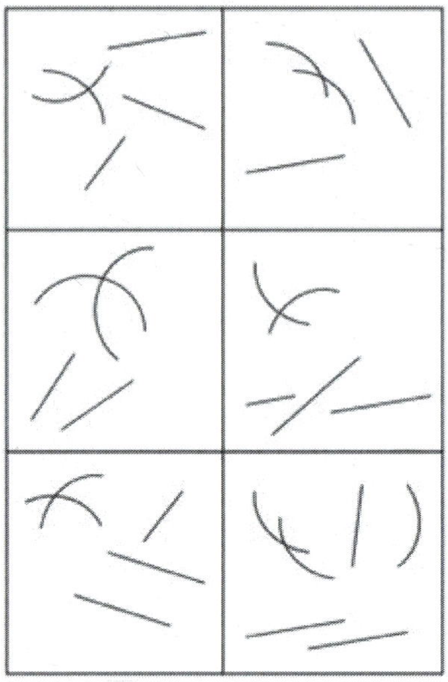

11
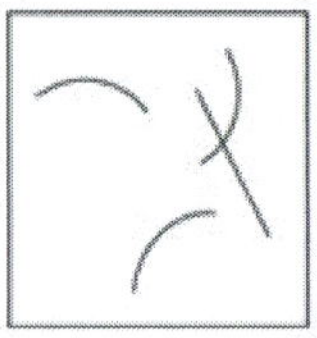
Set A
Set B
Neither

12
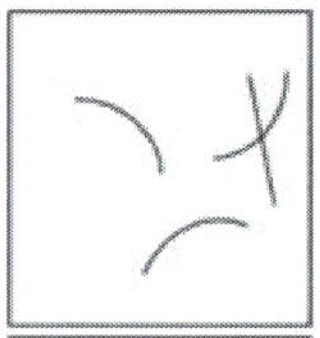
Set A
Set B
Neither

13
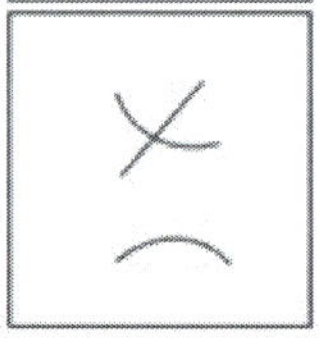
Set A
Set B
Neither

14
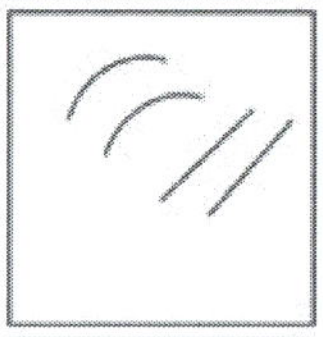
Set A
Set B
Neither

15
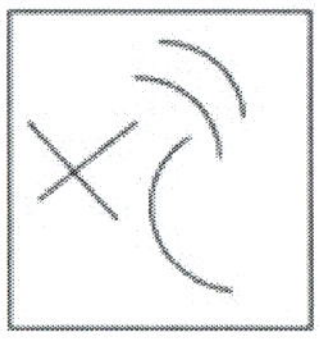
Set A
Set B
Neither

To which of the two sets do the following shapes belong?

Set A

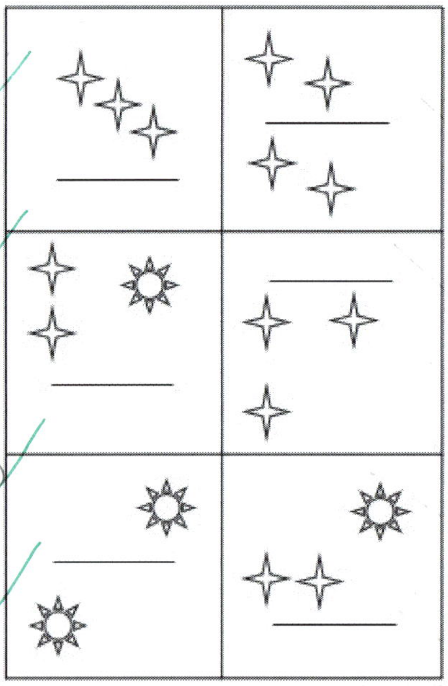

Set B

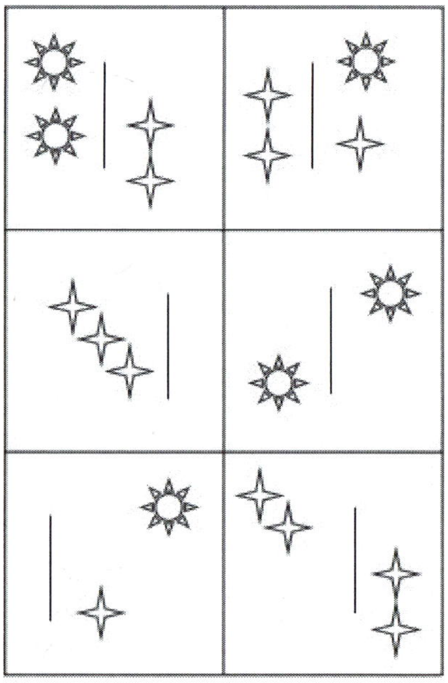

16

Set A
Set B
Neither

17
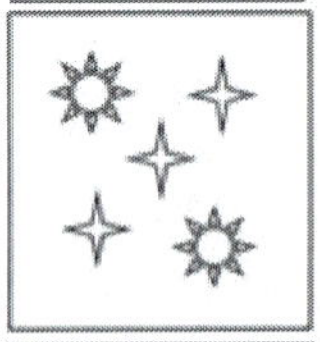
Set A
Set B
Neither

18
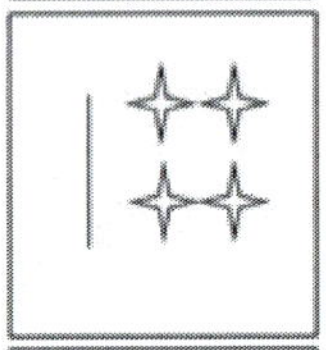
Set A
Set B
Neither

19
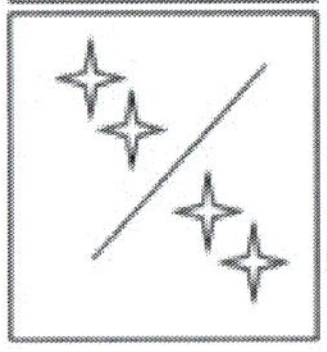
Set A
Set B
Neither

20

Set A
Set B
Neither

Set A | Set B

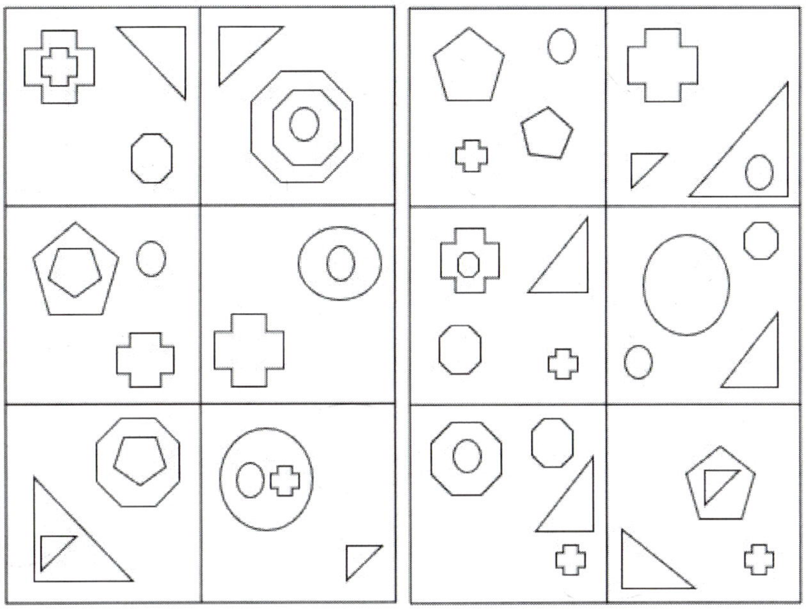

21
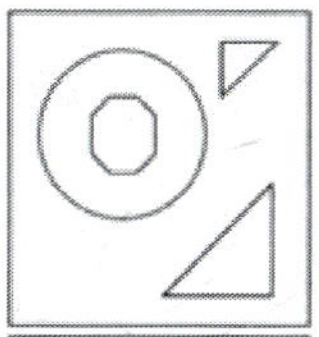
Set A
Set B
Neither

22
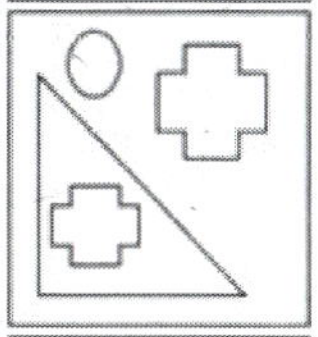
Set A
Set B
Neither

23
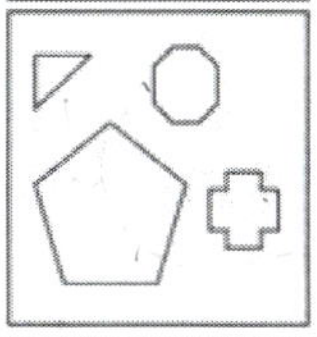
Set A
Set B
Neither

24
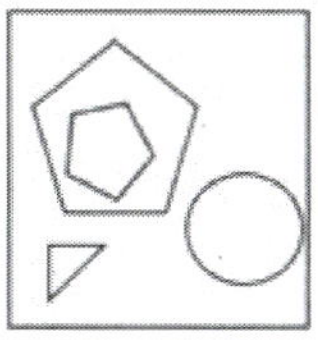
Set A
Set B
Neither

25
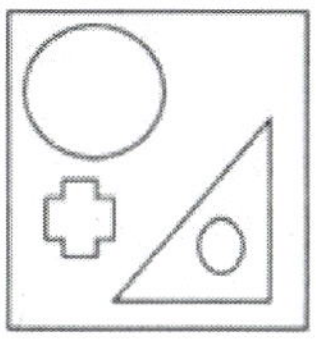
Set A
Set B
Neither

To which of the two sets do the following shapes belong?

Set A | Set B

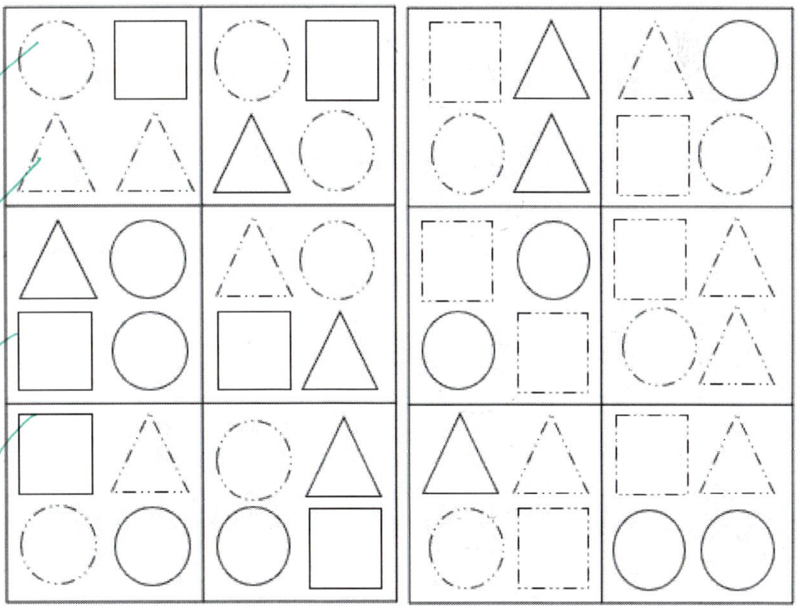

26
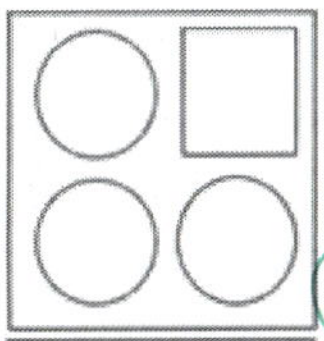
Set A
Set B
Neither

27
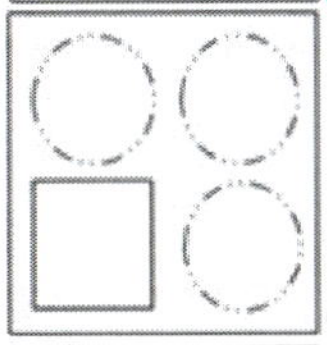
Set A
Set B
Neither

28
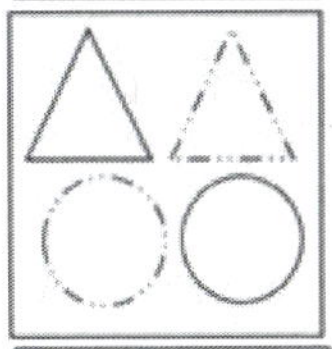
Set A
Set B
Neither

29
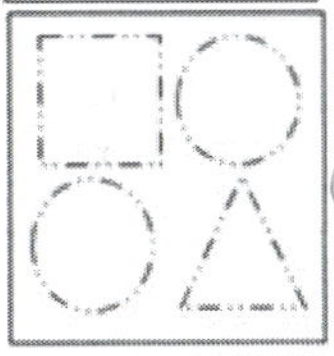
Set A
Set B
Neither

30
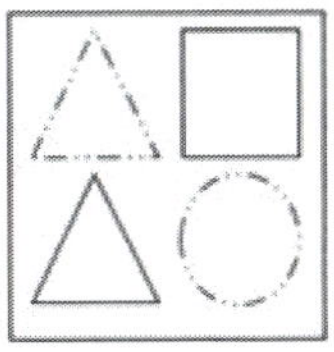
Set A
Set B
Neither

Set A

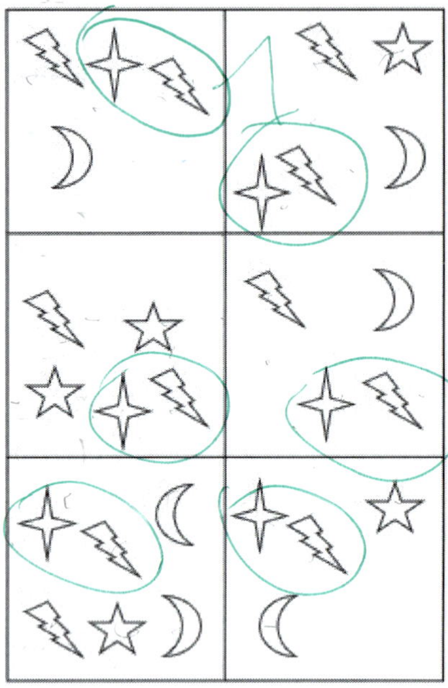

Set B

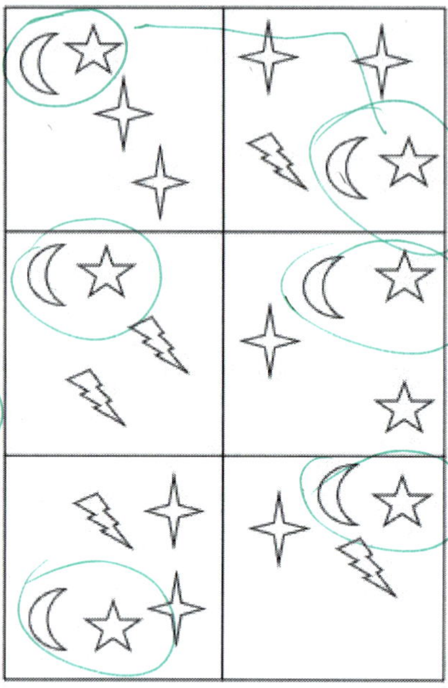

31 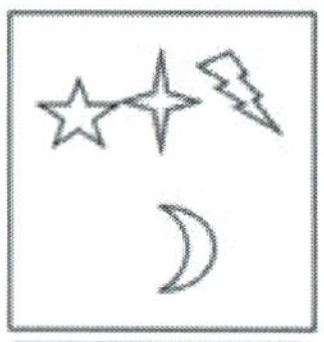
Set A
Set B
Neither

32 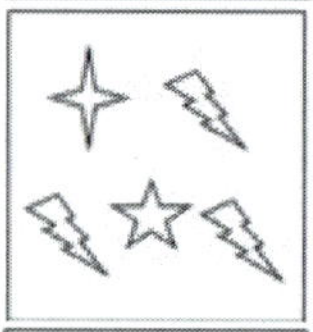
Set A
Set B
Neither

33 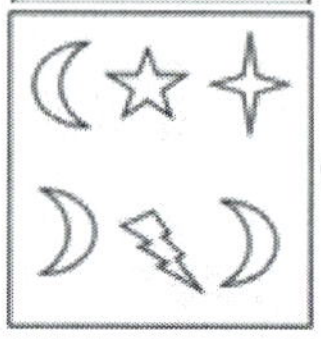
Set A
Set B
Neither

34 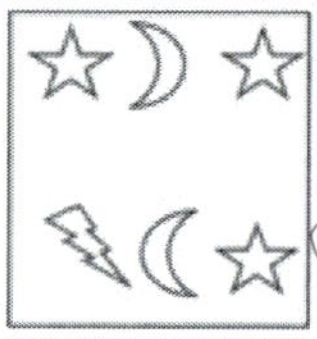
Set A
Set B
Neither

35 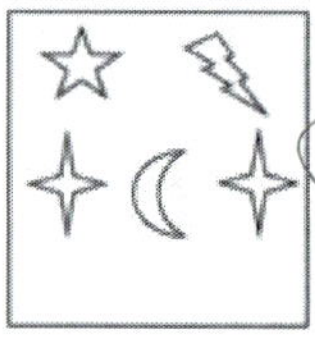
Set A
Set B
Neither

To which of the two sets do the following shapes belong?

Set A

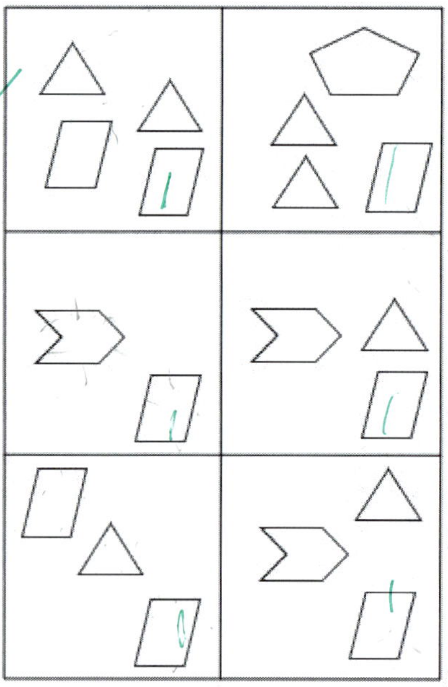

Set B

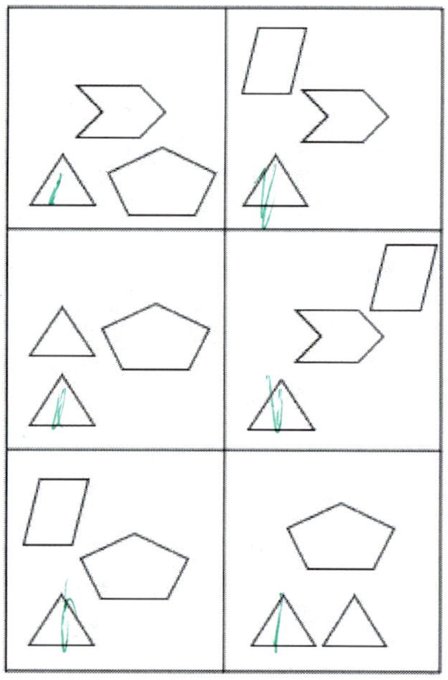

36 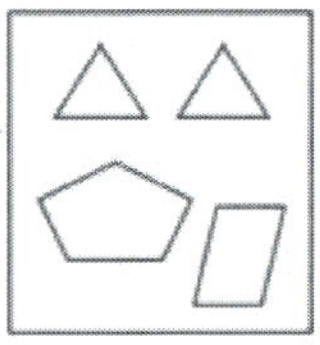
Set A
Set B
Neither

37 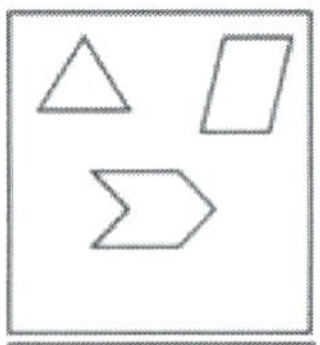
Set A
Set B
Neither

38 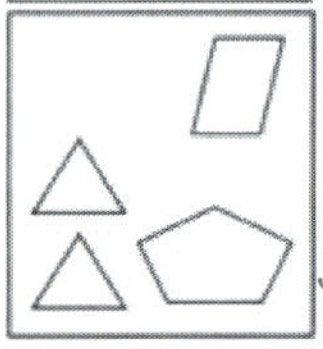
Set A
Set B
Neither

39 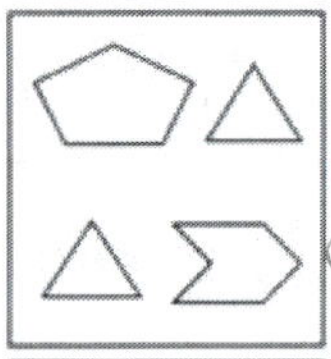
Set A
Set B
Neither

40 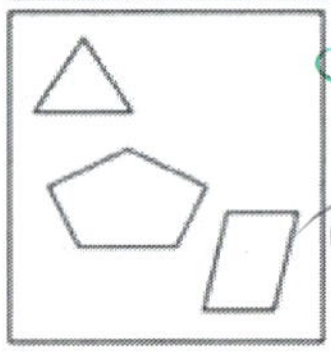
Set A
Set B
Neither

Set A | Set B

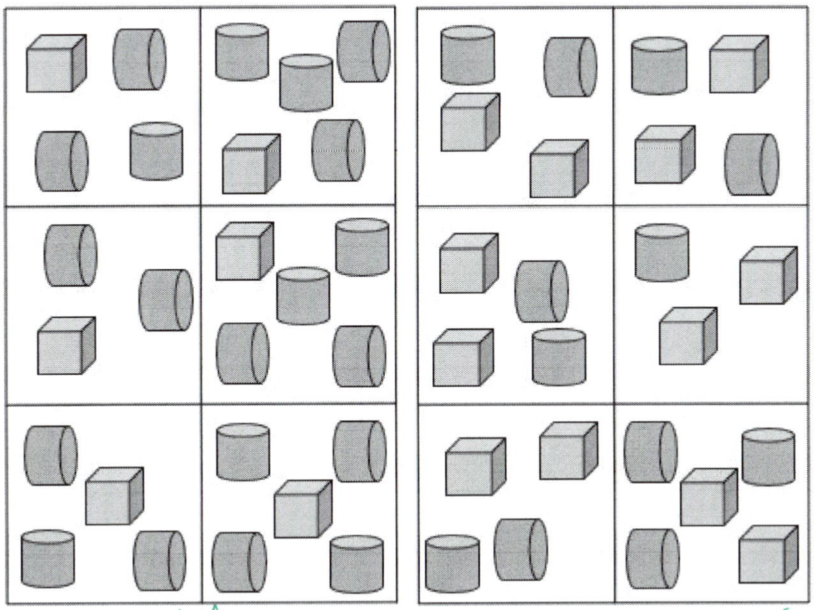

1x cube
2x segment

1x cylinder
2x cube

41
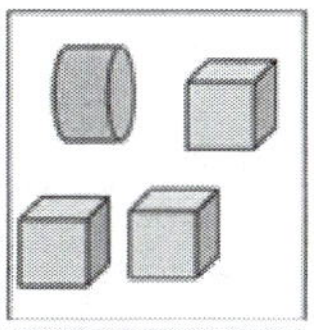
Set A
Set B
Neither

42
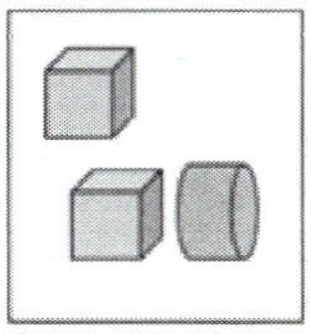
Set A
Set B
Neither

43
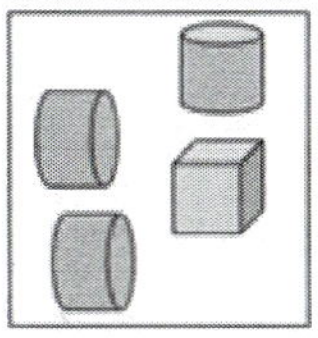
Set A
Set B
Neither

44
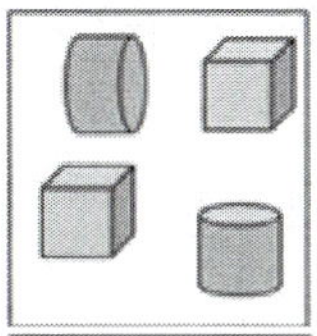
Set A
Set B
Neither

45
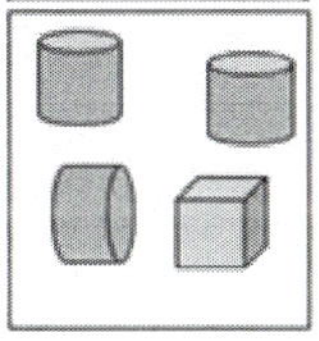
Set A
Set B
Neither

To which of the two sets do the following shapes belong?

Set A | Set B

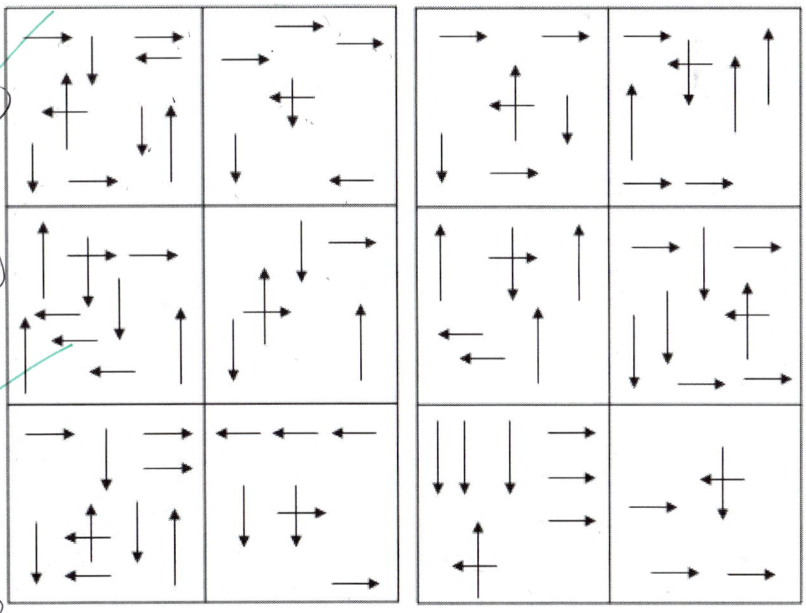

46
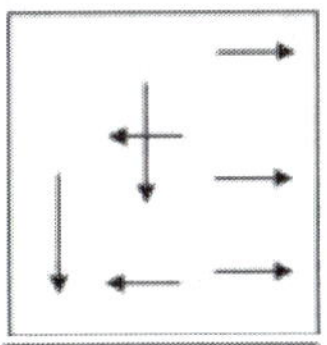
Set A
Set B
Neither

47
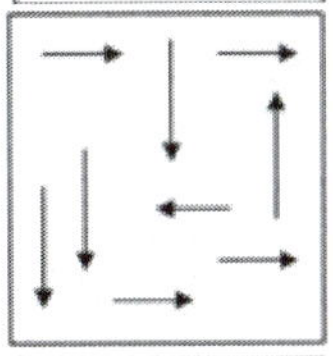
Set A
Set B
Neither

48
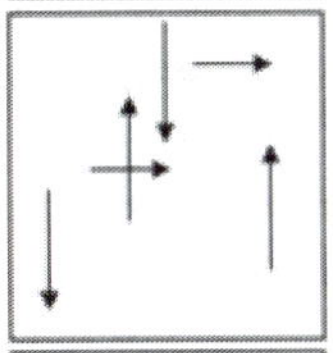
Set A
Set B
Neither

49
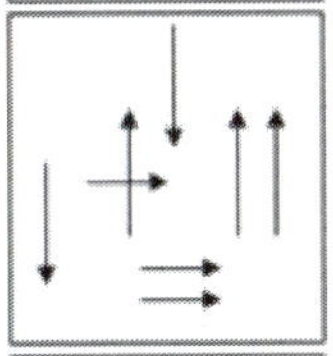
Set A
Set B
Neither

50
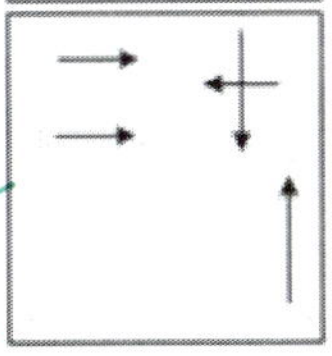
Set A
Set B
Neither

51

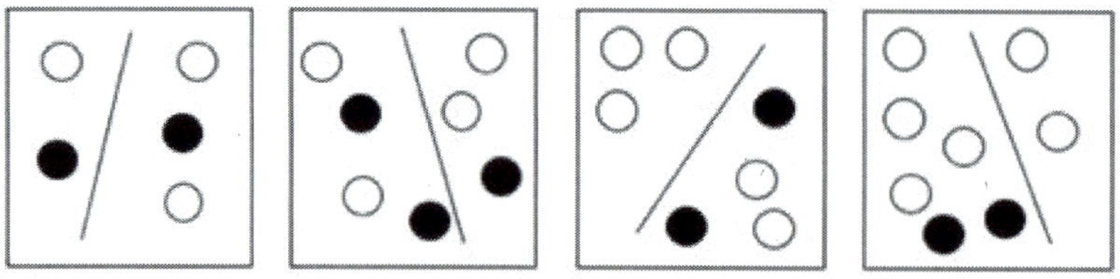

Which figure completes the series

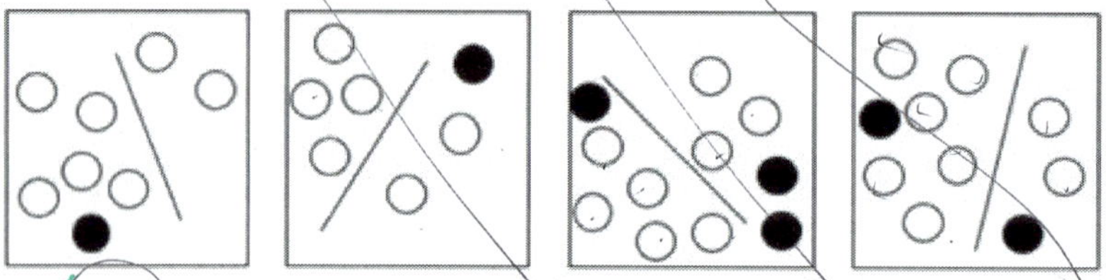

A B C D

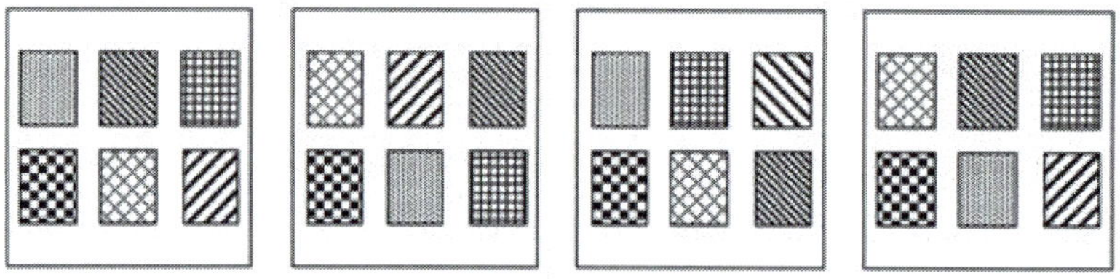

52

Which figure completes the series

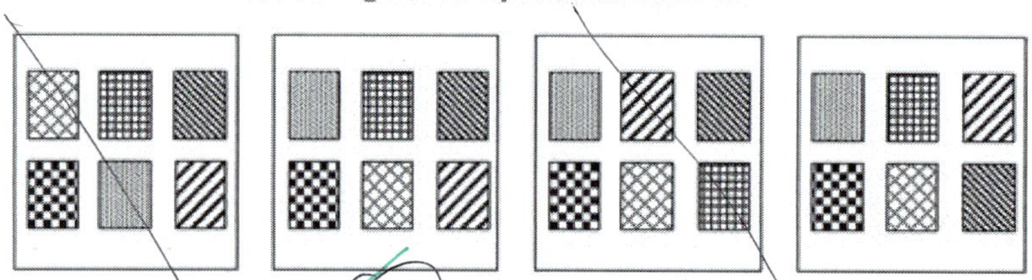

A B C D

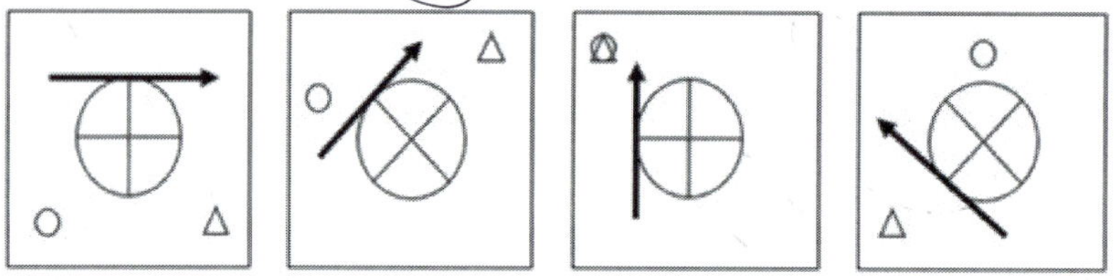

53

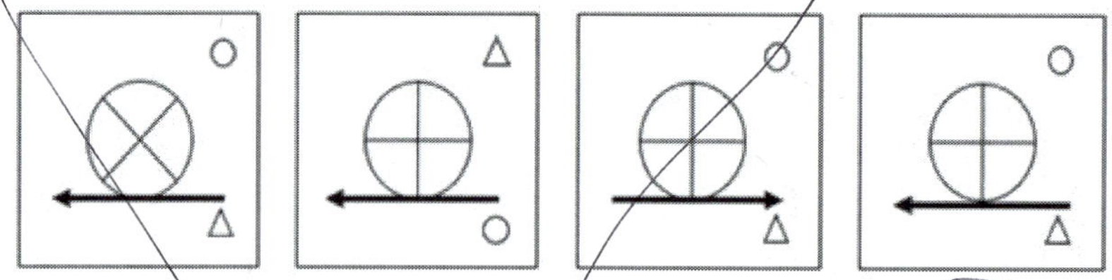

A B C D

Set A Set B

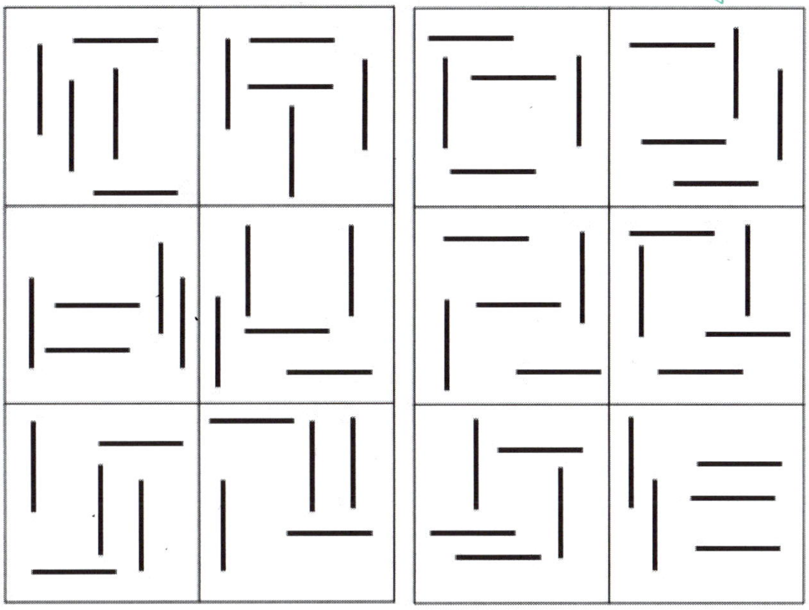

54 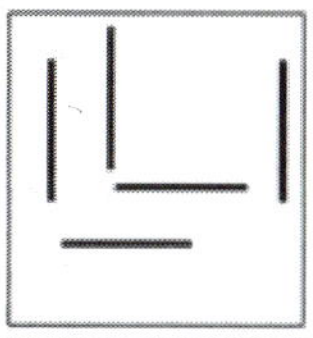
Set A
Set B
Neither

55 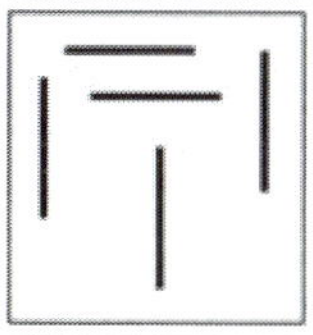
Set A
Set B
Neither

56 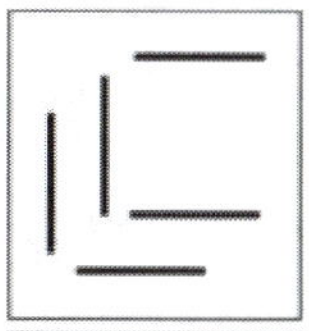
Set A
Set B
Neither

57 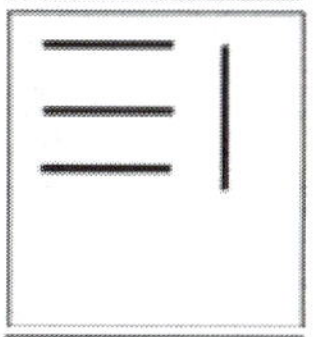
Set A
Set B
Neither

58 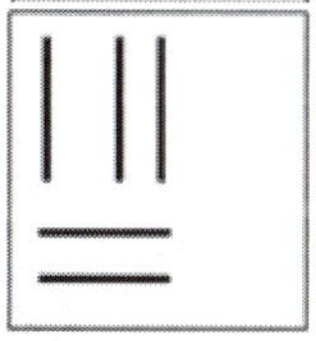
Set A
Set B
Neither

To which of the two sets do the following shapes belong?

Set A Set B

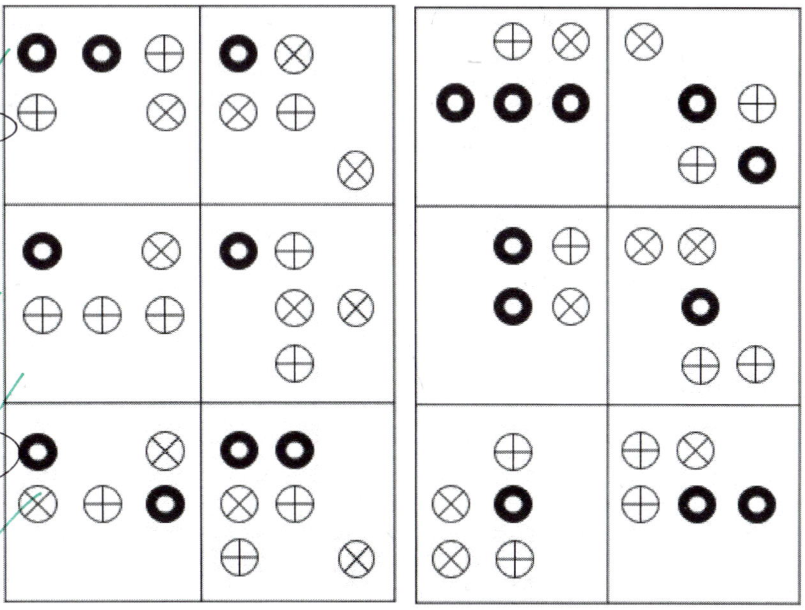

59 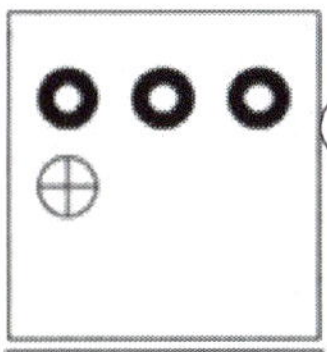
Set A
Set B
Neither

60 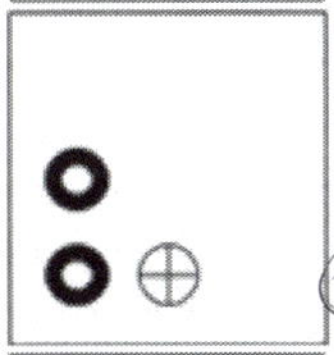
Set A
Set B
Neither

61 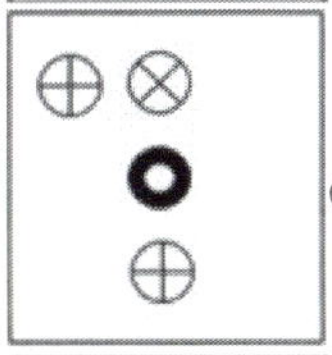
Set A
Set B
Neither

62 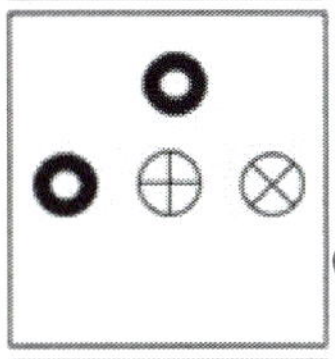
Set A
Set B
Neither

63 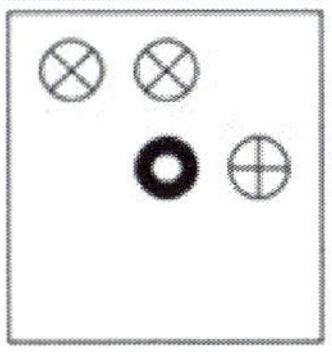
Set A
Set B
Neither

Set A

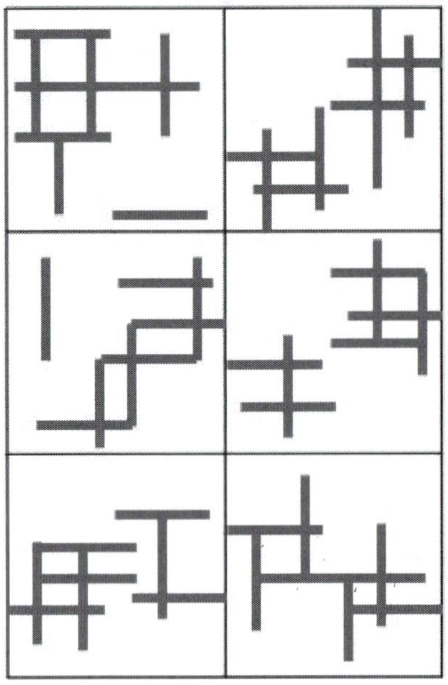

Set B

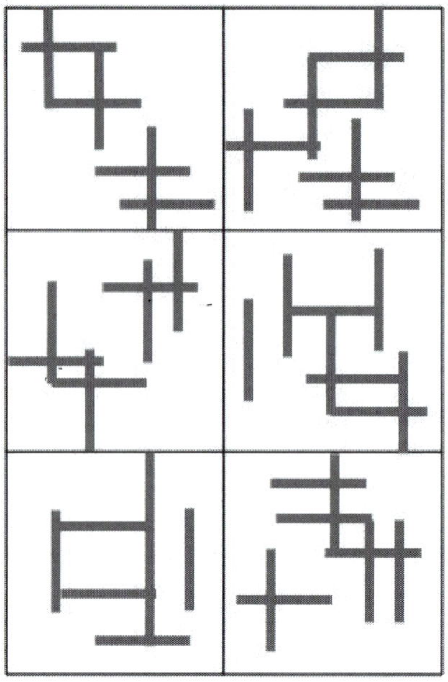

64 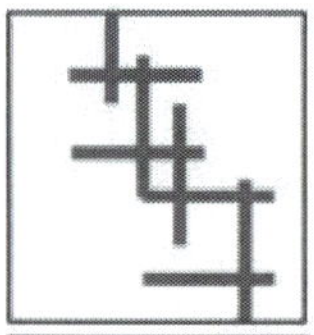
Set A
Set B
Neither

65 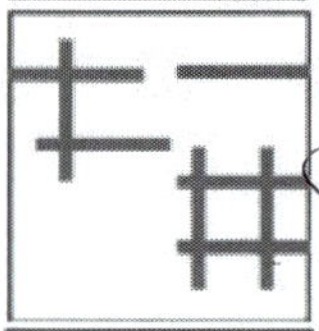
Set A
Set B
Neither

66 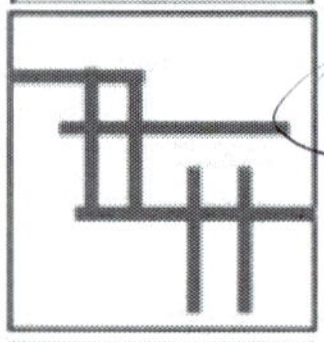
Set A
Set B
Neither

67 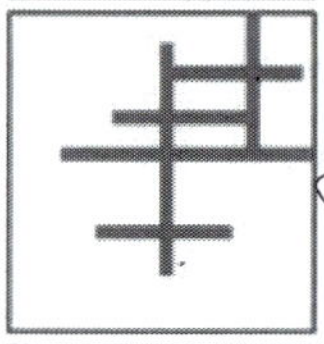
Set A
Set B
Neither

68 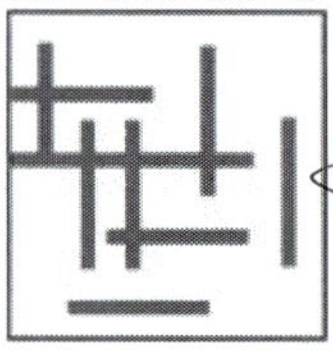
Set A
Set B
Neither

To which of the two sets do the following shapes belong?

Set A

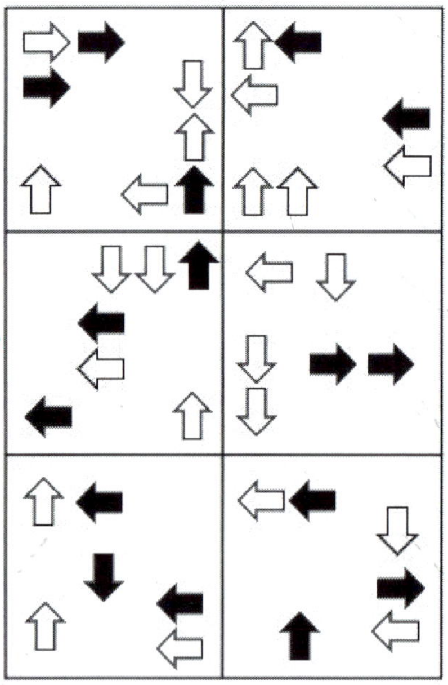

2x horizontal black

Set B

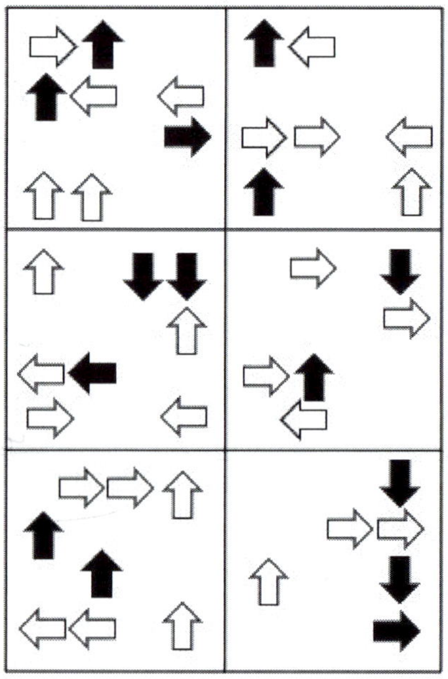

2x vertical black

69 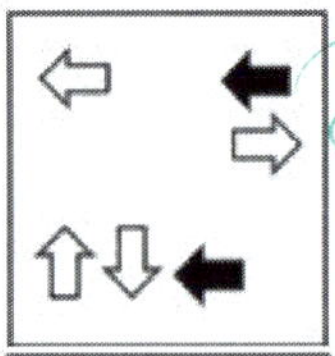
Set A
Set B
Neither

70 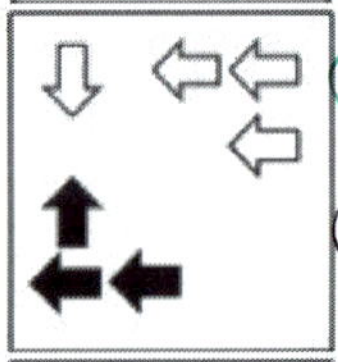
Set A
Set B
Neither

71 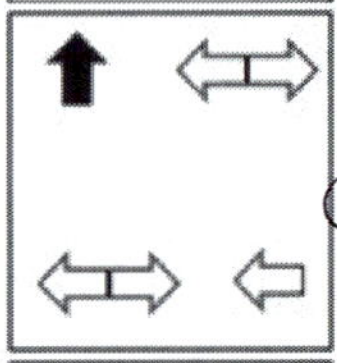
Set A
Set B
Neither

72 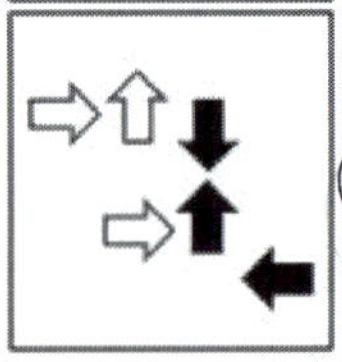
Set A
Set B
Neither

73 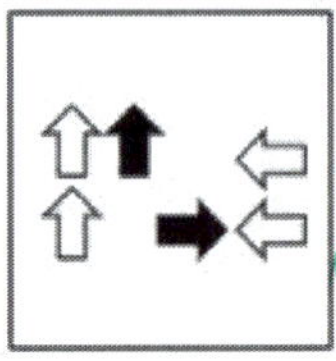
Set A
Set B
Neither

74

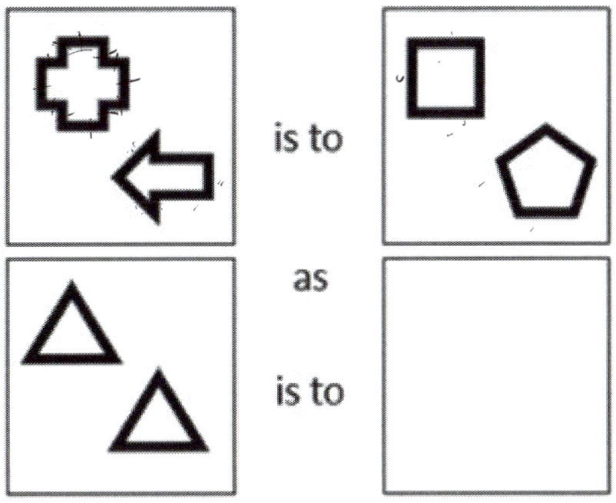

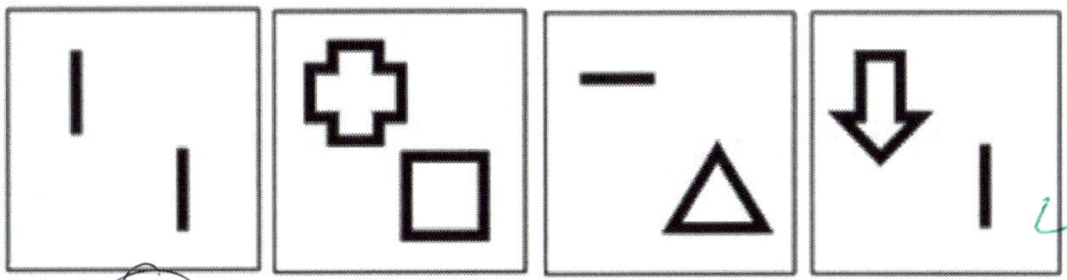

A B C D

75

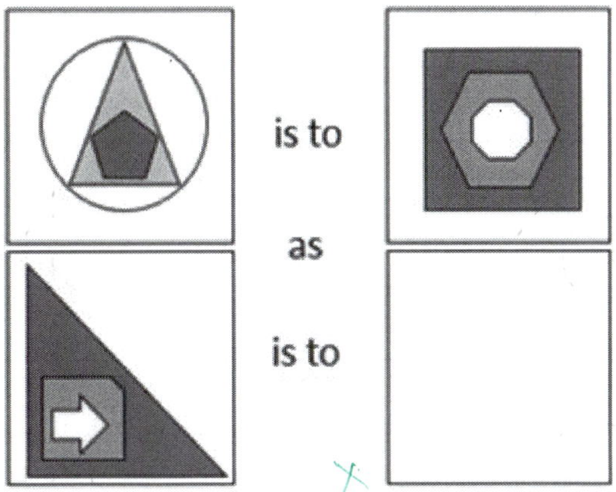

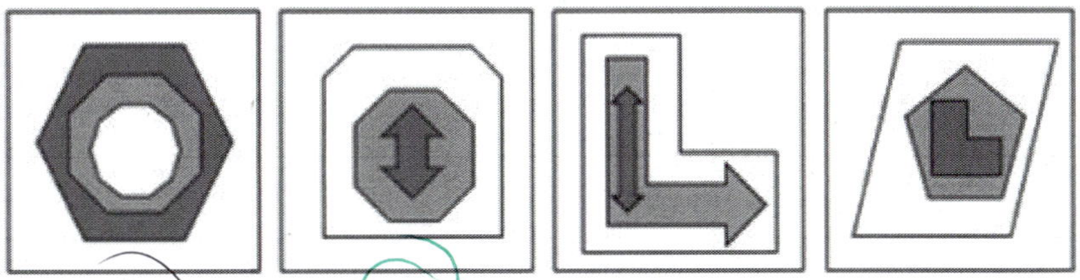

A B C D

Set A

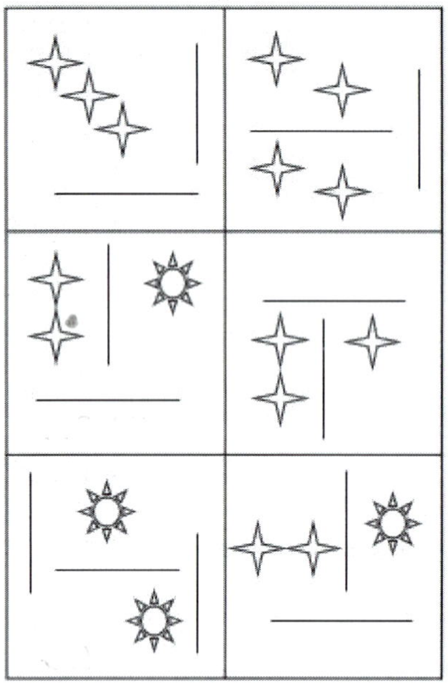

Set B

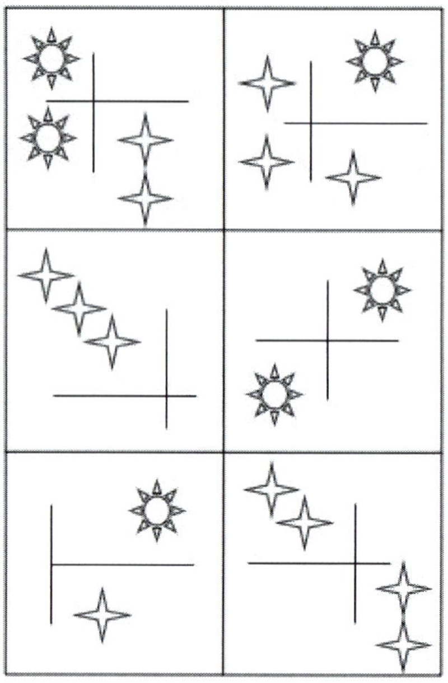

76 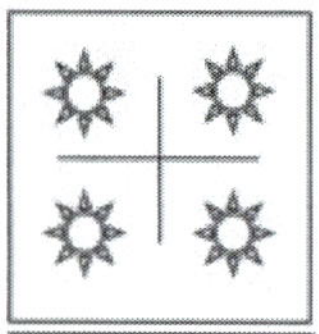
Set A
Set B
Neither

77 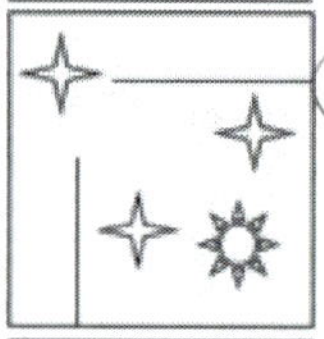
Set A
Set B
Neither

78 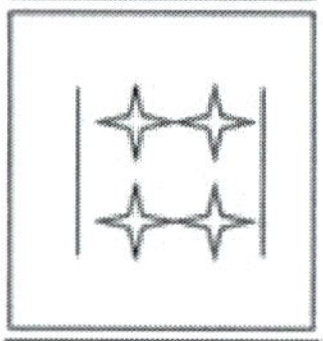
Set A
Set B
Neither

79 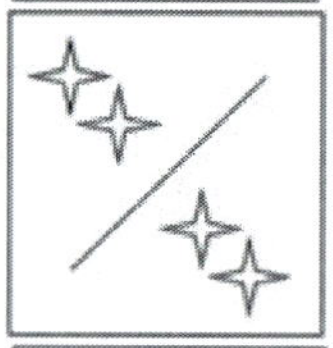
Set A
Set B
Neither

80 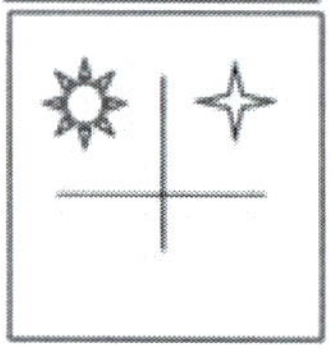
Set A
Set B
Neither

To which of the two sets do the following shapes belong?

Set A

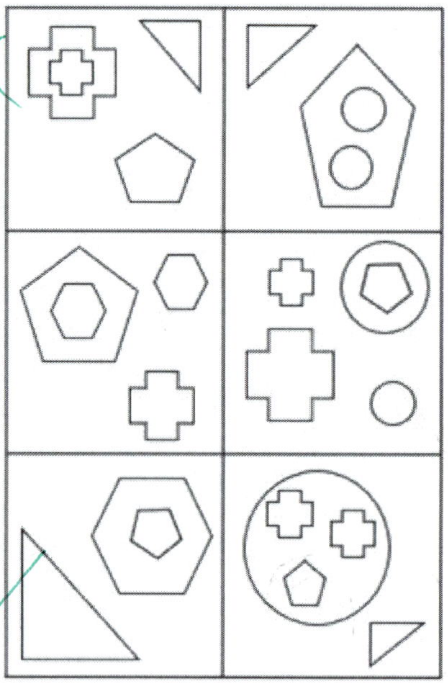

Set B

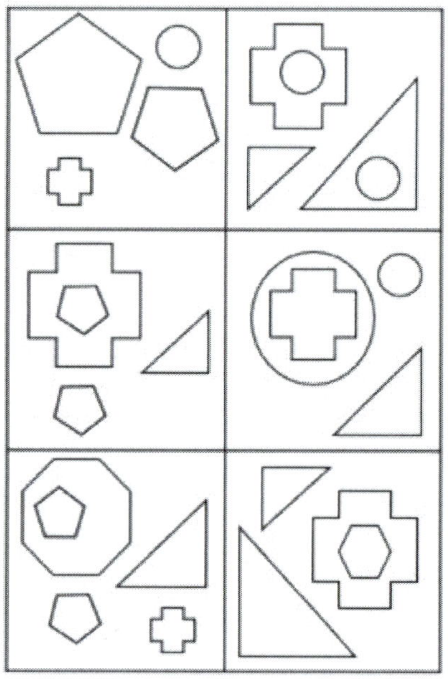

81 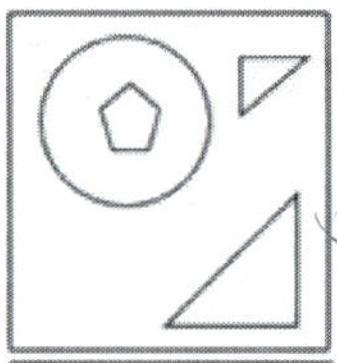
Set A
Set B
Neither

82 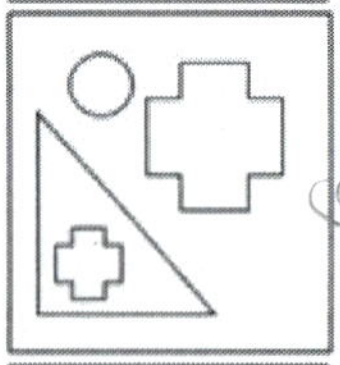
Set A
Set B
Neither

83 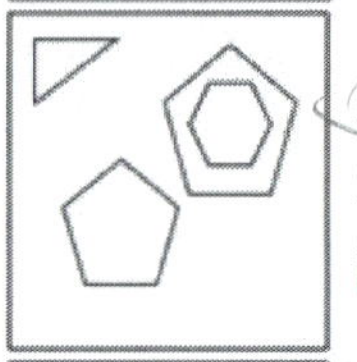
Set A
Set B
Neither

84 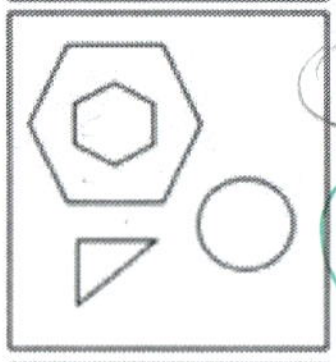
Set A
Set B
Neither

85 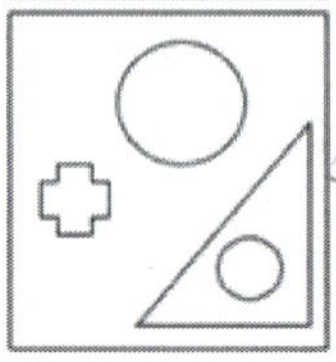
Set A
Set B
Neither

Set A | Set B

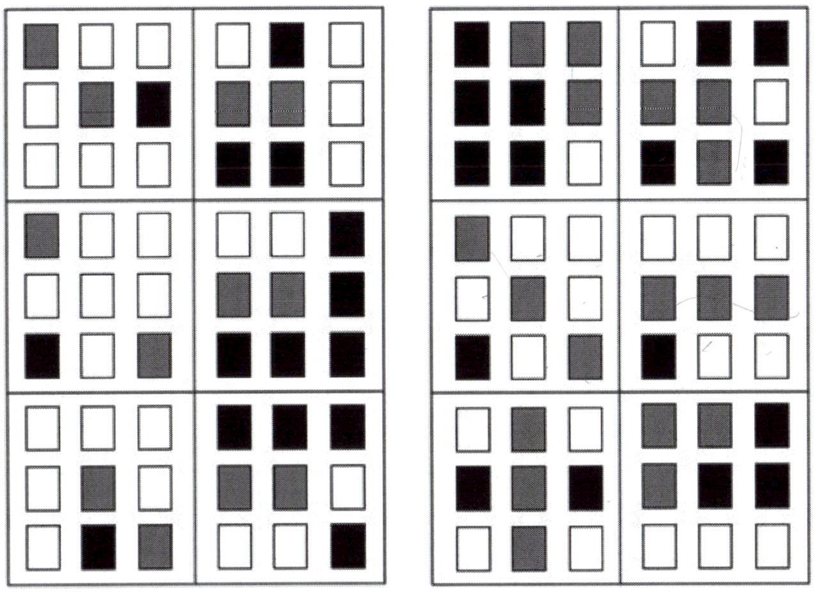

86 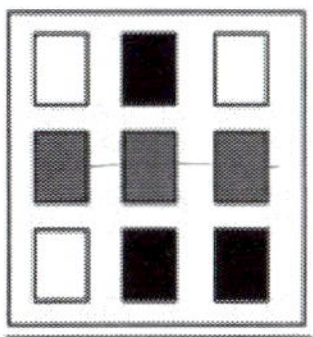

Set A
Set B
Neither

87 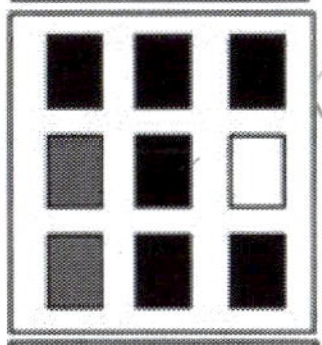

Set A
Set B
Neither

88 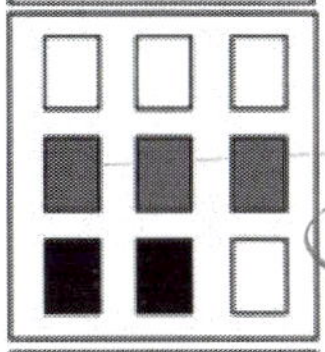

Set A
Set B
Neither

89 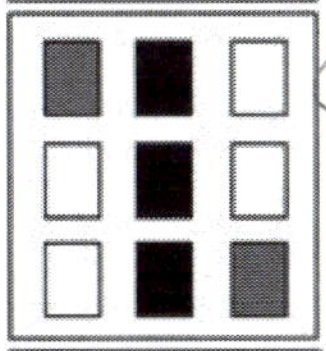

Set A
Set B
Neither

90 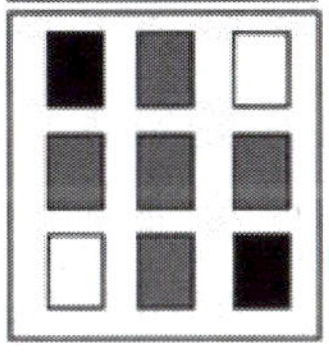

Set A
Set B
Neither

To which of the two sets do the following shapes belong?

Set A | Set B

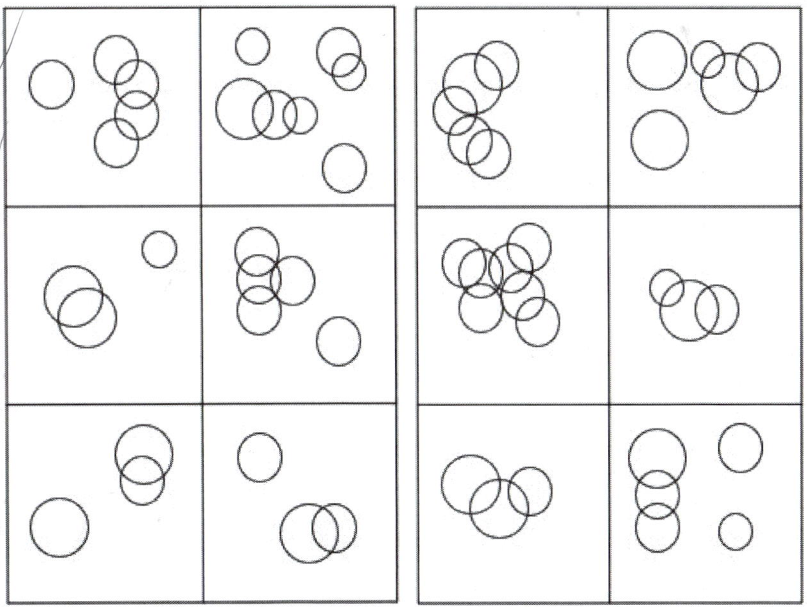

91 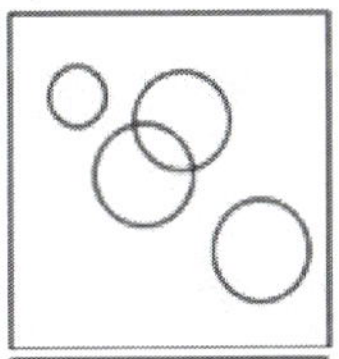

Set A
Set B
Neither

92 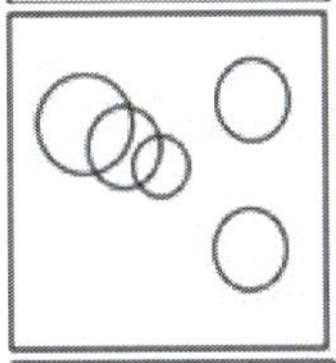

Set A
Set B
Neither

93 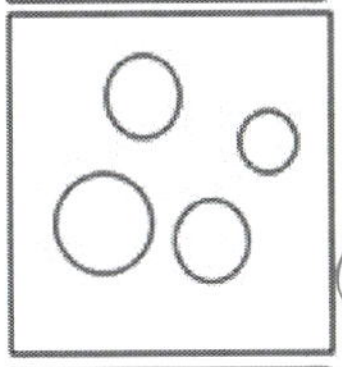

Set A
Set B
Neither

94 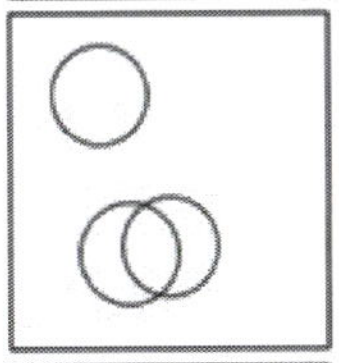

Set A
Set B
Neither

95 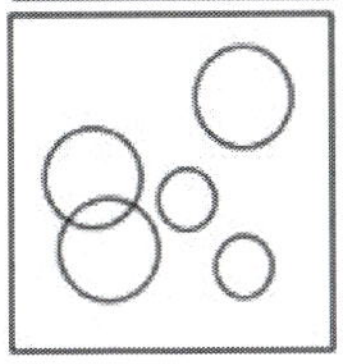

Set A
Set B
Neither

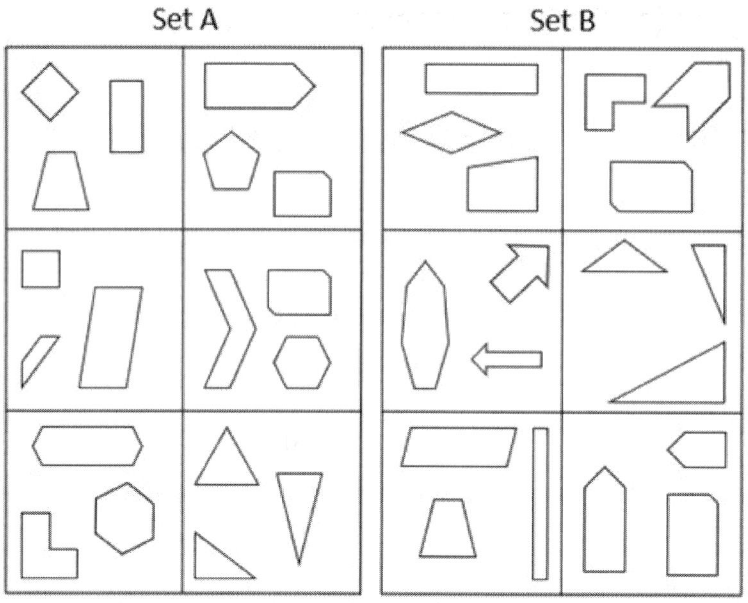

96 Which belongs in Set A?

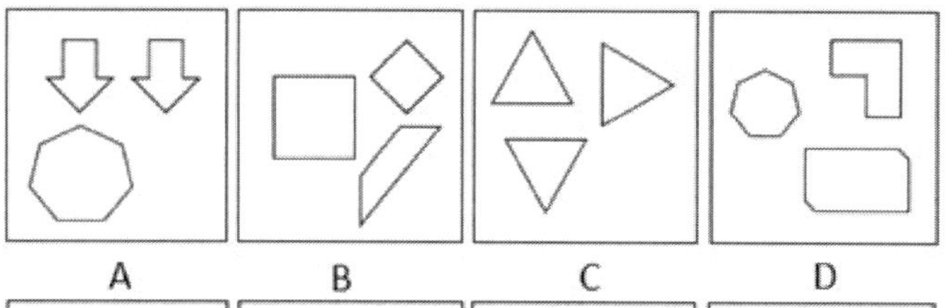

97 Which belongs in Set B?

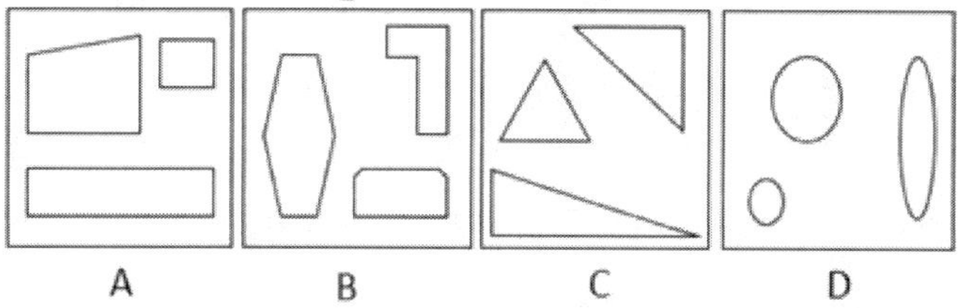

98 Which belongs in Set A?

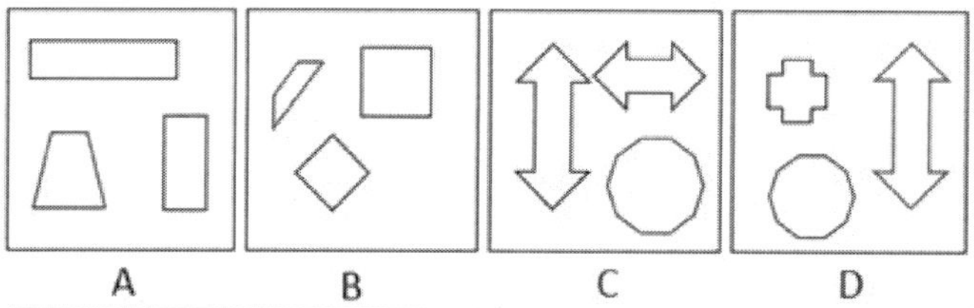

99 Which belongs in Set B?

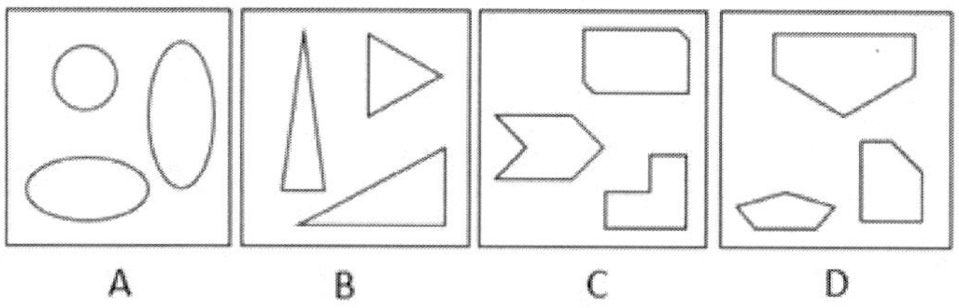

100 Which belongs in Set A?

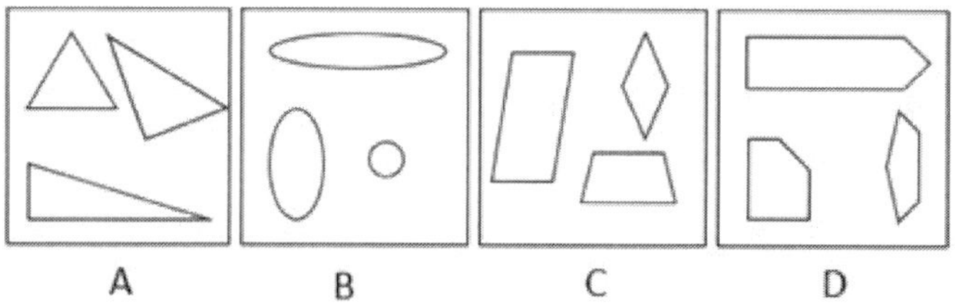

100 Abstract Reasoning Question Answers

Question Set 1 (questions 1 – 5)
Set A always contains three horizontal and three vertical arrows. Set B always contains four horizontal and two vertical arrows.

1. B
2. Neither
3. Neither
4. A
5. A

Question Set 2 (questions 6 – 10)
Set A always has one horizontal line. Set B always contains exactly three vertical lines.

6. A
7. B
8. A
9. Neither
10. B

Question Set 3 (questions 11 - 15)
Set A always contains a straight line intersecting a curved line. Set B always contains two curved lines intersecting each other.

11. B
12. A
13. A
14. Neither
15. Neither

Questions Set 4 (questions 16 - 20)
Set A always contains a horizontal line. Set B always contains a vertical line.

16. B
17. Neither
18. B
19. Neither
20. B

Question Set 5 (questions 21 - 25)
Set A always contains a pair of similar shapes – the smaller one inside the larger one. Set B always contains a pair of similar shapes – the shapes are independent of each other.

21. B
22. B
23. Neither
24. A
25. B

Question Set 6 (questions 26 - 30)
Set A always contains one solid square and a triangle. Set B always contains one dashed square and at least one circle.

26. Neither
27. Neither
28. Neither
29. B
30. A

Question Set 7 (questions 31 – 35)
Set A: Each four-pointed star has a lightning symbol to the right of it. Set B: Each moon with tips pointing right has a 5 pointed star to the right of it.

31. A
32. A
33. B
34. B
35. Neither

Question Set 8 (questions 36-40)
Set A: Has a parallelogram in the bottom right hand corner. Set B: Has a triangle in the bottom left hand corner.

36. A
37. Neither
38. B
39. B
40. A

Question Set 9 (questions 41-45)
Set A always contains a cube and two tube segments. Set B always contains a cylinder and two cubes.

41. Neither
42. Neither
43. A
44. B
45. Neither

Question Set 10 (questions 46-50)
Set A – has one intersecting pair and one other arrow pointing in each of the same directions as the intersecting pair. Set B – has one intersecting pair, and no other arrows pointing in the same directions.

46. A
47. Neither
48. A
49. Neither
50. B

51. A - In each of the boxes an extra white circle is added to the left of the line. There are always two white circles on the right side of the line. Ignore all black circles.

52. B - The top left and bottom middle shapes swap each time. The bottom left remains in place. The other three shapes move one space in a clockwise direction each time.

53. D - The arrow is moving anti-clockwise around the central large circle. The cross within the circle alternates between being set straight or and at an angle. The small circle moves half a length clockwise. The small triangle moves a whole length anti clockwise.

Question Set 11 (questions 54 – 58)
Set A contains three vertical and two horizontal lines. Set B always contains three horizontal and two vertical lines.

54. A
55. A
56. B
57. Neither
58. A

Question Set 12 (questions 59 – 63)
Set A always contains a circle with a straight cross and a circle with a diagonal cross and a black right. There is always a black ring in the upper left corner. Set B always has all three shapes with a black ring in the centre.

59. Neither
60. Neither
61. B
62. Neither
63. B

Question Set 13 (questions 64 – 68)
Set A – lines are always arranged to create two enclosed spaces. Set B – lines are always arranged to create one enclosed space.

64. A
65. A
66. B
67. B
68. Neither

Question Set 14 (questions 69 – 73)
Set A always contains two horizontal black arrows and Set B always contains two vertical black arrows.

69. A
70. A
71. Neither
72. B
73. Neither

74. A – the number of sides from the first shape is divided by three from the first to the second picture. The number of sides from the second shape has two subtracted from it

75. B – the relationship between the concentric shapes is 1. The shapes in the second picture have three more edges than those in the first. 2. The colour patter is reversed.

Question Set 15 (questions 76 – 80)
Set A always contains one horizontal and one vertical line that do not touch each other or the edge. Set B always contains one horizontal and one vertical line that do touch each other but don't touch the edge.

76. B
77. Neither
78. Nether
79. Neither
80. B

Question Set 16 (questions 81 – 85)
Set A always contains exactly one pentagon and Set B always contains at exactly one cross shape.

81. A
82. Neither
83. Neither
84. Neither
85. B

Question Set 17 (questions 86 – 90)
Set A always has two grey rectangles, Set B always has three grey rectangles.

86. B
87. A
88. B
89. A
90. Neither

Question Set 18 (questions 91 – 95)
Set A - Odd number of circles and odd number of overlap areas. Set B - Odd number of circles and even number of overlap areas.

91. Neither
92. B
93. Neither
94. A
95. A

Question Set 19 (questions 96 – 100)
In Set A there are always three shapes with an equal number of sides. One of these shapes has equal length edges whilst the other two have unequal length edges. In Set B there are always three shapes with an equal number of sides but none of the shapes has all equal length edges. Also - the two corners on the right have right angles positioned adjacent.

96. A
97. B
98. C
99. D
100. A

100 Situational Judgement Questions (answers begin on page 219)

GP receptionist answers a phone call from a hospital doctor enquiring about a patient registered at the surgery. She says she has an appointment later in the week with the patient but that the hospital computer has crashed, and she cannot access their recent test results. The receptionist doesn't recognise the name of the hospital doctor.

How appropriate are the following responses by the receptionist in this situation?

1. She decides to access the patient's records to see if there is any record of recent tests or an upcoming appointment before disclosing personal information.

A very appropriate thing to do

Appropriate but not ideal

Inappropriate but not awful

A very inappropriate thing to do

2. The receptionist refuses to check the patient's notes and says she will ask the GP to call the hospital doctor later

A very appropriate thing to do

Appropriate but not ideal

Inappropriate but not awful

A very inappropriate thing to do

3. The receptionist accesses the patient's files and tells the caller the test results

A very appropriate thing to do

Appropriate but not ideal

Inappropriate but not awful

A very inappropriate thing to do

4. The receptionist suggests that the doctor email their request in the hope that the email will come from an authentic hospital email address. If it does she responds quickly with the relevant information.

A very appropriate thing to do

Appropriate but not ideal

Inappropriate but not awful

A very inappropriate thing to do

A junior doctor is approached in a waiting area by an angry man who demands to know why his mother is being kept waiting. Their appointment should have been twenty minutes ago and they 'have places to be'.

How appropriate are the following responses by the junior doctor in this situation?

5. The junior doctor goes to the reception desk to ask them to bump the man's mother up the list and ensure she is seen next as the commotion is disturbing the other patients.

A very appropriate thing to do

Appropriate but not ideal

Inappropriate but not awful

A very inappropriate thing to do

6. The junior doctor goes to check why the clinic is running late and feeds the information back to the man with an estimate of when the appointment is likely to happen.

A very appropriate thing to do

Appropriate but not ideal

Inappropriate but not awful

A very inappropriate thing to do

7. The junior doctor apologises for the wait and suggests that the man ask the reception desk about the delay.

A very appropriate thing to do

Appropriate but not ideal

Inappropriate but not awful

A very inappropriate thing to do

8. The junior doctor apologises and then discreetly calls security and asks them to be on standby should things escalate.

A very appropriate thing to do

Appropriate but not ideal

Inappropriate but not awful

A very inappropriate thing to do

A GP accidentally leaves their intercom on whilst a consultation is in progress. The whole waiting room hears what the GP says, and some of the patient's responses as well. The next patient tells the GP what happened when they enter the consultation room.

How appropriate are the following responses by the GP in this situation?

9. The GP looks embarrassed and ensures the intercom is off and reassures them that their consultation won't be overheard.

A very appropriate thing to do

Appropriate but not ideal

Inappropriate but not awful

A very inappropriate thing to do

10. The GP immediately leaves the room to tell the Practice Manager to arrange to send a letter of apology to the patient concerned

A very appropriate thing to do

Appropriate but not ideal

Inappropriate but not awful

A very inappropriate thing to do

11. The GP laughs and says, "It's a good job it wasn't a sexual health matter!"

A very appropriate thing to do

Appropriate but not ideal

Inappropriate but not awful

A very inappropriate thing to do

12. The GP apologises and jokes that he is "too old and stupid" for modern technology

A very appropriate thing to do

Appropriate but not ideal

Inappropriate but not awful

A very inappropriate thing to do

A medical student is sitting in on a clinic at the hospital. When a patient comes in he realises that he went to school with her. She seems not to recognise him and has consented to a student sitting in on her appointment.

How appropriate are the following responses by the medical student?

13. The medical student halts the consultation and asks if the patient remembers him and is still happy for him to sit in on the consultation.

A very appropriate thing to do

Appropriate but not ideal

Inappropriate but not awful

A very inappropriate thing to do

14. The medical student decides that as they weren't good friends, and she doesn't seem to recognise him then he'll let the consultation carry on without interrupting.

A very appropriate thing to do

Appropriate but not ideal

Inappropriate but not awful

A very inappropriate thing to do

15. The medical student can't think what to do so pretends to feel suddenly ill and leaves the room.

A very appropriate thing to do

Appropriate but not ideal

Inappropriate but not awful

A very inappropriate thing to do

16. The medical student halts the consultation and explains the situation to the doctor.

A very appropriate thing to do

Appropriate but not ideal

Inappropriate but not awful

A very inappropriate thing to do

A medical student visits their GP, who has been the family doctor for their entire life, about a GUM matter. The student, who has been learning about procedures regarding chaperones, notices that their GP doesn't follow those procedures when examining them. The medical student is personally unconcerned given the history between the GP and patient.

How appropriate are the following responses by the medical student?

17. The medical student assumes that the GP usually follows correct procedures but, like them, considers it less necessary when there is a long-standing relationship between doctor and patient.

A very appropriate thing to do

Appropriate but not ideal

Inappropriate but not awful

A very inappropriate thing to do

18. The medical student reports the matter to the Practice Manager emphasising that whilst they were not concerned, they wished to ensure that procedures were usually followed.

A very appropriate thing to do

Appropriate but not ideal

Inappropriate but not awful

A very inappropriate thing to do

19. The medical student uses the incident as an example of 'bad practice' in his assignment on the matter.

A very appropriate thing to do

Appropriate but not ideal

Inappropriate but not awful

A very inappropriate thing to do

20. The student asks a friend, also a patient at the surgery, to go in with a fake complaint to see if proper procedures are followed.

A very appropriate thing to do

Appropriate but not ideal

Inappropriate but not awful

A very inappropriate thing to do

A medical student is feeling very under pressure and stressed by the number of assignments, and the placements, she must do and is concerned that her health is in danger. She shared her concerns with a friend who told her she'd have to get used to pressure if she was going to be a doctor and advised her to try harder and just 'push through it', also suggesting that the tutors would think poorly of her if she admitted that she was struggling.

How appropriate are the following responses by the medical student?

21. The medical student decides her friend's advice is sound and tries to ignore her symptoms and get everything done.

A very appropriate thing to do

Appropriate but not ideal

Inappropriate but not awful

A very inappropriate thing to do

22. The medical student voices her concerns to her tutor and asks for advice on managing her time

A very appropriate thing to do

Appropriate but not ideal

Inappropriate but not awful

A very inappropriate thing to do

23. The medical student decides she is not cut out for a high-pressure career as a doctor and leaves the course.

A very appropriate thing to do

Appropriate but not ideal

Inappropriate but not awful

A very inappropriate thing to do

24. The medical student spends a day devising a tight schedule, identifying inefficient use of time and prioritising her work load.

A very appropriate thing to do

Appropriate but not ideal

Inappropriate but not awful

A very inappropriate thing to do

A newly qualified doctor has a formal complaint made against him by a patient who claims he was rude and prejudiced during a consultation. The hospital assured the doctor that it is unlikely the complaint will be taken further as the patient is a 'serial complainer' and there is little evidence that what the patient claimed was actually said. The doctor concerned is however, quite upset and shaken.

How appropriate are the following responses by the newly qualified doctor?

25. The doctor insists on having a third person in his consultations from now on.

A very appropriate thing to do

Appropriate but not ideal

Inappropriate but not awful

A very inappropriate thing to do

26. The doctor asks for counselling and a debrief from the hospital complaints department to help him move on.

A very appropriate thing to do

Appropriate but not ideal

Inappropriate but not awful

A very inappropriate thing to do

27. The doctor insists on a transfer to a job where no private consultations are required.

A very appropriate thing to do

Appropriate but not ideal

Inappropriate but not awful

A very inappropriate thing to do

28. The doctor seeks out other victims of the serial complainer to find out what happened to them.

A very appropriate thing to do

Appropriate but not ideal

Inappropriate but not awful

A very inappropriate thing to do

A phlebotomist trips whilst carrying a tray of blood samples. Several of the vials smash and blood splashes on to the footwear of two admin staff members who are nearby.

How important is it to consider the following?

29. The lost blood samples and the need to ensure that patients are informed; and new samples are taken

Very important

Important

Of minor importance

Not important

30. The need to treat / assess admin staff for blood borne diseases

Very important

Important

Of minor importance

Not important

31. Safe and appropriate clearing up of smashed glass and organic material

Very important

Important

Of minor importance

Not important

32. Any trip hazards in the path of the phlebotomist which might have contributed to the fall.

Very important

Important

Of minor importance

Not important

A medical student is on placement in a pregnancy advice unit. As she looks down the patient list she notices that her 15-year-old sister is coming in for a termination of pregnancy. The medical student was not aware that her sister was even sexually active and is sure that their parents do not know.

How important is it to consider the following?

33. The patient has a right to confidentiality

Very important

Important

Of minor importance

Not important

34. The student doesn't think a 15-year-old should have an abortion without her parents knowing

Very important

Important

Of minor importance

Not important

35. The patient has clearly had inadequate sex education at school.

Very important

Important

Of minor importance

Not important

36. The student is sure her parents would want the patient to receive more counselling before the procedure takes place

Very important

Important

Of minor importance

Not important

37. The medical student disapproves of her sister's behaviour and actions

Very important

Important

Of minor importance

Not important

38. The patient is likely to feel uneasy if she sees her sister

Very important

Important

Of minor importance

Not important

A medical student, who is a fluent Polish speaker, is on placement in A&E. An urgent case comes in and the patient, a Polish man, requires immediate surgery. He is conscious, and a senior doctor asks the med student to 'consent him'.

How important is it to consider the following?

39. A Polish man may not qualify for NHS treatment

Very important

Important

Of minor importance

Not important

40. Just because someone is Polish doesn't mean he cannot speak or understand English

Very important

Important

Of minor importance

Not important

41. Consent gained by a med student may not be sufficient

Very important

Important

Of minor importance

Not important

42. The surgery is urgent

Very important

Important

Of minor importance

Not important

A medical student receives a 'friend request' on Facebook from a patient who they met on a recent placement.

How important is it to consider the following?

43. The medical student liked the patient in question

Very important

Important

Of minor importance

Not important

44. The doctor patient relationship requires a certain amount of professional distance

Very important

Important

Of minor importance

Not important

45. The treatment is now finished and there is no longer a doctor / patient relationship ongoing

Very important

Important

Of minor importance

Not important

46. Facebook isn't the same as a normal friendship as filters and permissions can be applied to protect privacy

Very important

Important

Of minor importance

Not important

A newly qualified doctor finds that the child he is treating on an oncology ward is the nephew of a famous footballer and his film actress wife. The couple come to visit and offer to donate signed merchandise to the ward which can be raffled or auctioned.

How important is it to consider the following?

47. The hospital could always do with extra funding and equipment

Very important

Important

Of minor importance

Not important

48. Organising a raffle or auction may use up valuable staff time

Very important

Important

Of minor importance

Not important

49. Accepting the gift shouldn't lead to preferential treatment for the patient

Very important

Important

Of minor importance

Not important

50. The wealthy celebrities should consider paying for private medical care for their relative and free up NHS resources

Very important

Important

Of minor importance

Not important

51. The child's parents should be involved in any decision about the donation.

Very important

Important

Of minor importance

Not important

52. The associated publicity will need to be well managed

Very important

Important

Of minor importance

Not important

An admin staff worker makes an error and the wrong test results and letters are inadvertently sent to about 20 patients. Some of the results were sensitive and were about serious illnesses.

How important is it to consider the following?

53. It is unlikely that the patients will know the intended recipient of the letter

Very important

Important

Of minor importance

Not important

54. Admin staff are underpaid

Very important

Important

Of minor importance

Not important

55. Patients should be able to trust the medical profession with their confidential details and deserve an apology

Very important

Important

Of minor importance

Not important

56. The admin worker was probably stressed and over worked

Very important

Important

Of minor importance

Not important

A medical student is practising taking blood pressure measurements on one of his friends and finds that his friend's blood pressure is incredibly inconsistent over the twenty measurements made in an hour.

How important is it to consider the following?

57. The friend may be seriously ill and should seek urgent medical attention

Very important

Important

Of minor importance

Not important

58. Practice makes perfect

Very important

Important

Of minor importance

Not important

59. The medical student is new to this procedure

Very important

Important

Of minor importance

Not important

60. Blood pressure readings are usually taken by nurses

Very important

Important

Of minor importance

Not important

A medical student realises that the information given by one of his lecturers is out of date when he compares it both to his up-to-date textbook and online resources. The old information has been shown to be harmful to patients in some instances.

How important is it to consider the following?

61. Even up-to-date advice becomes obsolete eventually

Very important

Important

Of minor importance

Not important

62. The lecturer may not have practiced medicine for many years but should make an effort to stay current

Very important

Important

Of minor importance

Not important

63. The lecturer's errors should be brought to their attention

Very important

Important

Of minor importance

Not important

64. The lecturer may be angry if his errors are pointed out

Very important

Important

Of minor importance

Not important

65. The incorrect information could be harmful if applied

Very important

Important

Of minor importance

Not important

A medical student is at a social occasion when a friend of a friend engages him in conversation about a series of health worries she has. Although each symptom described is minor, when taken as a whole the med student is concerned that they could indicate a serious condition which he learned about that week in lectures.

How important is it to consider the following?

66. This individual could be seriously ill.

Very important

Important

Of minor importance

Not important

67. The med student is uncertain about the condition they're thinking of

Very important

Important

Of minor importance

Not important

68. The symptoms being suffered by this person are only minor

Very important

Important

Of minor importance

Not important

69. Whether it is impolite for an individual to speak of their health at a social occasion

Very important

Important

Of minor importance

Not important

A doctor on a medical ward diagnoses the same rare condition twice in one day on patients in adjoining bays on the same ward. The condition only occurs in about one in 1,000,000 people so to find two people on the same day in the same place with it is very noteworthy and may mean that prevalence is increasing.

How appropriate are the following responses?

70. Tell the patients concerned as they may wish to keep in touch with one another given the unusual nature of their condition

A very appropriate thing to do

Appropriate but not ideal

Inappropriate but not awful

A very inappropriate thing to do

71. Write a paper about the case for a medical journal

A very appropriate thing to do

Appropriate but not ideal

Inappropriate but not awful

A very inappropriate thing to do

72. Ask the patients if they wish to be put in touch with other people with the condition and, depending on their answers, introduce them.

A very appropriate thing to do

Appropriate but not ideal

Inappropriate but not awful

A very inappropriate thing to do

73. Post about it on Facebook and Twitter given how unusual and exciting it is

A very appropriate thing to do

Appropriate but not ideal

Inappropriate but not awful

A very inappropriate thing to do

A newly qualified doctor is working in A&E. Every Friday and Saturday evening the unit is filled with intoxicated people and one man has been in 14 times in the last 8 weeks. On the next Friday night he attends again, once more drunk and with facial bruising. He claims a policeman punched him.

How appropriate are the following responses?

74. Investigate procedures for reporting abuses by the police

A very appropriate thing to do

Appropriate but not ideal

Inappropriate but not awful

A very inappropriate thing to do

75. Privately think that the man probably deserved it and don't even note his accusation

A very appropriate thing to do

Appropriate but not ideal

Inappropriate but not awful

A very inappropriate thing to do

76. Note the accusation but state alongside the note that they don't believe the man

A very appropriate thing to do

Appropriate but not ideal

Inappropriate but not awful

A very inappropriate thing to do

77. Treat any injuries and report the accusation to a senior member of staff

A very appropriate thing to do

Appropriate but not ideal

Inappropriate but not awful

A very inappropriate thing to do

Lewis is studying dentistry. Another student on his course, Frankie, asks to speak to him after lectures. Frankie confides that she is really struggling with the workload, is worried no-one else likes her and is having second thoughts about her career choice.

How appropriate are the following actions for Lewis?

78. Offer to help Frankie with her workload

A very appropriate thing to do

Appropriate but not ideal

Inappropriate but not awful

A very inappropriate thing to do

79. Offer to lend Frankie his lecture notes

A very appropriate thing to do

Appropriate but not ideal

Inappropriate but not awful

A very inappropriate thing to do

80. Invite Frankie to join his study group

A very appropriate thing to do

Appropriate but not ideal

Inappropriate but not awful

A very inappropriate thing to do

81. Reassure Frankie that it's normal to feel overwhelmed by university

A very appropriate thing to do

Appropriate but not ideal

Inappropriate but not awful

A very inappropriate thing to do

82. Suggest Frankie speak to her academic supervisor about how she feels

A very appropriate thing to do

Appropriate but not ideal

Inappropriate but not awful

A very inappropriate thing to do

83. Tell Frankie that dentistry is very demanding as a career and she should consider other options if she doesn't feel as though she is coping

A very appropriate thing to do

Appropriate but not ideal

Inappropriate but not awful

A very inappropriate thing to do

Julie is studying medicine. She is browsing the internet reading a blog written by a junior doctor. She is able to identify the author as John, an F1 working on the ward where she completed work experience last summer, because of a number of identifying details about patients.

How appropriate are the following actions for Julie?

84. Report John's blog to the senior consultant on the ward where she completed her placement.

A very appropriate thing to do

Appropriate but not ideal

Inappropriate but not awful

A very inappropriate thing to do

85. Report her concerns about the blog to her academic supervisor.

A very appropriate thing to do

Appropriate but not ideal

Inappropriate but not awful

A very inappropriate thing to do

86. Report the blog to the GMC

A very appropriate thing to do

Appropriate but not ideal

Inappropriate but not awful

A very inappropriate thing to do

87. Contact John via Facebook to explain her concerns about patient confidentiality

A very appropriate thing to do

Appropriate but not ideal

Inappropriate but not awful

A very inappropriate thing to do

Elvira, an Albanian immigrant, has just embarked on a medical degree in a UK university. Her English is very good, but she is finding that the speed of lectures and the complexity of academic text books is more taxing than she imagined. She thinks her fellow students are getting frustrated with her not understanding things quickly and with her accent.

How appropriate are the following course of action?

88. Elvira should sign up for extra English coaching to bring her skills up a level

A very appropriate thing to do

Appropriate but not ideal

Inappropriate but not awful

A very inappropriate thing to do

89. Elvira should ask fellow students for copies of their lecture notes so she can catch up on the bits she didn't understand

A very appropriate thing to do

Appropriate but not ideal

Inappropriate but not awful

A very inappropriate thing to do

90. Elvira should ask the lecturers to speak more slowly

A very appropriate thing to do

Appropriate but not ideal

Inappropriate but not awful

A very inappropriate thing to do

91. Elvira should defer her place and start again next year when her English is better

A very appropriate thing to do

Appropriate but not ideal

Inappropriate but not awful

A very inappropriate thing to do

92. Elvira should look for elocution lessons to make her accent less pronounced

A very appropriate thing to do

Appropriate but not ideal

Inappropriate but not awful

A very inappropriate thing to do

Stephanie and Michael met at medical school, began a relationship and are about to qualify. They are filling in their application forms for the FY1 year. Stephanie wants to remain in the city where they studied but Michael wants to apply to more prestigious hospitals in the area where his family live and where he eventually wants to settle.

How important is it for Stephanie to consider:

93. Michael has already lived for 5 years away from his family and if they want to be together she should compromise

Very important

Important

Of minor importance

Not important

94. She is not confident she would get a job at a prestigious hospital as her grades are not as high as Michael's.

Very important

Important

Of minor importance

Not important

How important is it for Michael to consider:

95. Even if the couple fill in their forms identically there is no guarantee that they'll end up living and working in the same area.

Very important

Important

Of minor importance

Not important

96. If the couple end up marrying and having a family then his career will most likely be the main one

Very important

Important

Of minor importance

Not important

Alastair has just started studying dentistry. He has always felt very pressured to become a dentist because his father, Iain, is a dentist. Early in the course he realises that he has no enthusiasm for the subject and wants to leave the course. He telephones his Dad to discuss it.

How important is it for Alastair to consider:

97. He has already demonstrated he has the ability to follow this career as he has gained a place on a competitive course

Very important

Important

Of minor importance

Not important

98. Dentistry is a good career and, in the absence of other ideas, it is worth persevering with it

Very important

Important

Of minor importance

Not important

99. Not wanting to disappoint his father

Very important

Important

Of minor importance

Not important

100. Most children don't follow the professional path of their parents

Very important

Important

Of minor importance

Not important

100 Situational Judgement Question Answers

1. A very appropriate thing to do – 2 points (1 point for Appropriate but not ideal)
It is appropriate to check the veracity of the caller's claims by looking at the patient's file.

2. Inappropriate but not awful – 2 points (1 point for Appropriate but not ideal or A very inappropriate thing to do)
This inconveniences both the hospital doctor and the GP but doesn't risk compromising the patient's confidentiality.

3. A very inappropriate thing to do – 2 points (1 point for Inappropriate but not awful)
She should make every effort to confirm the identity of the hospital doctor before disclosing any information.

4. A very appropriate thing to do – 2 points (1 point for Appropriate but not ideal)
This way the receptionist protects the confidentiality of the patient and buys herself some time to check that the patient has, in fact, got an appointment with the doctor on the telephone. One serious flaw in the plan, however, is that if the hospital computer system is down it is also possible that the doctor would not be able to email - at least not from their official hospital account.

5. A very inappropriate thing to do – 2 points (1 point for Inappropriate but not awful)
Although the motivation of protecting the other patients is noble it simply isn't fair to give preferential treatment to someone just because they're making a noise

6. Appropriate but not ideal – 2 points (1 point for A very appropriate thing to do or Inappropriate but not awful)
This is a good thing to do - but is not a good use of the doctor's time

7. A very appropriate thing to do – 2 points (1 point for Appropriate but not ideal)
This is a good response as it doesn't waste the junior doctor's time but takes the complaint seriously

8. Appropriate but not ideal – 2 points (1 point for A very appropriate thing to do or Inappropriate but not awful)

An apology is always appropriate and sadly, the presence of security is often necessary when people get agitated. However - there are other, better, things to do to try and calm the situation which could have also been done.

9. A very appropriate thing to do – 2 points (1 point for Appropriate but not ideal)
The GP certainly needs to ensure it won't happen again but reassuring the following patients is as much as they can do at that time.

10. Appropriate but not ideal – 2 points (1 point for A very appropriate thing to do or Inappropriate but not awful)
Although this is undoubtedly a good thing to do it could be done later, after the surgery is finished

11. A very inappropriate thing to do – 2 points (1 point for Inappropriate but not awful)
This breach of confidentiality is no laughing matter, regardless of the content of the consultation

12. Inappropriate but not awful – 2 points (1 point for Appropriate but not ideal or A very inappropriate thing to do)
Although an apology is entirely appropriate it may make a patient, who traditionally has a great deal of faith in the intelligence of their doctor, nervous to hear something so self-deprecating.

13. A very appropriate thing to do – 2 points (1 point for Appropriate but not ideal)
It is possible that a person who has previously consented to a medical student may feel differently if that student knows them personally.

14. Inappropriate but not awful – 2 points (1 point for Appropriate but not ideal or A very inappropriate thing to do)
The patient should really be given any 'new' information which pertains to consent.

15. A very inappropriate thing to do – 2 points (1 point for Inappropriate but not awful)
Whilst this gets him out of the situation it is also dishonest and means they miss out on a learning opportunity - either to see the consultation happen or to learn about the appropriate response to this situation.

16. Appropriate but not ideal – 2 points (1 point for A very appropriate thing to do or Inappropriate but not awful)
Although the key issue about the patient's confidentiality is addressed here it is rather rude for the med student to speak about the situation to the doctor and not to the patient, who is sitting in the room.

17. Inappropriate but not awful – 2 points (1 point for Appropriate but not ideal or A very inappropriate thing to do)
It is important that such procedures are followed, even when the parties involved don't deem them necessary. An assumption that 'things are usually OK' is unfounded and potentially dangerous.

18. Appropriate but not ideal – 2 points (1 point for A very appropriate thing to do or Inappropriate but not awful)
The student may wish to avoid embarrassing the GP and this is a way that they can ensure that no further action needs to be taken (or otherwise) without doing so.

19. Appropriate but not ideal – 2 points (1 point for A very appropriate thing to do or Inappropriate but not awful)
Using personal examples (especially if the parties are named, or traceable) in assignments can be problematic. However, if the example is carefully used it could lead to an interesting and informative discussion.

20. A very inappropriate thing to do – 2 points (1 point for Inappropriate but not awful)
This is a waste of the doctor's time, the friend's time and NHS resources.

21. Inappropriate but not awful – 2 points (1 point for Appropriate but not ideal or A very inappropriate thing to do)
Compromising one's own health for a course doesn't do anyone any favours but this course of action does, at least, show a degree of tenacity and determination.

22. A very appropriate thing to do – 2 points (1 point for Appropriate but not ideal)
A tutor will be concerned for the health and academic progress of a student and is almost certainly experienced in helping students deal with pressure and stress.

23. A very inappropriate thing to do – 2 points (1 point for Inappropriate but not awful)
This is a very poor course of action. Learning to deal with pressure and stress is as much a part of medical training as any other.

24. A very appropriate thing to do – 2 points (1 point for Appropriate but not ideal)
Good time management is a skill which needs to be learned by anyone wishing a demanding career such as medicine. Good self-discipline and time management can often alleviate stress and pressure.

25. Inappropriate but not awful – 2 points (1 point for Appropriate but not ideal or A very inappropriate thing to do)
This could be a waste of hospital resources and manpower, but not so much as the loss of a trained doctor

26. A very appropriate thing to do – 2 points (1 point for Appropriate but not ideal)
This is a good course of action and will enable the doctor to ask questions about his permanent record and good ways to avoid similar incidents in the future.

27. A very inappropriate thing to do – 2 points (1 point for Inappropriate but not awful)
The majority of doctors have to spend some time alone with their patients. It is unrealistic to expect a job where this won't happen.

28. Inappropriate but not awful – 2 points (1 point for Appropriate but not ideal or A very inappropriate thing to do)
This course of action may be understandable and provide reassurance for the doctor but does call his professional integrity into mind as it is likely the patient's confidentiality is at stake.

29. Very important – 2 points (1 point for Important)
Blood tests are always taken for a reason and whilst a re-test may be inconvenient for patients and staff it is imperative that, where the situation hasn't changed medically, the same tests are taken to gain the same information.

30. Of minor importance – 2 points (1 point for Important or Not important)
Serious blood borne disease such as HIV or hepatitis are unlikely to be an issue in this scenario given that the staff are wearing footwear.

31. Very important – 2 points (1 point for Important)
Shards of glass can be very dangerous (especially when they are covered in unknown blood) and proper procedures should be followed when cleaning it up.

32. Important – 2 points (1 point for Very important or Of minor importance)
Trips sometimes just happen, but sometimes can be prevented or the risk minimised. It is always worth checking if this is an avoidable risk.

33. Very important – 2 points (1 point for Important)

The patient's right to confidentiality is of primary importance in medicine. In this situation the confidentiality is coincidentally compromised but regardless of her personal feelings the medical student must maintain her sister's confidentiality.

34. Not important – 2 points (1 point for Of minor importance)
The procedure has been arranged and other, qualified, professionals must have assessed the patient and decided she was old enough to give proper consent. There is a legal framework to refer to and personal opinions cannot influence their application.

35. Of minor importance – 2 points (1 point for Important or Not important)
An unwanted pregnancy does indicate that something went wrong. It may be worth investigating if the patient needs family planning or sexual health information for the future, but this may not be due to a lack of education from school.

36. Not important – 2 points (1 point for Of minor importance)
The fact that it says 'more counselling' indicates that counselling has been offered / given before an appointment was made and the clinician and patient's judgement as to the need for counselling is the overriding one in this instance
37. Not important – 2 points (1 point for Of minor importance)
Personal ethical opinions cannot be imposed on patients and disapproval should not even be implied

38. Important – 2 points (1 point for Very important or Of minor importance)
However much the med student assures her sister that her conduct is professional it is likely that the patient wished to keep this procedure away from the whole family including her sister. Advice about how to proceed should be sought.

39. Not important – 2 points (1 point for Of minor importance)
An urgently ill patient always receives treatment. Other details can be sorted out afterwards

40. Of minor importance – 2 points (1 point for Important or Not important)
Gaining consent in the usual way with an English speaker may be more straightforward but the issue is gaining the consent and who it is appropriate to ask to do this.

41. Very important – 2 points (1 point for Important)
Proper and valid consent is of primary importance and senior medical professionals should ensure that it is properly gained.

42. Very important – 2 points (1 point for Important)
In urgent cases the immediate wellbeing of the patient is always considered first.

43. Not important – 2 points (1 point for Of minor importance)
When it comes to being a professional then the amount you like (or otherwise!) a patient should have no bearing on your professionalism (i.e. no preferential treatment, no bending of rules etc)

44. Very important – 2 points (1 point for Important)
The doctor patient relationship requires a certain amount of professional distance

45. Important – 2 points (1 point for Very important or Of minor importance)
The student is still obliged to behave in a way that is professional and consider the appropriateness of a friendship is which may still be affected by the former doctor patient relationship.

46. Of minor importance – 2 points (1 point for Important or Not important)
Facebook isn't the same as a normal friendship as filters and permissions can be applied to protect privacy.

47. Important – 2 points (1 point for Very important or Of minor importance)
Hospitals do benefit from private and charitable donations. A significant offer should usually be considered.

48. Important – 2 points (1 point for Very important or Of minor importance)
It is important to ensure that any benefit to the hospital is not outweighed by the workload in organising an event or similar

49. Very important – 2 points (1 point for Important)
Any donation which comes 'with strings' attached must be very carefully weighed. Preferential treatment for any patient on anything but clinical grounds is totally unacceptable.

50. Not important – 2 points (1 point for Of minor importance)
A wealthy person, and their relatives, are entitled to NHS care and if they make that choice it shouldn't be questioned.

51. Of minor importance – 2 points (1 point for Important or Not important)
The connection may be the child, but subsequent arrangements would be between the couple and the hospital. However - it is possible, even likely, that their child may feature in subsequent publicity and information in which case the parents should be consulted.

52. Important – 2 points (1 point for Very important or Of minor importance)
Publicity for the couple, the hospital and, potentially, the young patient can be good or bad. It is naive to assume it will need no attention or management.

53. Of minor importance – 2 points (1 point for Important or Not important)
A breach of confidentiality is a serious event regardless of whether people find out about their neighbours. A proper investigation needs doing even if 'no harm is done'

54. Not important – 2 points (1 point for Of minor importance)
Whether this is true or not is irrelevant. Sending out the wrong letters is an error regardless of salary levels

55. Very important – 2 points (1 point for Important)
The doctor patient relationship is founded on trust. When the medical profession gets it wrong - even by association (i.e. an admin worker) an appropriate apology is due.

56. Important – 2 points (1 point for Very important or Of minor importance)
When an error like this occurs, it is important to consider why it happened. It may turn out that the error had nothing to do with stress or overwork, but the question needs to be asked.

57. Of minor importance – 2 points (1 point for Important or Not important)
In the absence of other symptoms, it is unlikely that urgent attention would be required and there are more plausible explanations about the inconsistent readings rather than a serious ill health issue.

58. Very important – 2 points (1 point for Important)
Any new skill needs to be practised many times until the person becomes competent. Taking a blood pressure reading is no exception.

59. Very important – 2 points (1 point for Important)
It is likely that the inconsistent readings are more to do with his inexperience than any illness in his friend

60. Not important – 2 points (1 point for Of minor importance)
A doctor needs to be able to accurately and consistently perform routine observations

61. Not important – 2 points (1 point for Of minor importance)
Whilst this is true it is important to apply current knowledge and practice whilst it is still current.

62. Very important – 2 points (1 point for Important)
It is imperative that students are taught up to date material

63. Important – 2 points (1 point for Very important or Of minor importance)
There may be good and bad ways to do this, but substandard teaching should not be allowed to continue unchecked

64. Not important – 2 points (1 point for Of minor importance)
Nobody enjoys being corrected; or angering someone by correcting them but in this instance, there is a higher principle at stake.

65. Very important – 2 points (1 point for Important)
As there is potential for harm to patients this is the most important consideration. Any scenario where there could be harm requires that patient safety be the most important consideration.

66. Very important – 2 points (1 point for Important)
There is every chance the individual is not seriously ill but if there is a credible possibility then the med student should, at least, recommend they see a doctor.

67. Important – 2 points (1 point for Very important or Of minor importance)
The uncertainty the student is feeling is important. They are only a student and this condition may need tests and investigations to confirm. The student should be careful to express anything they say and with this in mind use terms like 'it could be' or 'there is a possibility' rather than implying they're certain the person is well or otherwise.

68. Not important – 2 points (1 point for Of minor importance)
Lots of serious illnesses present with nonspecific and minor symptoms

69. Not important – 2 points (1 point for Of minor importance)
People speak about all sorts of things at social occasions.

70. A very inappropriate thing to do – 2 points (1 point for Inappropriate but not awful)
Although an event like this may seem exciting and noteworthy to doctors it is still the condition of the individual patients who may wish to preserve their confidentiality concerning the matter. The word 'tell' implies that confidentiality regarding 'the patient in the next bay' has already been breached and is rather 'bossy'.

71. A very appropriate thing to do – 2 points (1 point for Appropriate but not ideal)
If confidentiality is properly protected, then this is an excellent thing to do. The medical profession needs ongoing research and data to continue to improve.

72. A very appropriate thing to do – 2 points (1 point for Appropriate but not ideal)
It would be possible to ask the patients independently if they would like to be in touch with other people with the same condition. If both agreed, then mutual support could be a great value to both of them.

73. A very inappropriate thing to do – 2 points (1 point for Inappropriate but not awful)
It is very difficult, if not impossible, to protect confidentiality in Social Media. Sharing any details, regardless of how scant, would be most unprofessional. Additionally - there is no benefit to the medical community in such an act making the risk even less worthwhile.

74. Appropriate but not ideal – 2 points (1 point for A very appropriate thing to do or Inappropriate but not awful)
The issue here is with the exact wording of the question. Whilst it may be appropriate to investigate the man's claims further it may be prudent to report an 'incident' rather than an 'abuse'.

75. A very inappropriate thing to do – 2 points (1 point for Inappropriate but not awful)
Whilst the private thoughts of a doctor are private, in the interests of good patient care it is sensible for doctors to aim to be as non-judgemental as possible so any 'thoughts' like this do not compromise patient care.

76. Inappropriate but not awful – 2 points (1 point for Appropriate but not ideal or A very inappropriate thing to do)
The doctor's suspicion may be judgemental and inappropriate, but it is understandable. If the doctor has good reason to suspect the accusation being made is spurious then their opinion may help the policeman in question to avoid unnecessary sanctions.

77. A very appropriate thing to do – 2 points (1 point for Appropriate but not ideal)
This is a very sensible option. Patient care is put at the forefront, and a more senior member of staff who has more experience and a wider remit can look into the accusation.

78. Appropriate but not ideal – 2 points (1 point for A very appropriate thing to do or Inappropriate but not awful)
Although this is kind, it is not a good long-term solution. It will not help Frankie to cope better if she is relying on Lewis and Lewis' own work may suffer if he is helping Frankie.

79. A very appropriate thing to do – 2 points (1 point for Appropriate but not ideal)
Depending on their quality, Frankie may benefit from reading Lewis' lecture notes.

80. A very appropriate thing to do – 2 points (1 point for Appropriate but not ideal)
This is very appropriate as it addresses not only Frankie's difficulty with the workload, but it also gives her the opportunity to make friends with other students. This is likely to boost her confidence in her abilities and her career choice.

81. A very appropriate thing to do – 2 points (1 point for Appropriate but not ideal)
Although no practical solutions are offered, this addresses the emotional aspect of the situation and would provide some comfort to Frankie that there's nothing wrong with struggling or feeling low.

82. A very appropriate thing to do – 2 points (1 point for Appropriate but not ideal)
This is appropriate, the academic supervisor is well placed to support students and encourage them to achieve their full potential as well as exploring other options if Frankie decides she no longer wishes to pursue dentistry as a career.

83. A very inappropriate thing to do – 2 points (1 point for Inappropriate but not awful)
This is very inappropriate as it will make Frankie feel worse and could lead a promising student to drop out of university.

84. Inappropriate but not awful – 2 points (1 point for Appropriate but not ideal or A very inappropriate thing to do)
Julie no longer works on the ward concerned and would have to make a special visit to speak to John's boss. This seems an extreme course of action, although clearly some action needs to be taken.

85. A very appropriate thing to do – 2 points (1 point for Appropriate but not ideal)

This would be a very appropriate response. As a med student Julie may not be fully conversant with what classifies as an 'identifying' component. If she discusses the situation with someone with more experience and knowledge than her then the way forward may become clear.

86. A very inappropriate thing to do – 2 points (1 point for Inappropriate but not awful)
This is an extreme course of action and may unnecessarily jeopardise John's career

87. Inappropriate but not awful – 2 points (1 point for Appropriate but not ideal or A very inappropriate thing to do)
Although speaking to the person involved in a situation/issue is usually the best course of action. There are two reasons why this option is not appropriate. Firstly, Julie does not have an ongoing professional or personal relationship with John meaning that she should report the issue to someone with whom she does have a professional relationship. Secondly, Facebook is too informal a platform to raise an issue as serious as breaching patient confidentiality.

88. A very appropriate thing to do – 2 points (1 point for Appropriate but not ideal)
If Elvira is struggling to understand and keep up, then this is a great option. With practice and study, it is likely that she will quickly be able to improve her English.

89. Appropriate but not ideal – 2 points (1 point for A very appropriate thing to do or Inappropriate but not awful)
The scenario states that Elvira's fellow students are already frustrated with her and being asked to supply notes may compound that feeling. However - in the short term it may enable Elvira to keep up.

90. A very inappropriate thing to do – 2 points (1 point for Inappropriate but not awful)
There will be dozens, if not hundreds, of students in each lecture and a limited time period in which to fit in a large amount of information. Asking the lecturer to speak slowly is effectively asking them to teach less and thus compromising the learning of all the other students.

91. A very inappropriate thing to do – 2 points (1 point for Inappropriate but not awful)
This is a very extreme course of action to take so soon into a medical degree. If all students decided to defer / leave at the first hurdle we would have no doctors!

92. Inappropriate but not awful – 2 points (1 point for Appropriate but not ideal or A very inappropriate thing to do)
Being understood is a key part of interacting with patients and if Elvira's accent would make it hard for patients to understand her then finding ways of minimising it would be good. However - the scenario only states that her fellow students are frustrated with her accent - among other things. It may not be as difficult to understand as she has assumed. Seeking advice about this first would be valuable for her.

93. Of minor importance – 2 points (1 point for Important or Not important)
If the couple want to remain (geographically) together then one of them will have to compromise. However - it cannot be assumed that this should be Stephanie's role; and proximity to family, though important and nice for Michael, should not be the defining factor which makes Stephanie's career choices.

94. Important – 2 points (1 point for Very important or Of minor importance)
You must fill in your application for anything carefully - considering your own strengths and weaknesses. An unrealistic application is often a waste of time, and space on your form. However - aiming high is also an admirable course.

95. Very important – 2 points (1 point for Important)
If either of them compromises their own career plans to be together it may backfire. They both may end up in jobs they didn't really want and still not be in the same place.

96. Not important – 2 points (1 point for Of minor importance)
This may be true, but it shouldn't enter Michael's deliberations unless the couple are discussing and agreeing it together. The assumption is outdated and sexist.

97. Very important – 2 points (1 point for Important)
Alastair, and Iain, should be proud of achievement of simply gaining a place. If Alastair chooses not to pursue the career it would not be because he wasn't capable of it.

98. Of minor importance – 2 points (1 point for Important or Not important)
Although dentistry is a good career it is not the only career. Continuing in a career path which you don't think you want to pursue is unlikely to lead to personal satisfaction.

99. Not important – 2 points (1 point for Of minor importance)
Naturally no-one wants to disappoint their parents but when it comes to something as significant as a career choice, but such concerns must not prevent appropriate action.

100. Very important – 2 points (1 point for Important)
Parents can unconsciously expect their children to emulate their professions but it's not that common for children to follow their parents.

Full Mock Test 1 **Verbal Reasoning (21 minutes for this section)**

Camera controls are interrelated. The total amount of light reaching the film plane (the 'exposure') changes with the duration of exposure, aperture of the lens, and on the effective focal length of the lens. Changing any of these controls can alter the exposure. Many cameras may be set to adjust most or all of these controls automatically.

The duration of an exposure is referred to as shutter speed and is typically measured in fractions of a second. It is quite possible to have exposures of several seconds, usually for still-life subjects, and for night scenes exposure times can be several hours.

The effective aperture is expressed by an f-number or f-stop (derived from focal ratio), which is proportional to the ratio of the focal length to the diameter of the aperture. Longer lenses will pass less light even though the diameter of the aperture is the same due to the greater distance the light has to travel: shorter lenses (a shorter focal length) will be brighter with the same size of aperture.

The smaller the f/number, the larger the effective aperture. The present system of f/numbers to give the effective aperture of a lens was standardised by an international convention. Older cameras use different number sequences.

If the f-number is decreased by a factor of the square-root of 2, the aperture diameter is increased by the same factor, and its area is increased by a factor of 2. The f-stops that might be found on a typical lens include 2.8, 4, 5.6, 8, 11, 16, 22, 32, where going up 'one stop' (using lower f-stop numbers) doubles the amount of light reaching the film.

1. According to the text, which of the following statements is true?

[redacted] A faster shutter speed allows more light to reach the film [redacted]
[redacted] A slower shutter speed gives a longer exposure
[redacted] A larger f-number increases the amount of light reaching the film
[redacted] A longer lens will allow more light to eventually reach the film

2. Effective aperture is measured by an f-number. Using the same lens, which of the following f-numbers would allow the least amount of light to reach the film?

[redacted] 2.8
[redacted] 4
[redacted] 8 [redacted]
[redacted] 16

3. To increase exposure you could employ these three things:

A. Slow shutter speed, long focal length, smaller f-number
B. Slow shutter speed, short focal length, smaller f-number
C. Fast shutter speed, short focal length, smaller f-number
D. Fast shutter speed, long focal length, larger f-number

4. All of the following statements are true except:

A. Film exposure is affected by effective aperture and shutter speed
B. The effective aperture is affected by the focal length and the lens aperture
C. Doubling the f-number halves the amount of light that reaches the film
D. Moving up one f-stop doubles the amount of light that reaches the film

A tropical cyclone is a storm system characterised by a low-pressure centre and numerous thunderstorms that produce strong winds and heavy rain. Tropical cyclones strengthen when water evaporated from the ocean is released as the saturated air rises, resulting in condensation of water vapour contained in the moist air. The characteristic that separates tropical cyclones from other cyclonic systems is that at any height in the atmosphere, the centre of a tropical cyclone will be warmer than its surroundings; a phenomenon called "warm core" storm systems.

The term "tropical" refers both to the geographical origin of storms and to their formation in maritime tropical air masses. While tropical cyclones can produce extremely powerful winds and torrential rain, they are also able to produce high waves and damaging storm surge as well as spawning tornadoes. They develop over large bodies of warm water, and lose their strength if they move over land due to increased surface friction and loss of the warm ocean as an energy source. This is why coastal regions can receive significant damage from a tropical cyclone, while inland regions are relatively safe from receiving strong winds. Heavy rains, however, can produce significant flooding inland, and storm surges can produce extensive coastal flooding up to 40 km from the coastline. Although effects on human populations can be devastating, tropical cyclones can relieve drought conditions. They also carry heat energy away from the tropics making them an important part of global atmospheric circulation.

5. All of the following statements are true except:

A. Cyclones form outside the tropics
B. The air outside a tropical cyclone is cooler than that inside the system
C. Cyclones form over land mass
D. Human populations can be devastated by the effects of tropical cyclones

6. According to the passage which of the following statements is true?

A. Tropical cyclones help to maintain a relatively stable and warm temperature worldwide
B. Tropical cyclones have a negative effect on the global climate
C. Coastal regions are fairly safe from the winds cause by tropical cyclones
D. The damage from cyclones is limited to coastal regions

7. A cyclone is formed when:

[redacted] Water from the ocean evaporates and the saturated air rises, heats up and is released as rain
[redacted] Water from the ocean evaporates; when this saturated air reaches the colder atmosphere, the water vapour condenses
[redacted] Water from the ocean condenses into the air as water vapour, and then is released as rain
[redacted] Water from the ocean condenses into the air and as this saturated air rises, cools down and releases water

8. According to the passage which of the following statements is true?

A. Only populations living on the coast should be on alert for tropical cyclones
B. Only populations living on the coast are affected by flood waters
C. Cyclones can cause devastation for many populations
D. There are no positive side-effects of cyclones

Bob Dylan (born Robert Allen Zimmerman; 24 May 1941) is an American singer-songwriter and musician. He has been a major figure in popular music for five decades. Much of his most celebrated work dates from the 1960s when he was at first an informal chronicler, and later an apparently reluctant figurehead of social unrest. A number of his songs such as 'Blowin' in the Wind' and 'The Times They Are a-Changin'' became anthems for the civil rights and anti-war movements.

His early lyrics incorporated a variety of political, social and philosophical, as well as literary influences. They defied existing pop music conventions and appealed hugely to the then burgeoning counterculture. Dylan has both amplified and personalised musical genres, exploring numerous distinct traditions in American song-from folk, blues and country to gospel, rock and roll and rockabilly, to English, Scottish and Irish folk music, embracing even jazz and swing.

Dylan performs with guitar, keyboard, and harmonica. Backed by a changing line-up of musicians, he has toured steadily since the late 1980s on what has been dubbed the Never Ending Tour. His accomplishments as a recording artist and performer have been central to his career, but his greatest contribution is generally considered to be his song writing.

9. Robert Zimmerman is a musician.
   A. True
   B. False
   C. Can't tell

10. Robert Zimmerman was born in 1951
   A. True
   B. False
   C. Can't tell

11. Bob Dylan only found popularity in his thirties.
   A. True
   B. False
   C. Can't tell

12. Bob Dylan was still touring in his fifties.
   A. True
   B. False
   C. Can't tell

x no mention of stopping

The Boeing B-17 Flying Fortress is a four-engine heavy bomber aircraft developed for the United States Army Air Corps (USAAC) and introduced in the 1930s. Competing against Douglas and Martin for a contract to build 200 bombers, the Boeing entry outperformed both competitors and more than met the Air Corps' expectations. Although Boeing lost the contract because the prototype crashed, the Air Corps was so impressed with Boeing's design that they ordered 13 B-17s. The B-17 Flying Fortress evolved through numerous design advancements.

The B-17 was primarily employed by the United States Army Air Forces (USAAF) in the daylight precision strategic bombing campaign of World War II against German industrial, civilian, and military targets. The United States Eighth Air Force based in England and the Fifteenth Air Force based in Italy complemented the RAF Bomber Command's night-time area bombing in Operation Pointblank to help secure air superiority over the cities, factories and battlefields of Western Europe in preparation for Operation Overlord. The B-17 also participated to a lesser extent in the Pacific War where it conducted raids against Japanese shipping and airfields.

13. The B-17 has four engines.
   A. True
   B. False
   C. Can't tell

14. The B-17s were built in the United States.
   A. True
   B. False
   C. Can't tell

15. Germany was bombed by the United States in World War I.
    A. True
    B. False
    C. Can't tell

16. The United States had airbases in England and Italy.
    A. True
    B. False
    C. Can't tell

Tuberculosis, MTB, or TB (short for tubercle bacillus), previously known as phthisis, phthisis pulmonalis, or consumption; is a common, often fatal, infectious disease caused by various strains of mycobacteria, usually Mycobacterium tuberculosis. Tuberculosis typically attacks the lungs, but can also affect other parts of the body. It is spread when people who have an active TB infection cough, sneeze, or otherwise transmit respiratory fluids through the air. Most infections do not have symptoms, known as latent tuberculosis. About one in ten latent infections eventually progresses to active disease which, if left untreated, kills more than 50% of those so infected.

The classic symptoms of active TB infection are a chronic cough with blood-tinged sputum, fever, night sweats, and weight loss (the latter giving rise to the formerly common term consumption). Infection of other organs causes a wide range of symptoms. Diagnosis of active TB relies on radiology (commonly chest X-rays), as well as microscopic examination and microbiological culture of body fluids. Diagnosis of latent TB relies on the tuberculin skin test (TST) and/or blood tests. Treatment is difficult and requires administration of multiple antibiotics over a long period of time. Social contacts are also screened and treated if necessary. Antibiotic resistance is a growing problem in multiple drug-resistant tuberculosis (MDR-TB) infections. Prevention relies on screening programmes and vaccination with the bacillus Calmette-Guérin vaccine.

One third of the world's population is thought to have been infected with M. tuberculosis, with new infections occurring in about 1% of the population each year. In 2007, there were an estimated 13.7 million chronic active cases globally, while in 2010, there were an estimated 8.8 million new cases and 1.5 million associated deaths, mostly occurring in developing countries. The absolute number of tuberculosis cases has been decreasing since 2006, and new cases have decreased since 2002. The rates of tuberculosis in different areas varies across the globe; about 80% of the population in many Asian and African countries tests positive in tuberculin tests, while only 5-10% of the United States population tests positive. More people in the developing world contract tuberculosis because of a poor immune system, largely due to high rates of HIV infection and the corresponding development of AIDS.

17. All of the following statements are true except:
    A. Mycobacterium is the usual bacterial cause of TB
    B. 50% of TB infections are fatal if left untreated
    C. In 2007 there were an estimated 13.7 million chronic active cases of TB globally
    D. Diagnosis of latent TB requires blood tests

18. Which of the following statements is most likely to be true?
    A. Tuberculosis can be spread through faeces
    B. The absolute number of tuberculosis cases has been increasing since 2006
    C. Diagnosis of latent TB relies on the tuberculin skin test (TST) and/or blood tests
    D. Two thirds of the world's population is thought to have been infected with M. tuberculosis

19. Based on the text which of the following statements is the most likely scenario for the future of TB?
    - A. More people will become infected with TB or develop the disease
    - B. Treatment of TB will become more problematic due to antibiotic resistance
    - C. A smaller proportion of the world population will be infected with TB
    - D. The increasing prevalence of HIV will lead to an increasing incidence of TB

20. All of the following statements are true except:
    - A. More than half of the population of Asia and Africa test positive in tuberculin tests
    - B. Infection of other organs causes a wide range of symptoms
    - C. Microscopic examination and microbiological culture of body fluids can also diagnose active tuberculosis
    - D. Tuberculosis was previously known as phthisis pulmonalis

The geography and ecology of the Everglades involves the complex elements affecting the natural environment throughout its southern region of the US state of Florida. Before drainage, the Everglades was an interwoven mesh of marshes and prairies covering 4,000 square miles (10,000 km2). The Everglades is simultaneously a vast watershed that has historically extended from Lake Okeechobee 100 miles (160 km) south to Florida Bay (around one-third of the southern Florida peninsula), and many interconnected ecosystems within a geographic boundary.

It is such a unique meeting of water, land, and climate that the use of either singular or plural to refer to the Everglades is appropriate. When Marjory Stoneman Douglas wrote her definitive description of the region in 1947, she used the metaphor 'River of Grass' to explain the blending of water and plant life.

21. The Everglades is a nature reserve.
    - A. True
    - B. False
    - C. Can't tell

22. The Everglades are found in the southern region of Florida.
    - A. True
    - B. False
    - C. Can't tell

23. The Everglades were drained.
    - A. True
    - B. False
    - C. Can't tell

24. Marjory Stoneman Douglas lived in the Everglades region in 1947
    - A. True
    - B. False
    - C. Can't tell

Europe is, by convention, one of the world's seven continents. Comprising the westernmost peninsula of Eurasia, Europe is generally divided from Asia by the watershed divides of the Ural and Caucasus Mountains, the Ural River, the Caspian and Black Seas, and the waterways connecting the Black and Aegean Seas.

Europe is bordered by the Arctic Ocean to the north, the Atlantic Ocean to the west, the Mediterranean Sea to the south, and the Black Sea and connected waterways to the southeast. Yet the borders of Europe, a concept dating back to classical antiquity, are somewhat arbitrary, as the primarily physiographic term "continent" can incorporate cultural and political elements.

Europe is the world's second-smallest continent by surface area, covering about 10,180,000 km^2 (3,930,000 $miles^2$) or 2% of the Earth's surface and about 6.8% of its land area. Of Europe's approximately 50 countries, Russia is by far the largest by both area and population, taking up 40% of the continent (although the country has territory in both Europe and Asia), while Vatican City is the smallest. Europe is the third-most populous continent after Asia and Africa, with a population of 733-739 million or about 11% of the world's population. The most commonly used currency is the euro.

Europe, in particular ancient Greece and ancient Rome is the birthplace of Western culture. It played a predominant role in global affairs from the 15th century onwards, especially after the beginning of colonialism. Between the 16th and 20th centuries, European nations controlled at various times the Americas, most of Africa, Oceania, and large portions of Asia. The Industrial Revolution, which began in Great Britain around the end of the 18th century, gave rise to radical economic, cultural, and social change in Western Europe, and eventually the wider world. Demographic growth meant that, by 1900, Europe's share of the world's population was 25%.

Both world wars were largely focused upon Europe, greatly contributing to a decline in Western European dominance in world affairs by the mid-20th century as the United States and Soviet Union took prominence. During the Cold War, Europe was divided along the Iron Curtain between NATO in the west and the Warsaw Pact in the east. European integration led to the formation of the Council of Europe and the European Union in Western Europe, both of which have been expanding eastward since the revolutions of 1989 and the fall of the Soviet Union in 1991. The European Union nowadays has growing influence over its member countries. Many European countries are members of the Schengen Area, which abolishes border and immigration controls among its members.

25. All of the following statements are true except:
   A. Industrial revolution gave rise to economic growth
   B. Europe is north of the Mediterranean Sea
   C. The Iron Curtain divided NATO and Warsaw Pact countries
   D. The world population is more than 7 billion people

26. Which of the following statements is most likely to be true?
   A. The EU abolished border controls to make it easier for nationals to move around Europe
   B. Europe is a not a continent in a physical, geographical sense
   C. Europe is less densely populated than the world as a whole on average
   D. Europe was only dominant in world affairs for 500 years

27. Regarding the cultural, economic and political impact on the world by Europe it is not true that:
   A. Europe has growing influence
   B. Most of the world has, at some point, been part of European colonies
   C. The industrial revolution began in Europe
   D. The Cold War was demarked through Europe

28. Which of the following statements is most likely to be true?
   A. Asia is the largest country in Europe
   B. Europe is divided from Asia by mountain ranges
   C. Africa is home to more than 11% of the world's population
   D. Europe as a continent covers 6.8% of the Earth's surface

The term drug misuse is applied to any drug-taking which harms or threatens to harm the physical or mental health of an individual, or other individuals, or which is illegal. Thus drug misuse includes alcohol and nicotine and the deleterious over-prescription of medicines (e.g. benzodiazepines and stimulants), as well as the more obvious taking of illicit drugs.

Drug dependence is a term used when a person has a compulsion to take a drug in order to experience its psychic effects, and sometimes to avoid the discomfort of withdrawal symptoms.

The likelihood of drug misuse leading to dependence depends on many factors, including the type of drug, the route of administration, the pattern of drug taking and the individual.

Rapid delivery systems increase the dependence potential. Intravenous injections have the additional dangers of infection.

Drug dependence is often associated with tolerance, a phenomenon that may occur with chronic administration of a drug. It is characterised by the necessity to progressively increase the dose of drug to produce its original effect. Tolerance may be due, in part, to increased metabolism of the drug (pharmacokinetic tolerance), but it is mainly caused by neuroadaptive changes in the brain.

Source: Neal, M. J. (1997) *Medical Pharmacology at a Glance* (3rd edn.), Oxford, Wiley-Blackwell.

29. Which of the following statements is true, according to the text?
    A. Drug dependence always leads to drug misuse
    B. Tolerance is associated with long term use of a drug
    C. Drug misuse always involves the use of illegal drugs
    D. Tolerance always occurs with drug misuse

30. All of the following are true except:
    A. Intravenous drug users are at an increased risk of dependence
    B. Occasional or recreational users of illegal drugs would not be classified as drug misusers
    C. Drug dependence can be caused by a physical need to take the drug
    D. Tolerance requires the user to increase the dose or frequency of use

31. Which of the following statements is most likely to be true?
    A. Legal drugs do not lead to tolerance
    B. Some people are more likely to become dependent than others
    C. Tolerance and dependence are the only risks in drug misuse
    D. Prescription medications cannot be misused

32. The following statements are all true except:
    A. Tolerance may be caused by changes in the way the user's body metabolises the drug
    B. Tolerance may be caused by alterations in the user's brain
    C. Tolerance requires a decrease in the frequency or dose of the drug
    D. Tolerance means the user struggles to achieve the original effect of the drug

Peppa Pig is a children's television programme broadcasting in the UK, USA, Australia and Latin America. Each episode is approximately 5 minutes long. The show revolves around Peppa, an anthropomorphic female pig, and her family and friends. Each of her friends is a different species of mammal. Peppa's friends are the same age as her, and Peppa's younger brother George's friends are the same age as him. Episodes tend to feature everyday activities such as attending playgroup, going swimming, visiting their grandparents, playing with cousins, going to the playground, or riding bikes.

The characters wear clothes, live in houses, and drive cars, but still display some characteristics of the animals on which they are based. Peppa and her family snort like pigs during conversations in which they are speaking in English, the other animals make their respective noises when they talk, with some exhibiting other characteristics, such as the Rabbit family's enjoyment of carrots. The Rabbits are also the sole exception to the rule of human-like habitation, in that they live in a burrow in a hill, although it does have windows and is furnished in the same way as the other houses. The characters also blush when embarrassed and their mouths are used to express other emotions such as sadness, happiness, irritation, bewilderment and confusion.

Although the mammals are anthropomorphic, other animals are not, for example, the ducks, Tiddles the tortoise, and Polly Parrot.

Peppa and her family did not wear seat belts in the first two series. After receiving several complaints, Astley Baker Davies announced that all future animation would include characters wearing seat belts, and that the relevant scenes in the first two series would be re-animated to include them. Similar changes were also made to early episodes with characters riding bicycles to add cycle helmets, which were not included in the original versions.

Peppa was used to promote the Labour government's Sure Start programme but in April 2010, during the UK General Election campaign, E1 Entertainment confirmed Peppa would not be attending the launch of the UK Labour Party's families manifesto "in the interests of avoiding any controversy or misunderstanding".

33. All of the following scenarios are typical of an episode of Peppa Pig except:
   A. Visiting the zoo
   B. Celebrating a birthday
   C. Rescuing a kidnapped princess
   D. Having a picnic

34. Which of the following featured in the first two series of the show according to the text?
   A. Riding bikes and travelling in cars
   B. Going swimming
   C. Visiting grandparents for tea
   D. The first day of school

35. Which of the following is true of all animals in Peppa Pig?
   A. All animals express human emotions with facial expression
   B. All animals live in human style homes
   C. All animals maintain some characteristics of their species
   D. All animals have alliterative names

36. Which statement is most likely to be true regarding Peppa Pig and politics?
   A. Peppa Pig had appeared in a political manifesto prior to 2010
   B. Peppa Pig was used to promote services for young children given her wide appeal
   C. The makers of Peppa Pig stopped supporting the Labour Party
   D. Peppa Pig attended political events for a political party other than the Labour Party.

Radar (acronym for RAdio Detection And Ranging) is an object-detection system that uses radio waves to determine the range, altitude, direction, or speed of objects. It can be used to detect aircraft, ships, spacecraft, guided missiles, motor vehicles, weather formations, and terrain. The radar dish or antenna transmits pulses of radio waves or microwaves that bounce off any object in their path. The object returns a tiny part of the wave's energy to a dish or antenna that is usually located at the same site as the transmitter.

Radar was secretly developed by several nations before and during World War II. The term RADAR itself, not the actual development, was coined in 1940 by the United States Navy as an acronym for RAdio Detection And Ranging. The modern uses of radar are highly diverse, including air traffic control, radar astronomy, air-defence systems, anti missile systems; marine radars to locate landmarks and other ships; aircraft anti collision systems; ocean surveillance systems, outer space surveillance and rendezvous systems; meteorological precipitation monitoring; altimetry and flight control systems; guided missile target locating systems; and ground-penetrating radar for geological observations. High tech radar systems are associated with digital signal processing and are capable of extracting useful information from very high noise levels.

Other systems similar to radar make use of other parts of the electromagnetic spectrum. One example is "lidar", which uses visible light from lasers rather than radio waves

The information provided by radar includes the bearing and range (and therefore position) of the object from the radar scanner. It is thus used in many different fields where the need for such positioning is crucial. The first use of radar was for military purposes: to locate air, ground and sea targets.

In aviation, aircraft are equipped with radar devices that warn of aircraft or other obstacles in or approaching their path, display weather information, and give accurate altitude readings. The first commercial device fitted to aircraft was a 1938 Bell Lab unit on some United Air Lines aircraft. Such aircraft can land in fog at airports equipped with radar-assisted ground-controlled approach systems in which the plane's flight is observed on radar screens while operators radio landing directions to the pilot.

Meteorologists use radar to monitor precipitation and wind. It has become the primary tool for short-term weather forecasting and watching for severe weather such as thunderstorms, tornadoes, winter storms, precipitation types, etc. Geologists use specialised ground-penetrating radars to map the composition of the Earth's crust.

Police forces use radar guns to monitor vehicle speeds on the roads.

37. All of the following are possibly true except:

A. Radar was used before 1945
B. High tech radar systems can extract useful information from very high noise levels
C. The first use of radar was for marine life surveillance
D. Radar can be used at airports to help aircrafts land in fog

38. Which of the following is not cited as a contemporary use of radar technology:

A. Meteorological precipitation monitoring
B. Ocean surveillance systems
C. Air traffic control
D. Satellite detection

39. Which of the following is a similarity between radar and lidar?

A. Both use radio waves
B. Both are used for military applications
C. Both use the electromagnetic spectrum
D. Both can be used to locate air, ground, and sea targets

40. Which of the following statements are true?

A. Radio waves can travel through air, matter and vacuum
B. Radar is a monitoring system
C. The position of an object cannot be determined if you know its bearing and range
D. Radio waves are unaffected by weather conditions

The Supermarine Spitfire is a British single-seat fighter aircraft used by many other Allied countries throughout the World War II. The Spitfire continued to be used into the 1950s both as a front line fighter and in secondary roles. It was produced in greater numbers than any other British aircraft and was the only Allied fighter in production throughout the war.

The Spitfire was designed as a short-range high-performance interceptor aircraft by R. J. Mitchell, chief designer at Supermarine Aviation Works. He continued to refine the design until his death in 1937, whereupon his colleague Joseph Smith became chief designer and continued his work. The Spitfire's elliptical wing had a thin cross-section, allowing a higher top speed than the Hawker Hurricane and several contemporary fighters. Speed was seen as essential to carry out the mission of home defence against enemy bombers.

During the Battle of Britain there was a public perception that the Spitfire was the RAF fighter of the battle; in fact the more numerous Hurricane actually shouldered a greater proportion of the burden against Germany.

Much loved by its pilots, the Spitfire saw service in several roles, including interceptor, photo-reconnaissance, fighter-bomber, carrier-based fighter, and trainer; it was built in many different variants, with four different types of engine and several wing configurations.

41. Joseph Smith was chief designer for the Spitfire.

A. True
B. False
C. Can't tell

42. More Spitfires than Hurricanes flew during the Battle of Britain.

A. True
B. False
C. Can't tell

43. Spitfires were built in at least three variants.

A. True
B. False
C. Can't tell

44. Spitfires were used in bombing missions over Germany.

A. True
B. False
C. Can't tell

Full Mock Test 1 Decision Making (31 minutes for this section)

1. A sixth form college is planning its timetable for the new term. The college offers 10 courses. There are 8 class rooms available for teaching and each course needs 5 lessons per week. There are 4 lessons in the timetable each day.

Select the words 'Yes' or 'No' and drop them to the appropriate places if the conclusion does or doesn't follow

This college has enough space to fully deliver this programme	Yes / No
The college could treble the number of courses they offer and still be able to schedule the classes	Yes / No
Each course has a daily class of one hour	Yes / No
The college must employ at least 10 teachers	Yes / No
The college could decommission half of their classrooms without making timetabling impossible	Yes / No

2. The nurses break room is always well supplied with chocolates, biscuits, and flowers given by grateful patients. One quiet afternoon Sue tidies the room.
On the table there are four tubs of chocolates. One is 75% full. One is 50% full. One is 25% full and the other is unopened.
In the cupboard there are three boxes of biscuits. The chocolate biscuits for all three boxes have been eaten. The biscuit tin is empty.
On the shelf there are four vases. Two of them have dead flowers in – which Sue throws away. Of the other two – one has a combination of pink roses and yellow daffodils; the other has a mixture of carnations.
Select the words 'Yes' or 'No' and drop them to the appropriate places if the conclusion does or doesn't follow

Sue could empty all of the chocolates into two tubs	Yes / No
All of the boxes of biscuits have been opened	Yes / No
Sue could put all of the biscuits in the biscuit tin	Yes / No
There are at least three colours of flower on display after Sue finishes	Yes / No
More than one patient gave the nurses these gifts	Yes / No

3. It has been shown that soft fruit crop yields are up to 50% higher when there is above average rainfall in the spring in the UK
It was a very rainy winter and spring with rainfall 20% more than the average.
Select the words 'Yes' or 'No' and drop them to the appropriate places if the conclusion does or doesn't follow

Soft fruit yields were 50% higher	Yes / No
The rain in the winter had no impact on the crop yield of soft fruits	Yes / No
The relationship with above average rain and above average yields is directly proportional	Yes / No
In a dry year the crop yields will be below average	Yes / No
Average rainfall in spring will result in average crop yields	Yes / No

4. All cars need legal registration certificates
No legal registration certificates cost £20
Some legal registration certificates are issued electronically
Some legal registration certificates are not related to cars

Select the words 'Yes' or 'No' and drop them to the appropriate places if the conclusion does or doesn't follow

Some legal registration certificates for cars are issued electronically	Yes / No
No cars have legal registration certificates which cost £20	Yes / No
Legal registration certificates which are not for cars cost £20	Yes / No
Electronically issued certificates make up a proportion of certificate issues	Yes / No
Legal registration certificates are necessary for other vehicles as well as cars	Yes / No

5. A group of friends - Benjamin, Joel, Matthew and Beatrice - compared notes on the homework they had done the previous evening. They had been studying Biology, Chemistry, History and Psychology. Each spent a different amount of time studying with the shortest being 1 hour, the next being 1.5 hours, then 2 hours then the longest was 2.5 hours.

- The Psychology homework took the longest
- Joel worked for half an hour less than Benjamin
- Chemistry took an hour longer than History
- Beatrice worked the second longest

Which of the following statements must be true?

A. Ben is studying History
B. The Chemistry homework took 1.5 hours
C. Matthew worked the longest
D. Biology took an hour longer than History

6. Amanda is a busy mother of five children who all need to be taken to various after school clubs. Her children Jacob, Elizabeth, Daniel, Grace and Andrew go to activities on Monday to Friday. The activities are chess club, gymnastics, music lesson, St John Ambulance and swimming lesson.

- Amanda's final trip of the week is to gymnastics
- Grace doesn't attend her music lesson on Monday or Tuesday
- Jacob has his after-school activity on Thursday; it isn't chess club
- Elizabeth is taken to her activity the day before Daniel goes to St John Ambulance

Which of the following must be true?

A. Elizabeth goes to swimming lessons
B. Grace has her activity on Wednesday
C. Andrew does chess
D. St John Ambulance meet on a Thursday

7. A group of friends; Helen, Linda, Andy and Mona meet at one of their homes for a meal. They each bring a different item. One brings chicken, one brings rice, one brings salad and the final one brings drinks. They all arrive within 15 minutes of each other - one arrives at 6.50, the next at 6.55, the next at 7.00 and the final friend arrives at 7.05.

- The chicken arrived last
- Andy was earliest, but he didn't bring the drinks
- Mona arrived before Helen
- The person bringing rice came immediately after the person bringing drinks

Which of the following statements must be true?

A. The rice arrived at 6.55
B. Helen brought the chicken
C. The drinks arrived after the salad
D. The salad didn't arrive at 6.50

8. This dinner table shows where family P ate their dinner. The family consists of Alex, Ben, Ellen, John, Lydia, Mark, Tom and Vivienne.

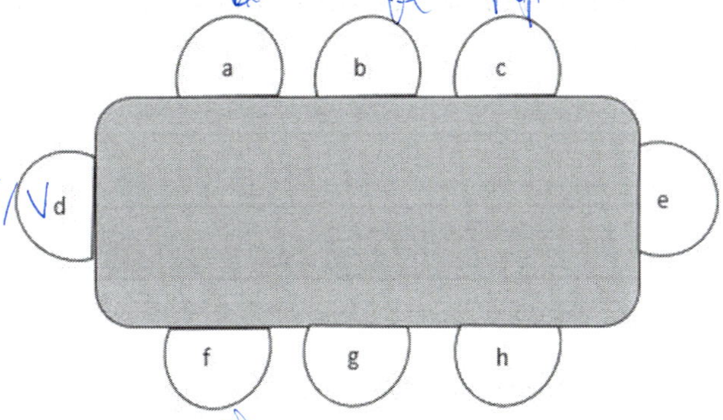

- The parents of the family are John and Vivienne and they sat at the two ends of the table
- Lydia and Ellen sat opposite each other
- Ben sat between Lydia and Mark
- Alex sat in seat c

Which of the following statements must be true?

A. Vivienne sat in seat d
B. John had Ellen on one side and Lydia on the other
C. Tom sits between Alex and Ellen
D. Mark is sitting next to Vivienne

9. Four universities (Andover, Bridlington, Carlisle and Doncaster) are building new facilities (A multi-media Suite, research lab, theatre and swimming pool) in partnership with various big businesses (Edward and Farley, General Engineering, Harlon and Son and Intergalactic).

- Harlon and Son are a Bridlington based business committed to help their local university, but not with a research lab
- Neither Doncaster nor Carlisle University need a new swimming pool as they already have modern sports centres. One of them got a new research lab thanks to General Engineering though
- The theatre (not at Andover or Doncaster) has been sponsored by Intergalactic – a creative arts company

Which of the following statements must be true?

A. Andover Uni got a new swimming pool
B. Harlon and Son funded a multi-media suite
C. Carlisle University got a new facility thanks to Intergalactic
D. The multi-media suite was funded by Edward and Farley

10. It is clear that the study of music will strongly complement the study of mathematics as both systems are fundamentally based on sequences, ratios and counting. Whilst it may not be evident to the conscious mind - the harmonies in music are based on ratios between the soundwaves of differently pitched notes - the subconscious mind can mathematically interpret music and be pleased. All serious mathematicians are also serious music appreciators and all students of mathematics should be students of music.

All maths students should learn to play a musical instrument alongside their mathematics studies.

Select the strongest argument from these options:

A. Yes - giving yourself something completely different to do will provide an emotional and physical break leaving the student refreshed for more study
B. Yes - applying mathematics to seemingly unrelated areas of human study will enable a broader picture to be appreciated and inspire further exploration
C. No - mathematics is a serious discipline and studying something which is essentially merely creative rather than academic can only lead to distraction
D. No - if a student wishes to embark on two disciplines that is their choice, but they won't complement the other in any meaningful way

11. Animal intelligence is notoriously difficult to classify as applying human standards is inevitable though inappropriate. In various tests of animal intelligence, it has been shown that dogs are far more receptive to training and can respond accurately to a large variety of human language commands. Cats rarely respond to human commands. However - cats have been shown to have greater problem-solving skills and also better memory skills.

Cats are cleverer than dogs

Select the strongest argument from these options:

A. Yes - the skills of problem-solving and memory are superior to following commands
B. Yes - cats may consciously choose to ignore human commands which shows self-awareness
C. No - language is the pinnacle of intelligence and dogs demonstrate they can understand it
D. No - there is no way to make a fair judgement

12. Factory farming keeps animals at high stocking densities and uses modern technology to facilitate faster animal growth, lower illness and death rates, and higher production outputs. Many people, particularly business owners and investors, think that factory farming is one of the best innovations of the modern times and has solved numerous problems in society. However, there are also those who say that factory farming is harmful to the environment as well as to the health of both animals and humans.

Should factory farming continue?

Select the strongest argument from these options:

A. Yes – lower costs and bigger outputs will enable poor people to buy enough food for themselves and their families
B. Yes – but efforts must be made to minimise the risk to health and the environment
C. No – it's mainly business owners and those who want to make profit who support it
D. No – factory farming creates more problems than it solves

13. Experience has shown that foreign aid cannot right all social wrongs or solve every economic problem of a developing country. It cannot bring about instant progress.

Should foreign aid should be de-prioritised in rich countries?

Select the strongest argument from the options below:

A. Yes – it is not the responsibility of rich countries to prop up poorer ones
B. Yes – it is much better to let the countries develop a robust economy without artificial inputs
C. No – foreign aid can do some good which is better than doing no good
D. No – rich countries must make humanitarian efforts to help the desperately poor

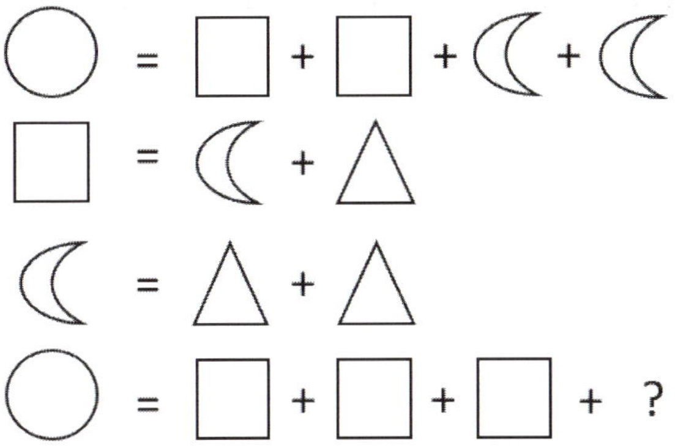

14. Which shape will make the last equation true?

A. Circle
B. Square
C. Crescent
D. Triangle

15. The introduction of e-cigarettes, which enable ex-smokers to stop smoking without withdrawal from nicotine, is a good thing as it will save lives that may have been lost due to smoking.

Select the strongest argument from these options:

A. Yes – e-cigarettes are not as antisocial and unpleasant smelling to the general public
B. Yes – the growth of the e-cigarette industry can counteract losses to the tobacco industry
C. No – nicotine itself may be a cancer-causing chemical so e-cigarettes are still dangerous
D. No – the wide range of e-cigarette flavours encourages young people who don't smoke to use them

16. As online shopping increases, there will be a gradual decline, and eventual death, of high street shops.

Select the strongest argument from these options:

A. Yes – the rise in online shopping will continue at current rates for a long time
B. Yes – the overheads of high street shops mean they can't compete on price
C. No – there are some products that people will always want to see before purchase so there will always be some high street shops
D. No – there are too many jobs dependent on retail so the sector must be protected

17. The Smith family have owned a number of pets over the years. There have been a total of 3 cats, 3 chickens, 4 hamsters, 2 rabbits and a goldfish. The garden coop held rabbits for some years before the chickens arrived. The family once owned 3 cats at once but now there are only 2. Two of the hamsters were tragically eaten by a family cat. The goldfish died shortly after arriving in the house. Currently the family only have 2 pets - both cats.

Select the words 'Yes' or 'No' if the conclusion does or doesn't follow

The family owned both rabbits at the same time	Yes / No
Two hamsters died of natural causes	Yes / No
The chickens and the rabbits lived with the family at the same time	Yes / No
The most pets the Smiths could have owned at once is 11	Yes / No
The family owned 2 rabbits and a goldfish at one time	Yes / No

18. It is better to give people who receive government assistance vouchers for just food and energy rather than giving them money.

Select the strongest argument from these options:

A. Yes – poor people may spend their welfare payments on things like cigarettes and alcohol and this ensures they use it sensibly.
B. Yes – luxury products should be reserved only for people who can pay for them with their own earnings
C. No – this takes away the dignity of poor people and allows the government to track their purchases
D. No – it is difficult to assess the needs of any household and these restrictions may cause unintended hardship

19. The oval represents ants

The rectangle represents black bugs
The triangle represents insects
The diamond represents red bugs
The arrow represents tropical parasites

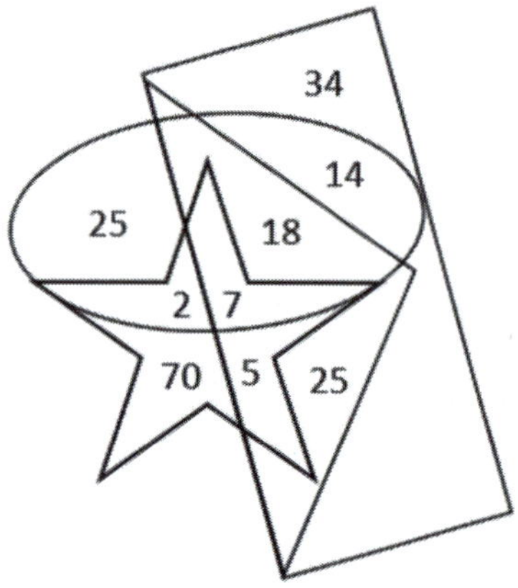

Which of the following statements is false?

A. There are 126 black insects represented in the chart
B. None of the tropical parasites are red bugs
C. There are a total of 147 non insects represented in the chart
D. There are 65 ants that are neither red nor black

20. The diagram shows the data on creatures in popular fantasy novels.
The oval represents novels with winged creatures.
The triangle represents novels with malevolent creatures.
The rectangle represents novels with mythical creatures.
The star represents novels with deadly creatures.

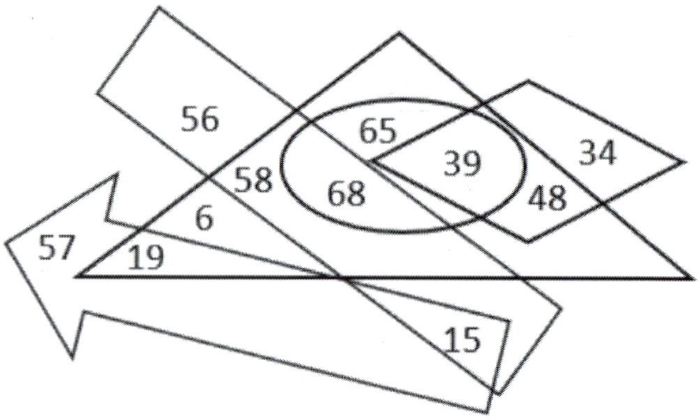

Which of the following statements is true?

A. All novels with malevolent creatures also contain winged creatures.
B. Out of all the novels that feature winged creatures, just over 10% also feature creatures which are deadly, malevolent and mythical.
C. Novels with malevolent and mythical creatures are equal to those that feature deadly creatures.
D. Novels with mythical, deadly and malevolent creatures are equal to novels with mythical, deadly, malevolent and winged creatures.

21. Four young people – David, Eleanor, Frank and Georgina all have part time jobs. They work at a cinema, a delivery firm, a factory and a shop. Each earns a different hourly rate. One earns £6.50 per hour, another earns £7.00 per hour, another £7.50 and the last earns £8.00 per hour.

- David earns 50p per hour less than Eleanor working in the shop
- The delivery firm employee earns the least
- Georgina does not earn the £7.00 per hour wages at the factory
- Frank does not work at the cinema or the shop
- The shop worker earns £1 per hour more than the factory worker

Which of the following statements must be true?

A. David works for £7.00 per hour
B. David doesn't work at the delivery company
C. Eleanor earns less than Frank
D. Georgina works at the cinema
E. Frank earns the least

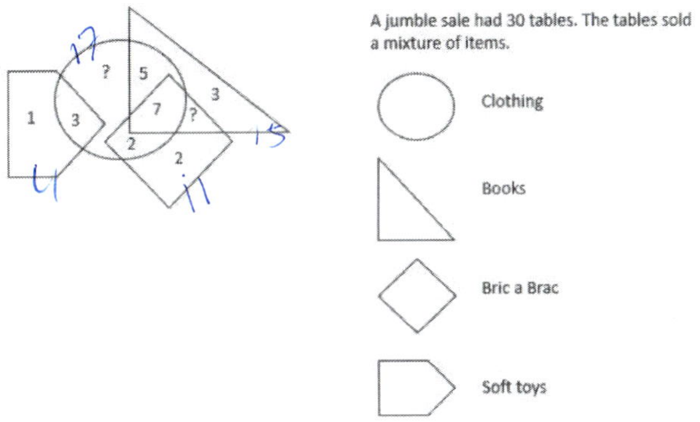

22. 14 tables were selling bric-a-brac. How many were selling clothing?

A. 17
B. 19
C. 21
D. 23

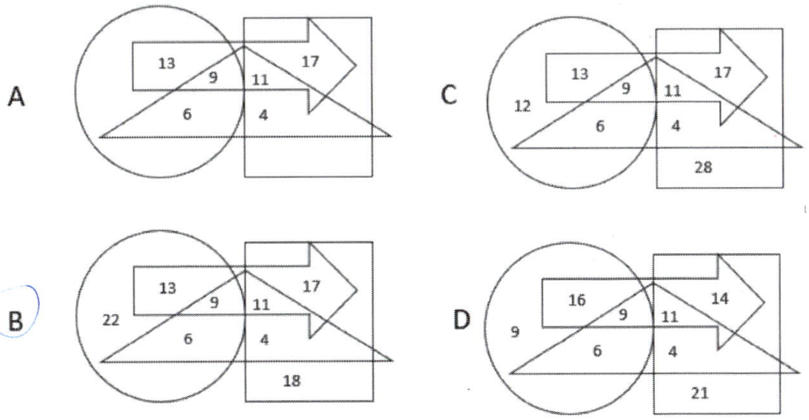

23. 100 top-rated photos of pets were analysed. There were 60 cat photos and 40 dog photos. In 6 of the cat photos the cat was asleep. In 17 of the dog photos the dog was walking or running. Twenty of the pets were wearing collars.

Which diagram represents this data set?

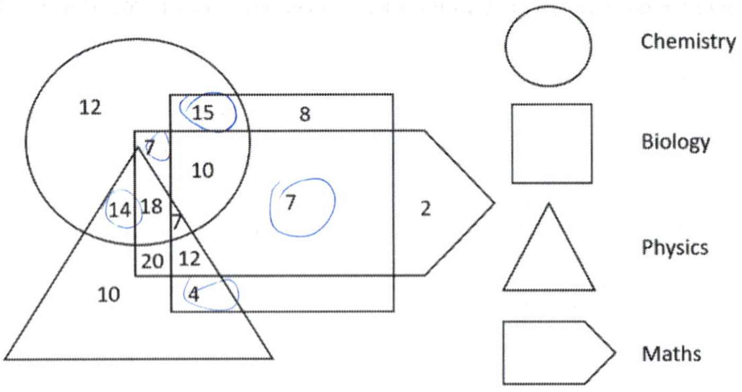

24. The Venn diagram shows which Science A-levels a group of new under graduates has.

How many students took any combination of two of these subjects?

A. 65
B. 66
C. 67
D. 68

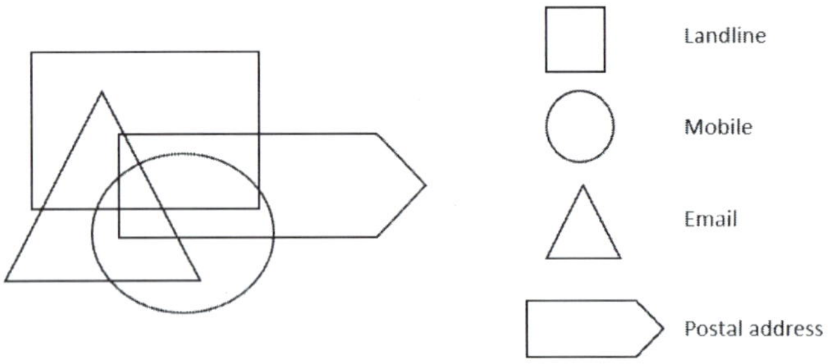

25. Satsev is updating her address book with her current contacts. She has incomplete information for many of them.

Which individual would be classified in the overlap of triangle and circle?

A. Ray Spencer, 19 Windsor Gardens, 0201555 5555
B. Mona Patel 0776955555, monapatel456@hotmail.com
C. Jo Knight, Jotheknight@gmail.co.uk, 45 Church View Grove
D. Adam Bird, 0778912345, adamjbird@yahoo.com, 02017412589

26. A drawer contains pairs of socks folded together in matching pairs. There is one pair of socks in each of the following colours: red, yellow, blue, green, black and white, and one pair of striped socks.
A pair of socks is chosen at random and replaced before choosing a second pair at random.
Is the probability of choosing a blue pair both times 0.07?
Select the strongest argument from these options:

A. Yes, the probability of choosing two pairs of any colour is 0.07
B. Yes, the probability of choosing a blue pair is 1 in 7
C. No, choosing a blue pair both times is more likely than 0.07
D. No, choosing a blue pair both times is less likely than 0.07

27. Five women go to antenatal class together. After the first couple of months two of the women have their babies; both are boys.
As there is an exactly 50% chance of any unborn baby being a boy there is a 1/32 chance that all five babies will be boys
Select the strongest argument from these options:

A. Yes - because 0.5 x 0.5 x 0.5 x 0.5 x 0.5 = 0.031
B. Yes - because any specific combination of babies would have a 1 in 32 chance of happening
C. No - because two babies have already been born
D. No - because there is a 31/32 chance that at least one of the babies will be a girl

28. The probability of a school child owning a laptop is 0.28, of owning a phone is 0.76 and of owning both is 0.21.

If a school child is chosen at random the probability that he or she owns only a laptop or phone is 0.83?

Select the strongest argument from these options:

A. Yes - this group and the group that own both are mutually exclusive
B. Yes - there are no children that own neither a laptop or a phone as 0.28 + 0.76 is more than 1
C. No - the correct probability is 1 minus 0.76 which is 0.23
D. No - the correct probability is 1 minus 0.21 which is 0.79

29. Two football teams, - City and United, - are playing against one another. In their previous 80 matches City have won 20 times, United have won 50 times and there have been 10 draws. United have had some players become ill just before the match. They think this increases their likelihood of losing by 10%.

United still have a more than 70% chance of winning this match based on past performance and this assumption

Select the strongest argument from these options:

A. Yes, because a 10% increase of the 25% loss rate take it to 27.5%
B. Yes, because they have won 75% of matches in the past
C. No, United have a 60% chance of winning based on these numbers
D. No, their chance of winning or drawing is over 70%

Full Mock Test 1 Quantitative Reasoning (24 minutes for this section)

In 2008 Mr and Mrs Singh decided to open a takeaway restaurant. They took out a bank loan for £125,000 to renovate an old corner shop and fit it out with a new kitchen. The cost of renovations came to a total of £78,458.47, which included the cost of a new sign of £950.42.

Before the first day of opening Mrs Singh went to the local wholesalers to buy food stock items and the bill came to £4768.20. However, the wholesaler was having a promotion for all new customers and she was able to get 20% off the total bill. On the same day Mr Singh went to the printers to collect the new menus and paid the £389 bill.

The next week on 2 January 2009, Mr and Mrs Singh opened their takeaway shop. In the first week they took £1764.23 in sales and served 138 customers. The most popular dish was the prawn delight which was priced at £7.36.

1. How much did Mrs Singh pay for the food stock items?

A. £953.64
B. £238.41
C. £3814.56
D. £4768.20
E. £1764.23

2. What was the average amount a customer spent in the first week of January?

A. £2.82
B. £7.36
C. £1015.68
D. £1764.23
E. £12.78

3. 60% of the first week's sales were from customers phoning in their order. How much money came from these phone orders? Give the answer in pounds, to the nearest penny.

A. £1058.54
B. £29.40
C. £1764.23
D. £1059
E. £705.69

4. If no other bills are received how much money should Mr and Mrs Singh have in their business account by the end of their first week of trading? Include any loan remaining. Give the answer in pounds, to the nearest penny.

A. £43151.78
B. £44102.20
C. £43148.56
D. £42198.14
E. £1764.23

Some statisticians calculated the probability of a series of events whilst driving down a 100 mile stretch of the M99 motorway:

- A. Likelihood of getting a speeding fine = 0.073
- B. Likelihood of passing a broken-down vehicle = 1/49 0.02
- C. Likelihood of seeing at least one motorbike = 7/10 0.7
- D. Likelihood of seeing light aircraft = 0.271
- E. Likelihood of being involved in an accident = 2/278 0.007

(The likelihood of multiple events happening can be calculated by multiplying probabilities together. The likelihood of alternative events (i.e. A or B) can be determined by adding probabilities together)

5. Which event is the most likely to happen whilst driving down the M99?

A. Event D (aircraft)
B. Event B (broken-down vehicle)
C. Event A (fine)
D. Event C (motorbike)
E. Event E (accident)

6. What is the probability that a driver would get a speeding fine AND see a light aircraft? Round the answer to 3 decimal places.

A. 0.020
B. 0.344
C. 0.269
D. 0.022
E. 0.019

7. What is the probability that a driver would pass a broken-down vehicle or see at least one motorbike? Give the answer as a fraction.

A. 8/59
B. 33/47
C. 353/490
D. 7/490
E. 490/7

8. What is the probability that the driver will see at least one motorbike and also see either an aircraft or broken-down car? Round the answer to 3 decimal places.

A. 0.991
B. 0.705
C. 0.204
D. 0.004
E. 0.291

	Income (Weekly)		Expenditure (Weekly)
ESA	£99.15	Rent	£150.00
Housing Benefit	£150.00	Council Tax	£14.27
Child Benefit	£33.70	Utilities & Bills	£70.00
Child Tax Credit	£20.96	Food	£40.00
Council Tax Benefit	£14.27		

The above table shows the regular weekly income and expenditure for a household. A parent has two children aged 13 and 15.

9. What is the household's weekly disposable income?

A. £65.22
B. £58.08
C. £52.67
D. £43.81
E. £29.54

10. The family live in a three-bedroom house and both children are the same sex. A change to housing benefit means the family's housing benefit is reduced by 14% because they are considered to have a spare bedroom. What fraction most closely represents the reduction in the family's disposable income?

A. 8 / 17
B. 12 / 25
C. 2 / 25
D. 21 / 44
E. 7 / 50

11. When the oldest child reaches 16, they leave home. Child benefit is paid at £20.30 for the eldest qualifying child in a household at any point and £13.40 for any other children. Tax credits are paid at £10.48 per child. Because of one of the children leaving the weekly expenditure on utilities drops by 15% and on food drops by 25%. What is the weekly disposable income for the household now?

A. £64.31
B. £50.83
C. £19.93
D. £40.43
E. £72.21

12. On the above income and expenditure, the family decide to save 12% of their weekly disposable income towards a washing machine which costs £315. How many weeks will it take them to save up for the new washing machine?

A. 54 weeks
B. 79 weeks
C. 67 weeks
D. 72 weeks
E. 60 weeks

Physicists use the following conversions when calculating astronomical distances:

- 1 light year = 5 874 601 673 400 miles
- 1 astronomical unit (AU) = 149 597 870.69 kilometres (km)
- 1 mile = 1.609 km

13. If the distance between two planets was 457 743 646 km, how many astronomical units would this be? Round the answer to 2 decimal places.

A. 0.33 AU
B. 3.06 AU
C. 308145775.31 AU
D. 0.34 AU
E. 2.59 AU

14. Which is the largest: 1 light year, 23 AU, 567 km or 998 867 654 567 miles?

A. 1 light year
B. 567 km
C. 998,867,654,567 miles
D. 23 AU
E. Cannot tell

15. If a light year is the distance that light can travel in a year, how far can light travel in 8 months?

A. 5 874 601 673 400 × 0.8
B. (5 874 601 673 400 / 12) × 0.8
C. 5 874 601 673 400 / 0.8
D. 5 874 601 673 400 / 0.12
E. (5 874 601 673 400 × 8)/12

16. Another astronomical unit used is the parsec, where 1 parsec = 3.263 light years. When expressed as a percentage of a light year, how big is a parsec?

A. 226.3 %
B. 326.3 %
C. 32.63 %
D. 3.263 %
E. 30.65 %

Bill	Direct Debit Amount
Gas	£35
Electricity	£84
Water	£26
Council Tax	£118
Satellite TV	£30
Rent	£675

Jamie's monthly bills

17. What proportion of the monthly bills is for utilities (gas, electricity and water)? Give the answer as a percentage.

A. 7%
B. 14%
C. 15%
D. 11%
E. 48%

18. What is the average cost of a bill each month? Give the answer to the nearest pound

A. £649
B. £35
C. £194
D. £118
E. £161

19. If Jamie's monthly income is £1,492.00, what percentage of his income is used to pay the monthly bills? Round the answer to 1 decimal place

A. 64.9%
B. 15.4%
C. 64.8%
D. 35.1%
E. 35.2%

20. In the following month, there were some changes to Jamie's bills: the satellite TV company charged extra for two ordered films at £2.99 per film, and the gas company returned £15.82 for unused gas in the previous month. What percentage of this following month's outgoings is for council tax if the bill remains at the previous month's rate? Round the answer to 2 decimal places.

A. 12.19%
B. 9.84%
C. 12.32%
D. 12.36%
E. 11.92%

Player	Score
Speedy 99	39,754
JoJo42	56,753
DaveP	24,787
Wayne1	64,665
Ozzie	87,664
Mhmd18	45,876

Leader's Board of individual scores for players of the Raceway computer game

21. What is the mean score? Give the answer to 2 significant figures.

A. 53,250
B. 62,877
C. 63,000
D. 53,000
E. 56,225.50

22. What is the range of the scores? Give the answer to the nearest whole number

A. 62,877
B. 53,249.83
C. 53,250
D. 63,000
E. 51,315

23. What is the median score? Give the answer to the nearest whole number.

A. 56,753
B. 51,315
C. 62,877
D. 53,250
E. 45,876

24. If the player with the lowest score plays another round in the game and increases his score by 5,842, and another player's score of 11,765 is added to the leader board, what is the new mean score?

A. 56,184
B. 47,323
C. 48,158
D. 42,138
E. 46,489

Brand	% Beef Meat
Mr Beefy	23.4%
Good Price	15.6%
Smiths	88.2%
Quality	59.5%
Organic Farm	96.9%
Speciality	68.3%
Farm Fresh	87.7%

Percentage of beef meat in a selection of sausage products

25. What proportion of the sausage products has low beef content (less than 60%)? Round the answer to three decimal places.

A. 0.286
B. 0.571
C. 0.429
D. 0.570
E. 0.428

26. If the weight of the Quality brand sausages is 370 g, what is the weight of beef meat?

A. 220.15 g
B. 6.22 g
C. 149.85 g
D. 310.50 g
E. 286.65 g

27. The Speciality brand sausage is twice the price of the Good Price brand sausage, but the Good Price brand is a fifth of the cost of Farm Fresh. If the Farm Fresh sausage is £5.90, how much is the Speciality brand?

A. £14.75
B. £1.18
C. £2.99
D. £2.36
E. £2.01

28. If the price of the Organic Farm sausages is £9.45 and they weigh 280 g, what is the price to the nearest penny per gram of beef meat?

A. £0.03
B. £0.06
C. £0.04
D. £0.05
E. £0.05

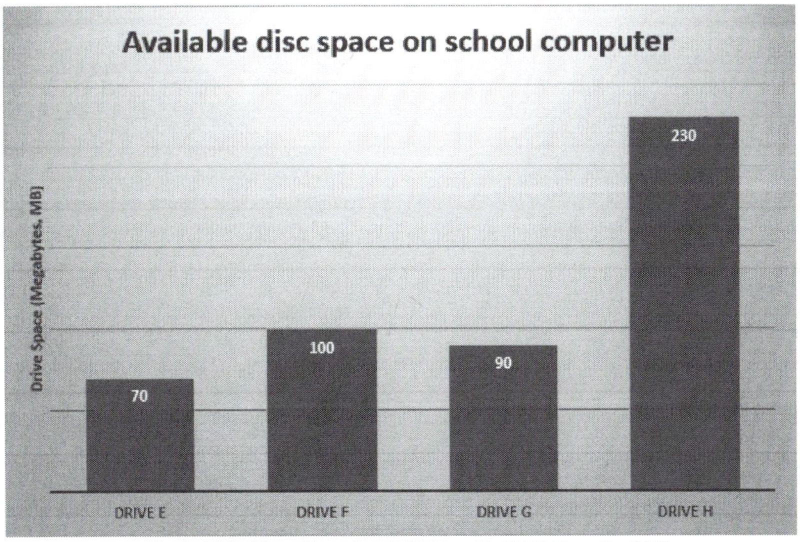

Typical File Sizes: Type A = 5 MB, Type B = 7 MB, Type C = 2 MB

29. How many files of Type A can be stored in Drive E?

A. 350
B. 70
C. 14
D. 0.07
E. 23

30. What percentage of the total available disk space is on Drive G? Give the answer to 2 decimal places.

A. 18%
B. 5.44%
C. 18.37%
D. 90%
E. 20.87%

31. The next day the available disk space on Drive H increased by of 69%. How much extra disk space was available? Give your answer to the nearest whole MB.

A. 158.7 MB
B. 388.7 MB
C. 389 MB
D. 159 MB
E. 71 MB

32. If six Type B files were put in Drive E, what percentage of the original available drive space is left? Give the answer to the nearest whole number.

A. 40 %
B. 60 %
C. 40 MB
D. 67 MB
E. 48 %

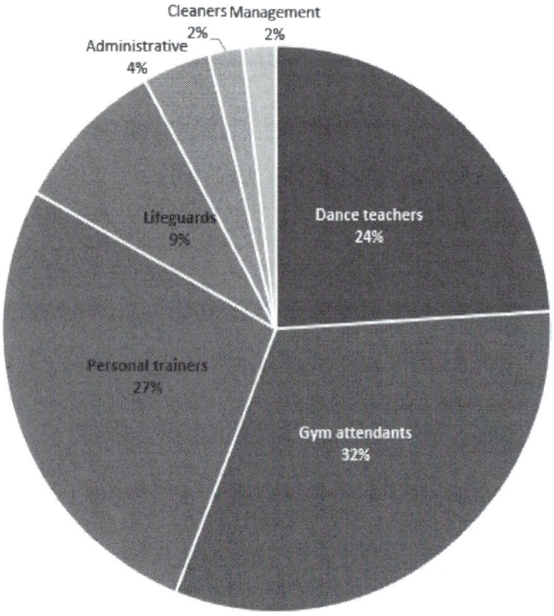

Total number of leisure centre employees = 6674

33. How many employees are personal trainers? Give the answer to the nearest whole number.

A. 247
B. 2002
C. 1802
D. 2003
E. 1738

34. How many more dance teachers are there than Lifeguards Give the answer to the nearest whole number.

A. 464
B. 1602
C. 1001
D. 961
E. 445

35. If 17% of the dance teachers are qualified to teach yoga, how many dance teachers is this? Give the answer to the nearest whole number.

A. 1135
B. 272
C. 393
D. 1134
E. 16

36. If the leisure centre decided to employ 50 more lifeguards, what percentage of the staff will be a lifeguard? Give the answer to 1 decimal place.

A. 9.9%
B. 9.8%
C. 9.0%
D. 9.6%
E. 9.7%

Full Mock Test 1 Abstract Reasoning (13 minutes for this section)

Set A | Set B

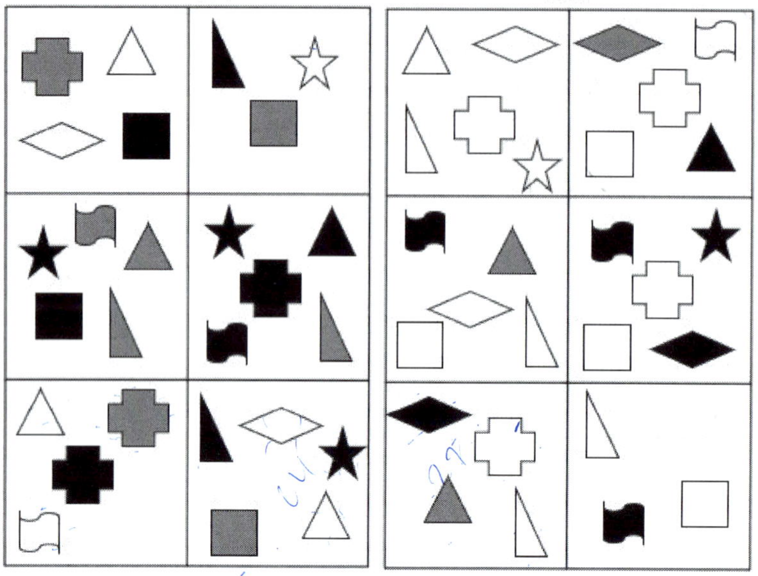

1 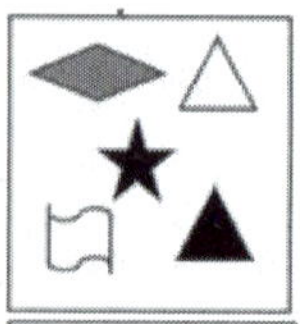
Set A
Set B
Neither

2 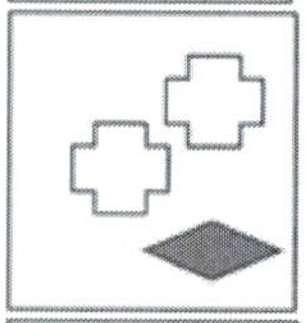
Set A
Set B
Neither

3 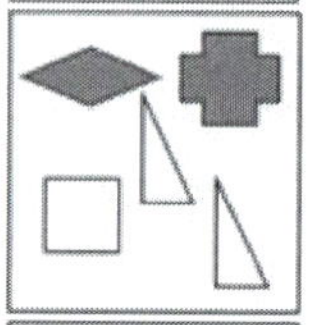
Set A
Set B
Neither

4 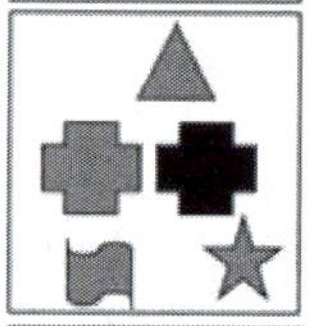
Set A
Set B
Neither

5 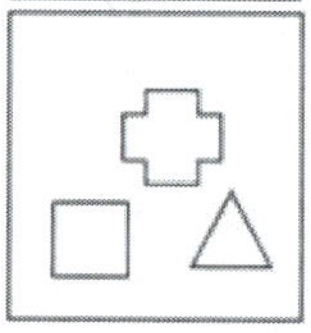
Set A
Set B
Neither

To which of the two sets do the following shapes belong?

Set A | Set B

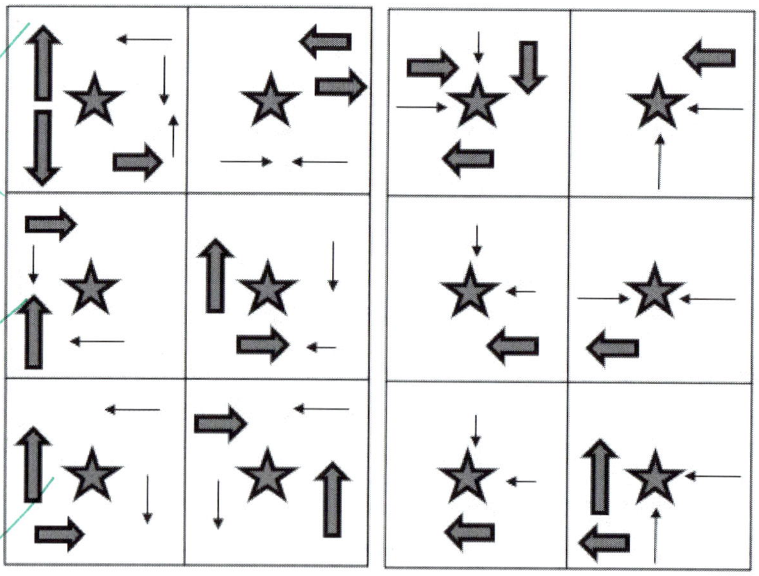

6 
Set A
Set B
Neither

7 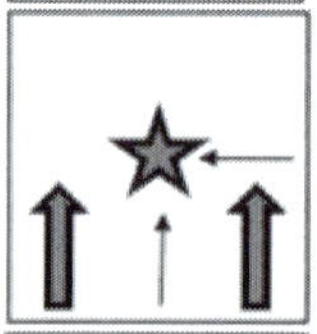
Set A
Set B
Neither

8 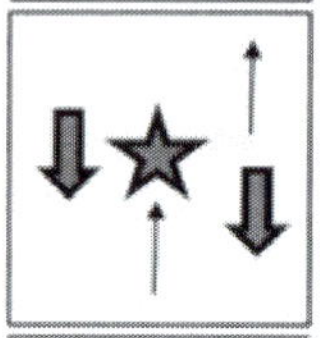
Set A
Set B
Neither

9 
Set A
Set B
Neither

10 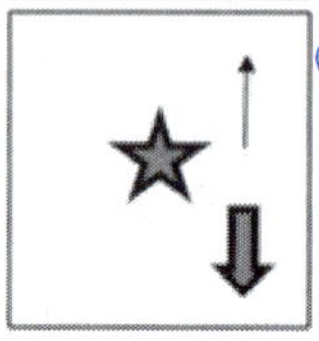
Set A
Set B
Neither

11 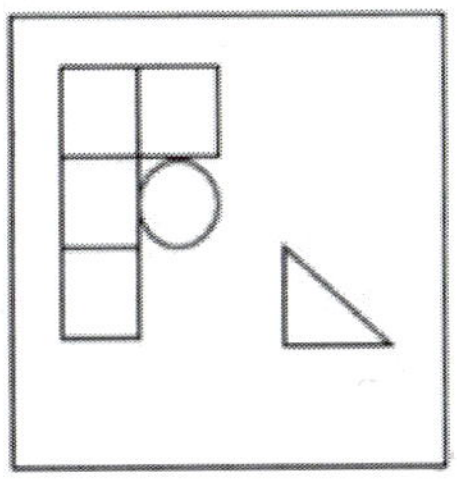 is to 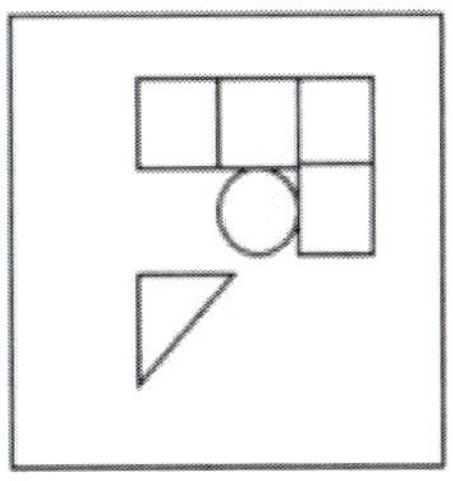

as

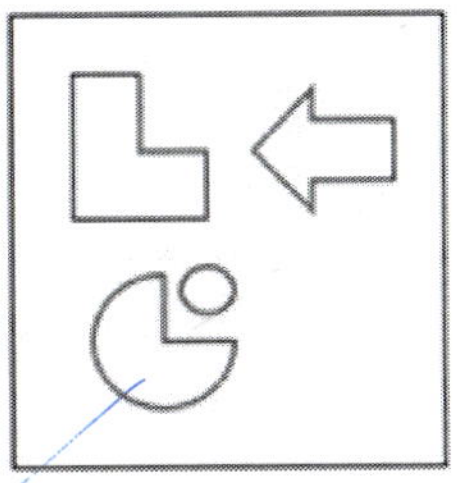 is to 

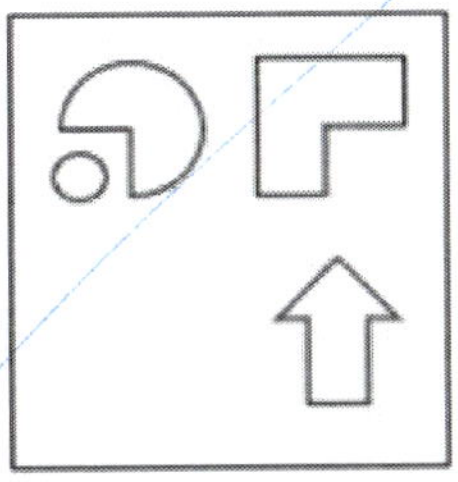
A

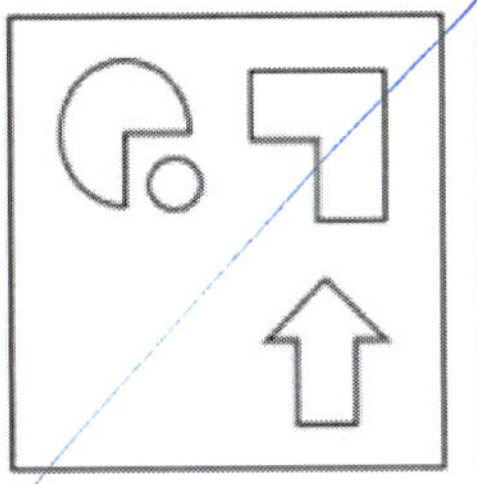
B

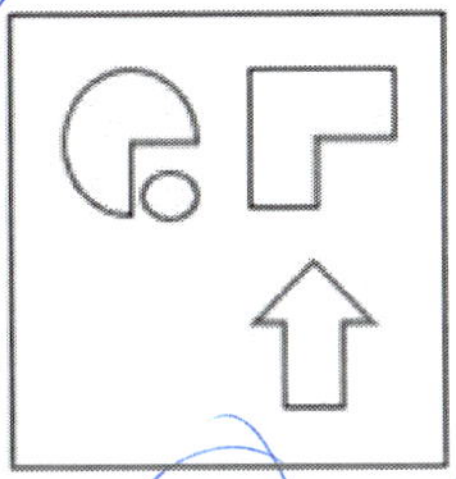
C

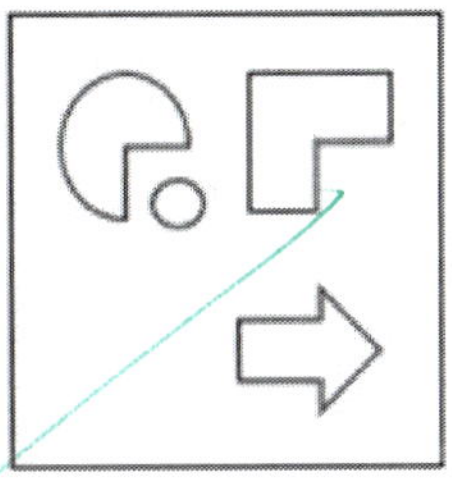
D

12 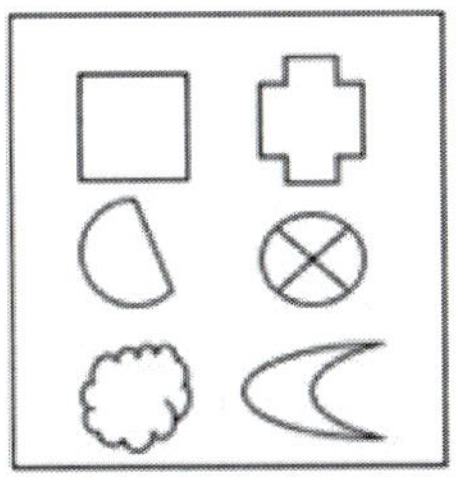 is to 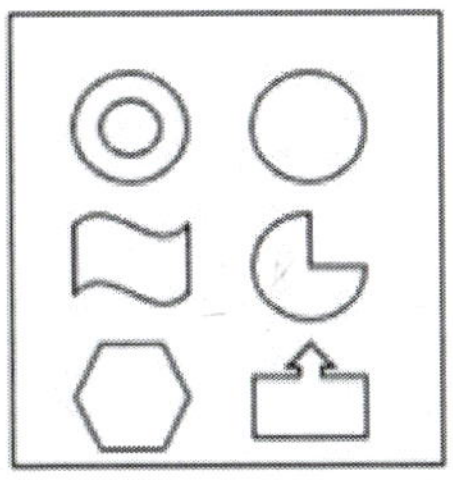

as

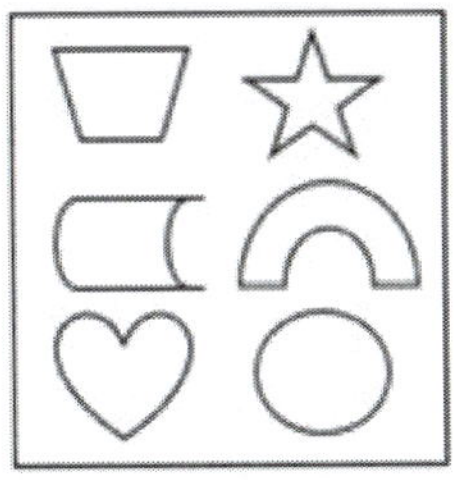 is to 

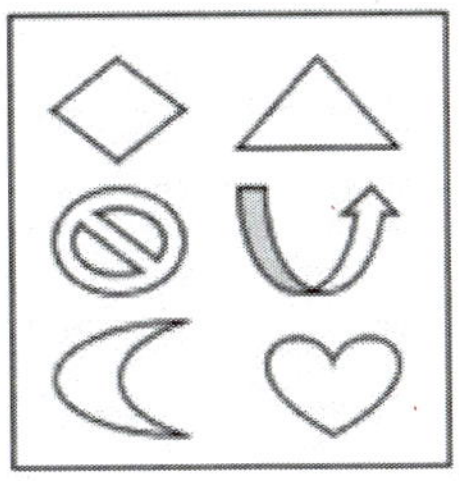
A

B

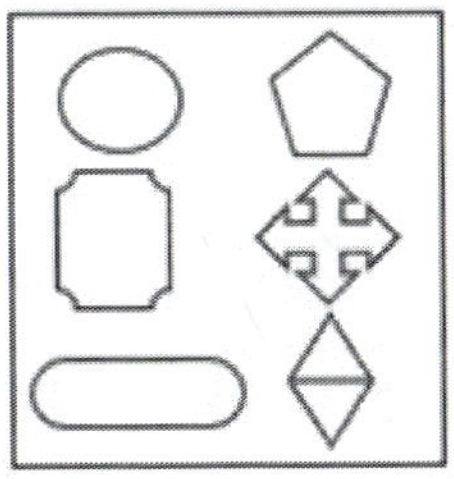
C

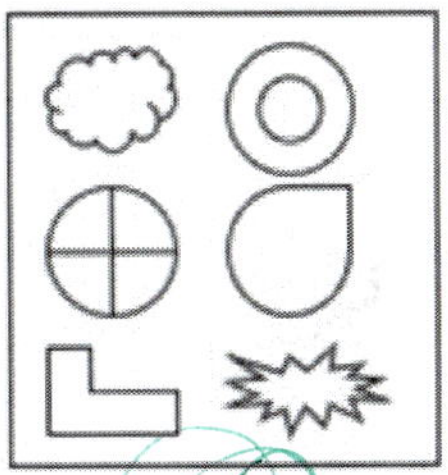
D

Set A

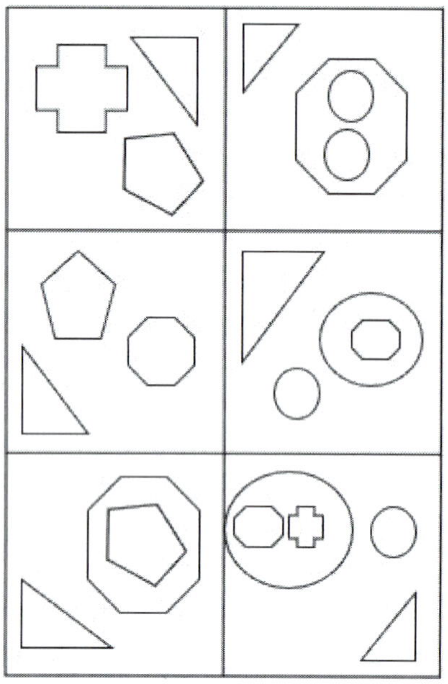

Set B

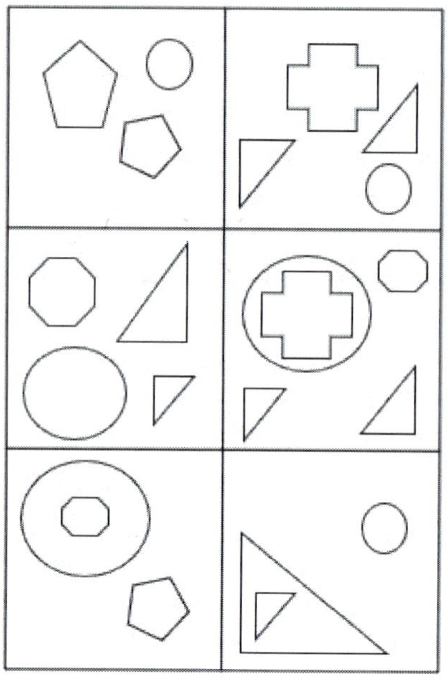

13 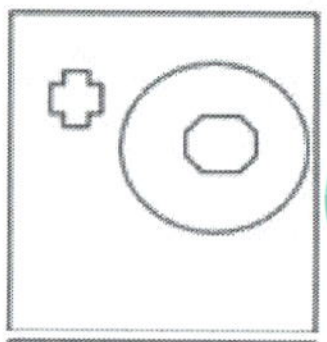
Set A
Set B
Neither

14 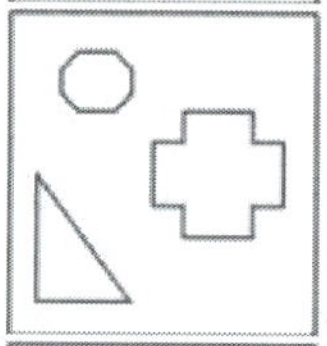
Set A
Set B
Neither

15 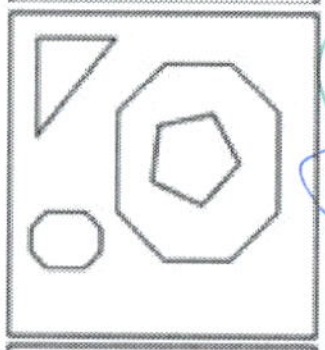
Set A
Set B
Neither

16 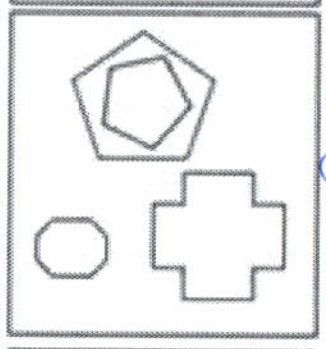
Set A
Set B
Neither

17 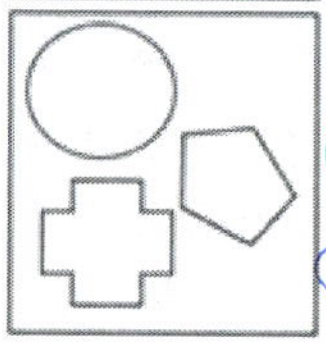
Set A
Set B
Neither

To which of the two sets do the following shapes belong?

18 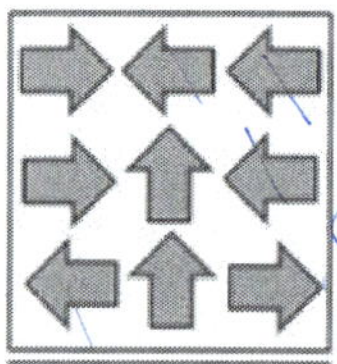
Set A
Set B
Neither

19 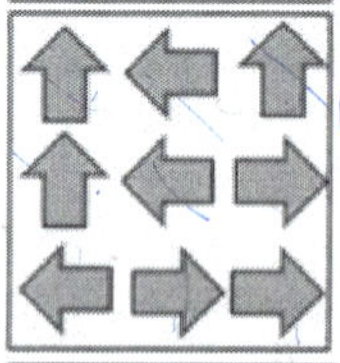
Set A
Set B
Neither

20 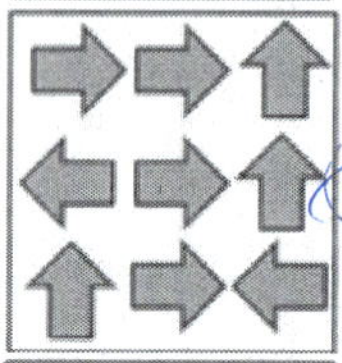
Set A
Set B
Neither

21 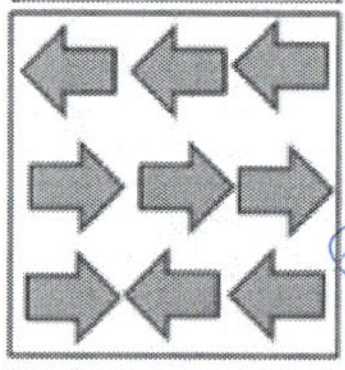
Set A
Set B
Neither

22 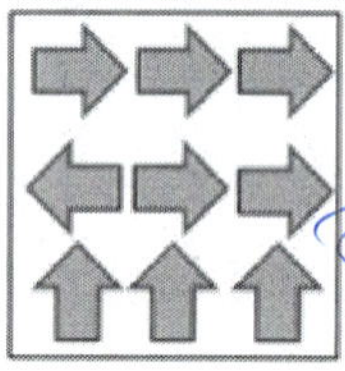
Set A
Set B
Neither

Set A

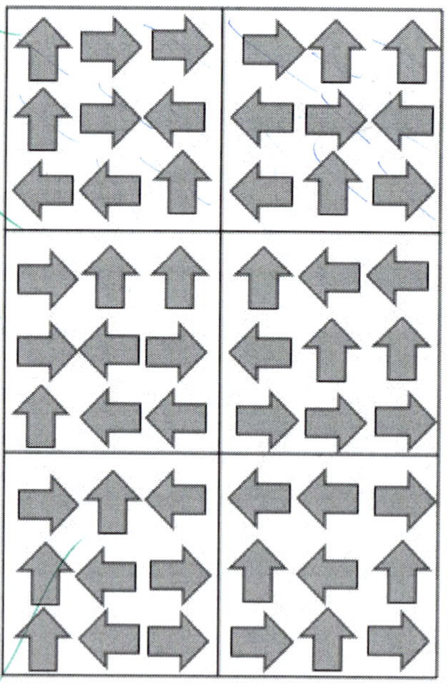

Set B

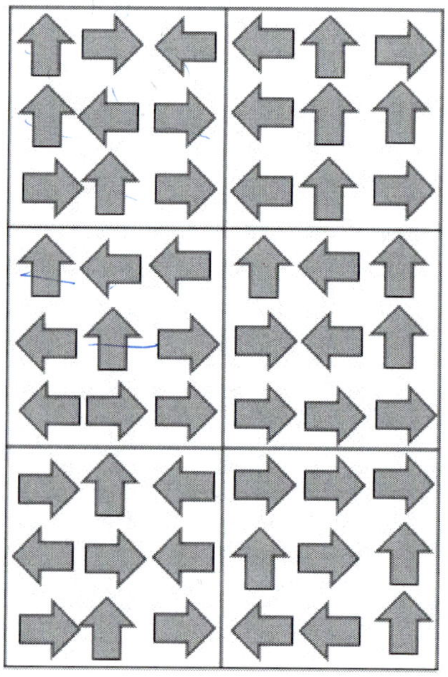

Set A Set B

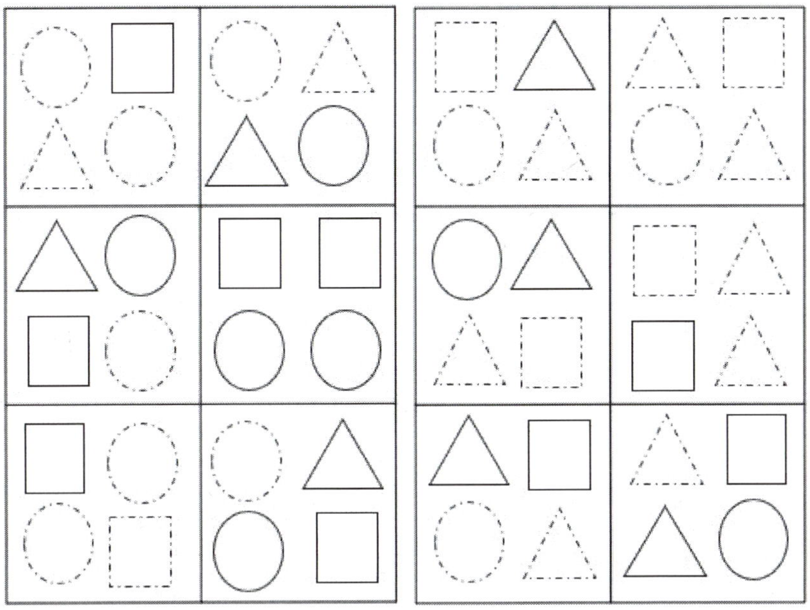

23 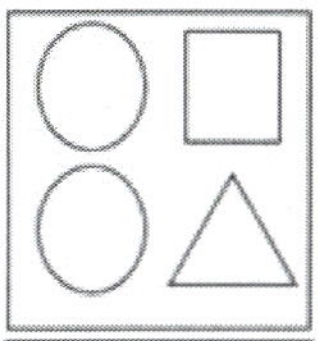
Set A
Set B
Neither

24 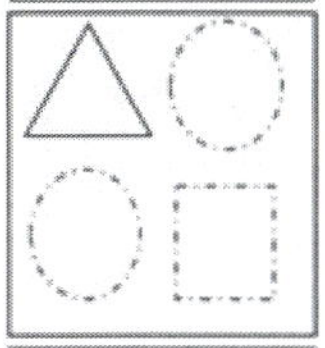
Set A
Set B
Neither

25 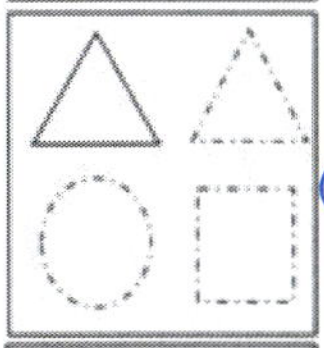
Set A
Set B
Neither

26 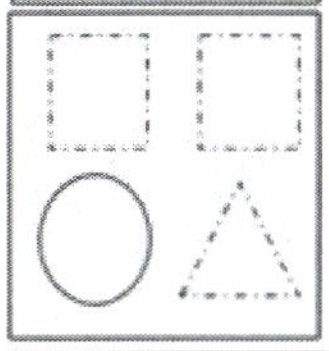
Set A
Set B
Neither

27 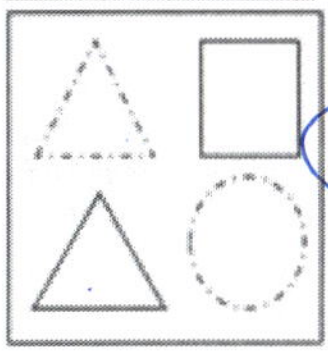
Set A
Set B
Neither

To which of the two sets do the following shapes belong?

Set A Set B

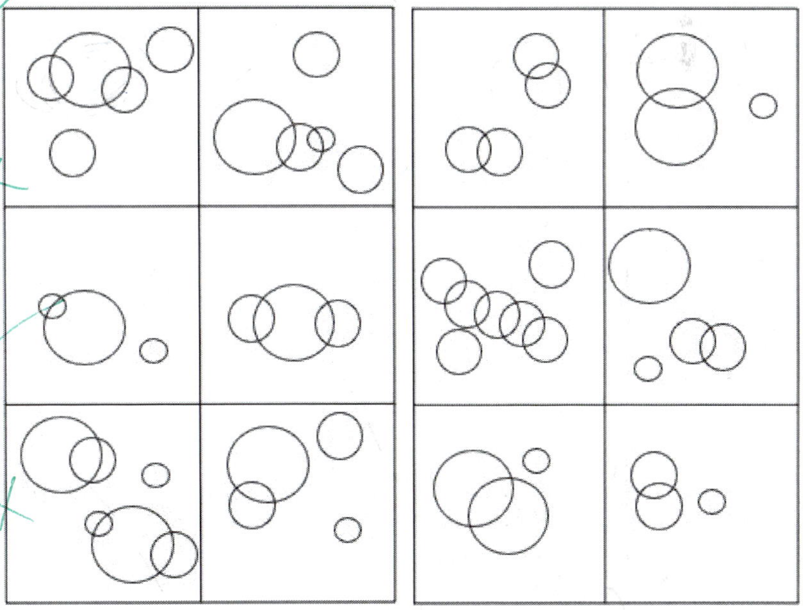

28 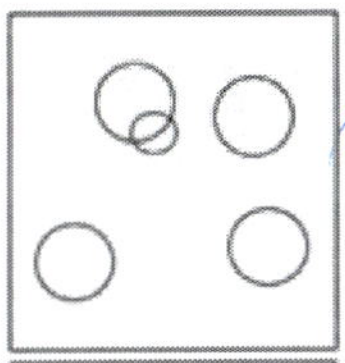
Set A
Set B
Neither

29 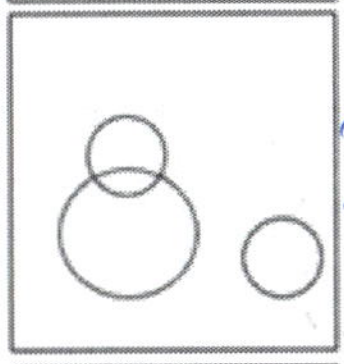
Set A
Set B
Neither

30 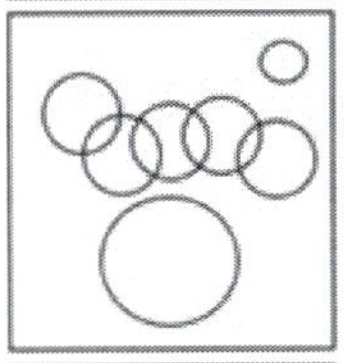
Set A
Set B
Neither

31 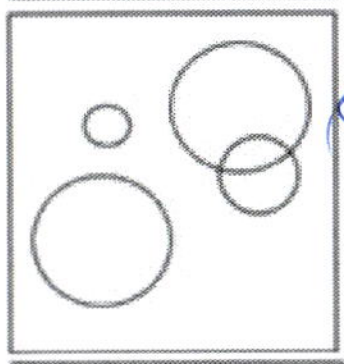
Set A
Set B
Neither

32 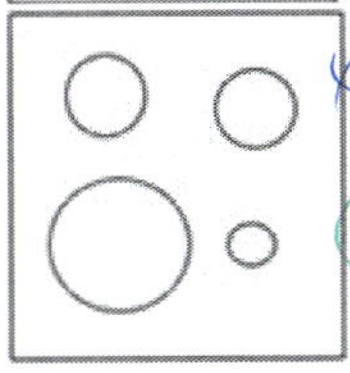
Set A
Set B
Neither

33 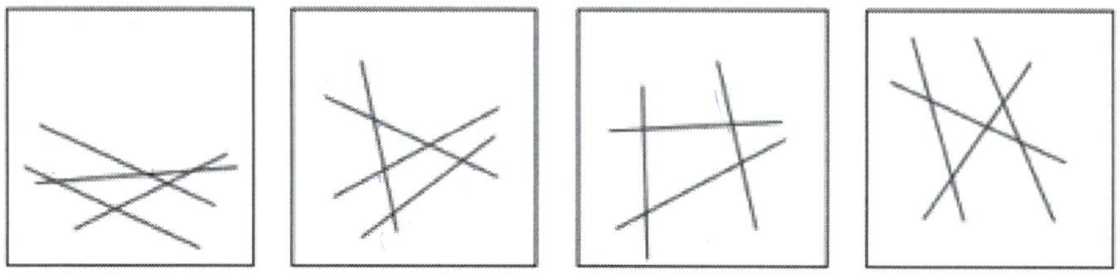

Which figure completes the series?

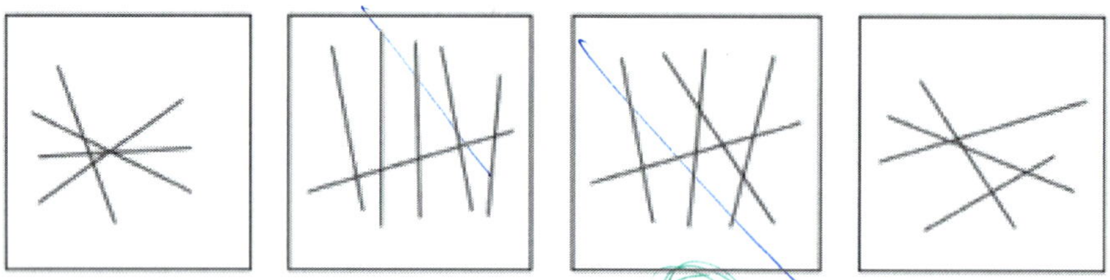

A B C D

34 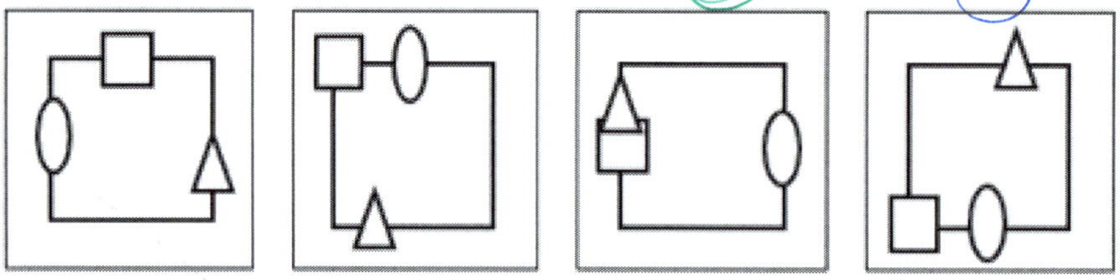

Which figure completes the series?

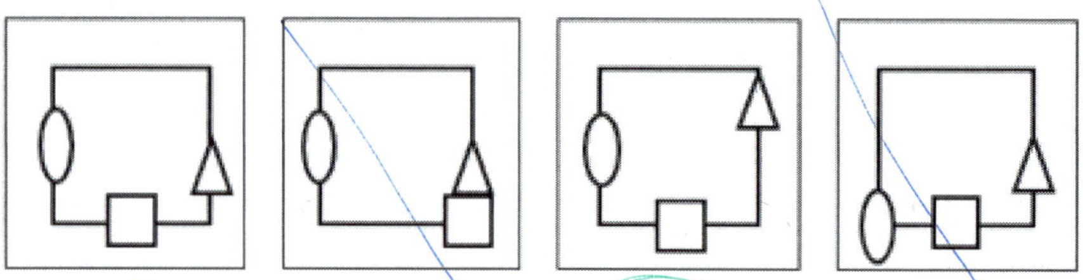

A B C D

35 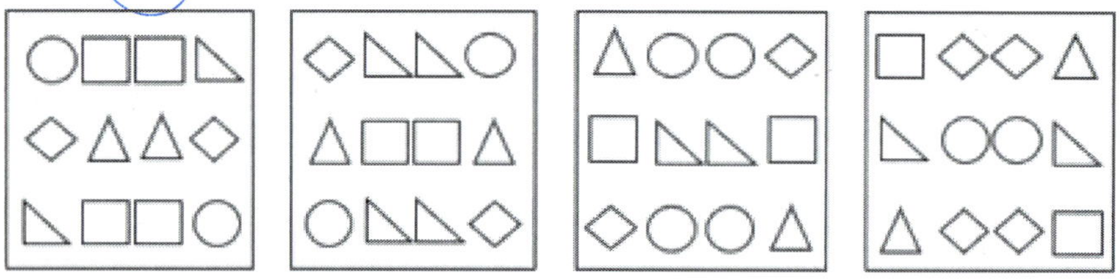

Which figure completes the series?

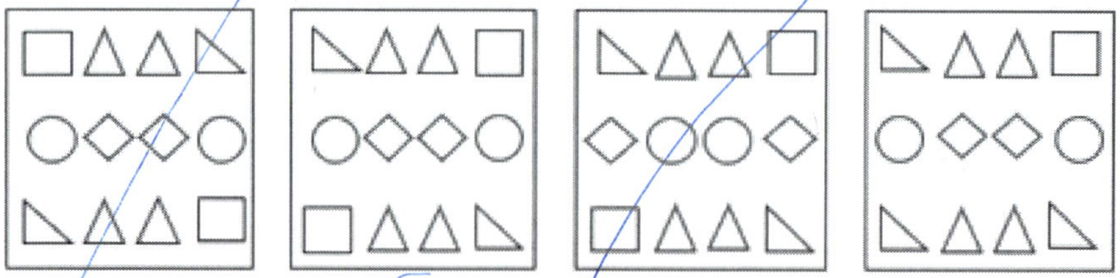

A B C D

Set A

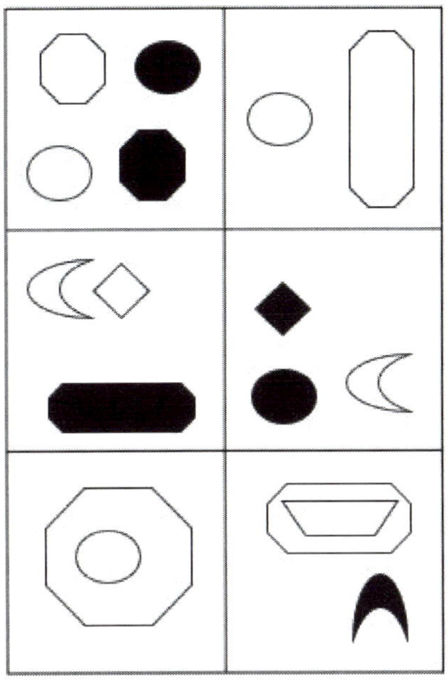

Set B

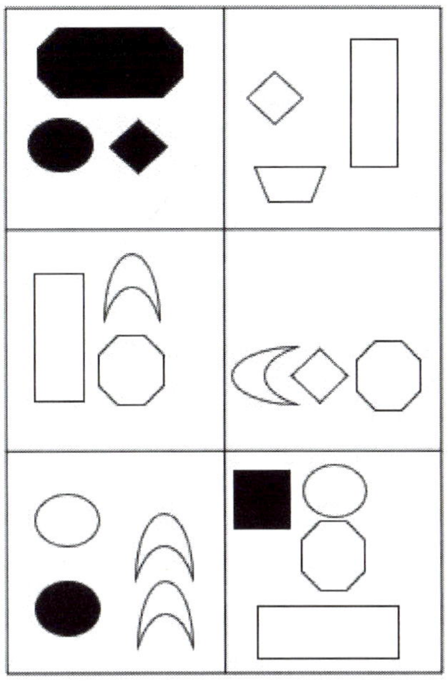

36 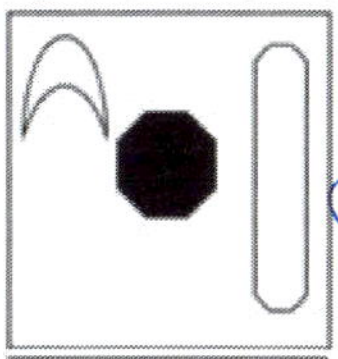
Set A
Set B
Neither

37 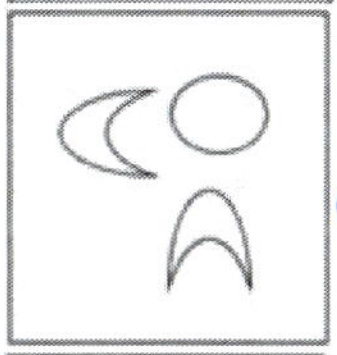
Set A
Set B
Neither

38 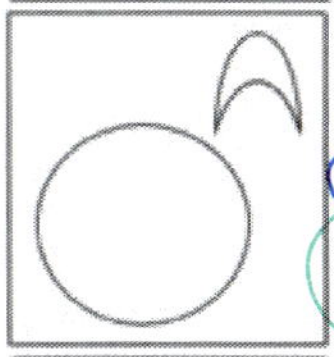
Set A
Set B
Neither

39 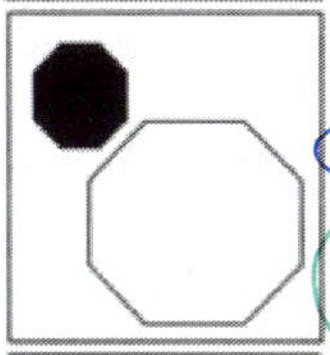
Set A
Set B
Neither

40 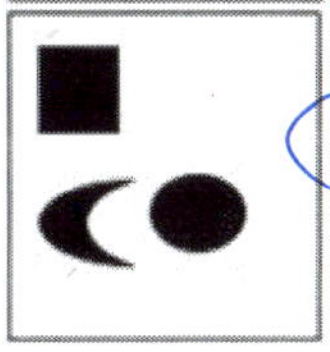
Set A
Set B
Neither

To which of the two sets do the following shapes belong?

Set A

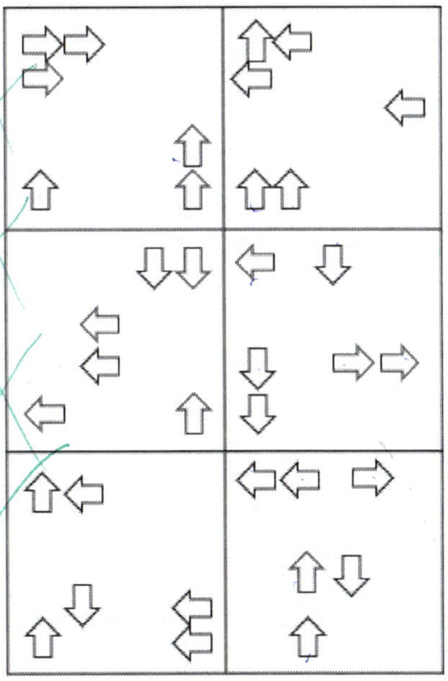

Set B

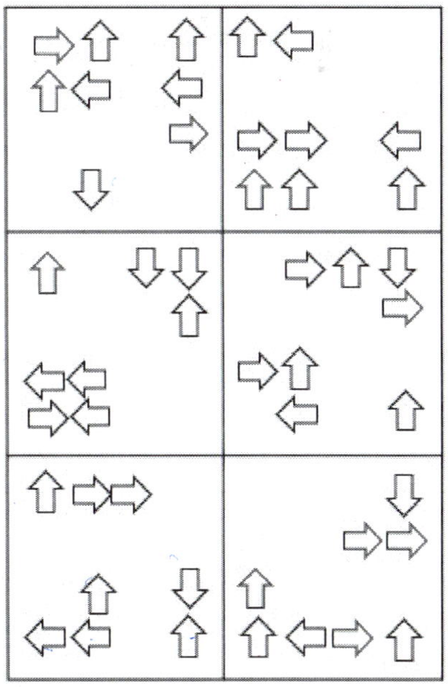

41 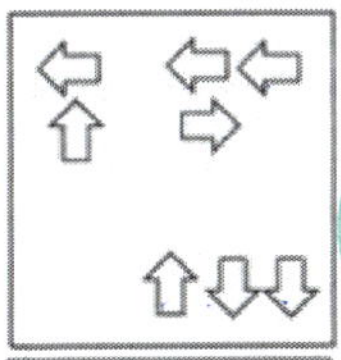
Set A
Set B
Neither

42 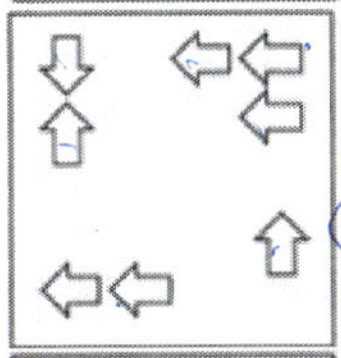
Set A
Set B
Neither

43 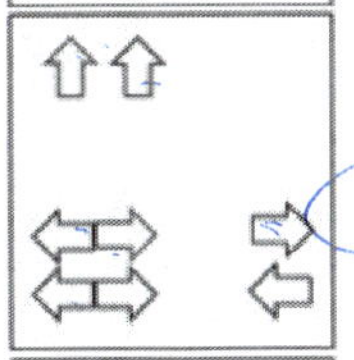
Set A
Set B
Neither

44 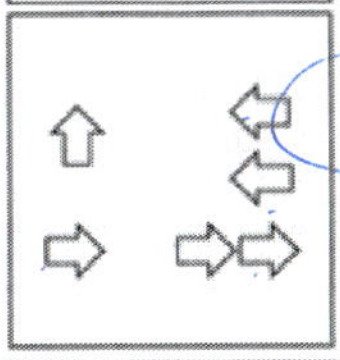
Set A
Set B
Neither

45 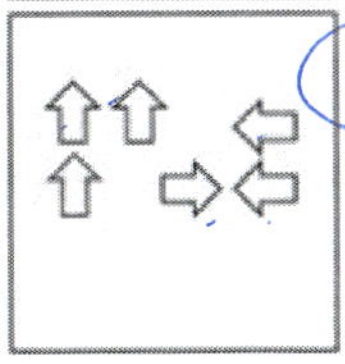
Set A
Set B
Neither

Set A

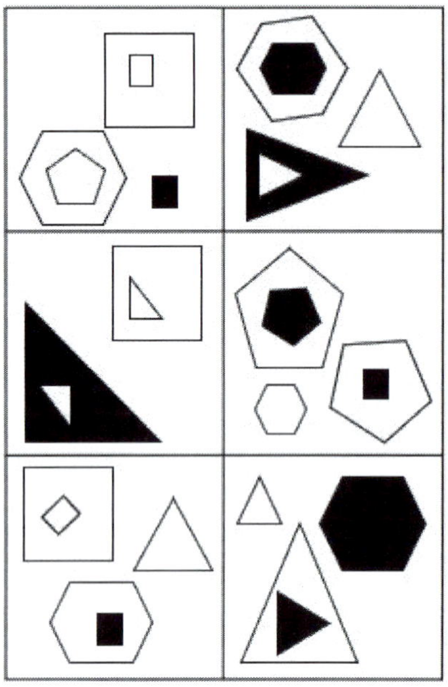

Set B

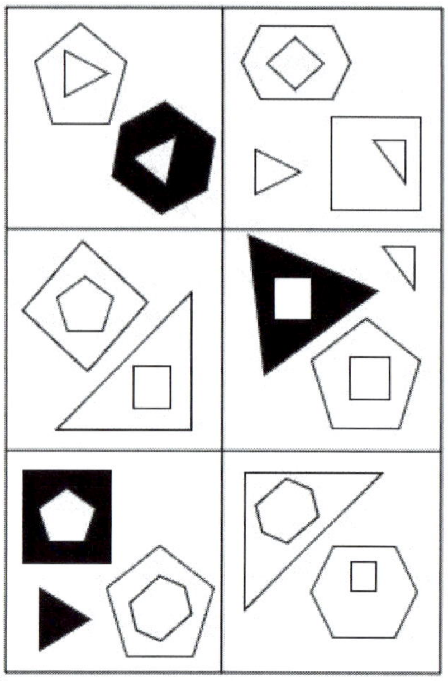

46
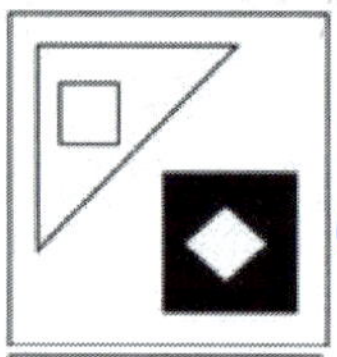
Set A
Set B
Neither

47
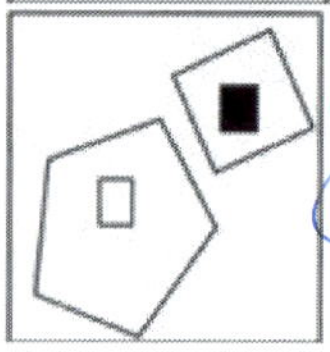
Set A
Set B
Neither

48
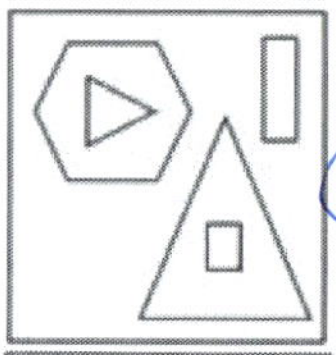
Set A
Set B
Neither

49
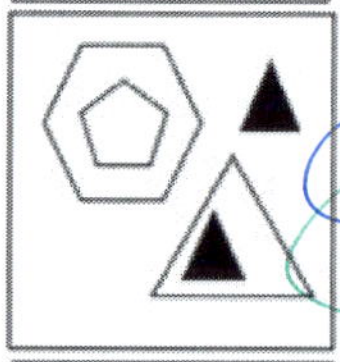
Set A
Set B
Neither

50
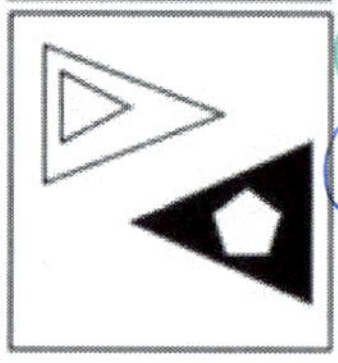
Set A
Set B
Neither

To which of the two sets do the following shapes belong?

Set A

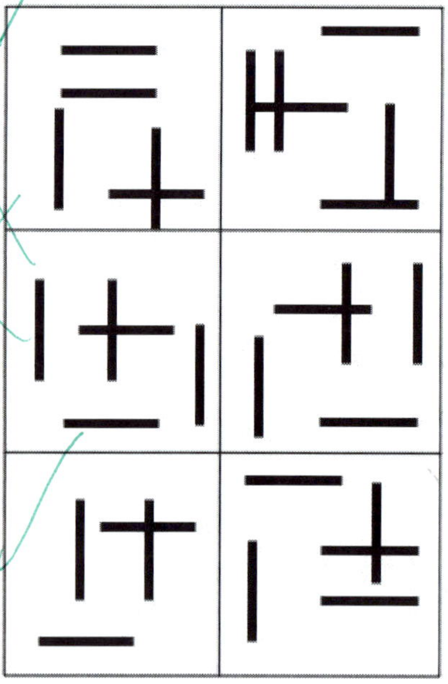

Set B

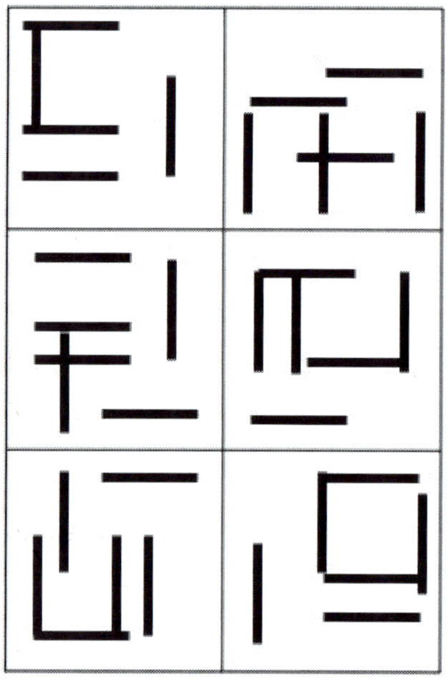

51
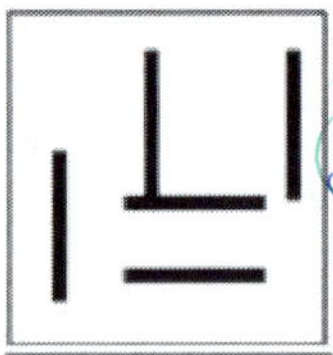
Set A
Set B
Neither

52
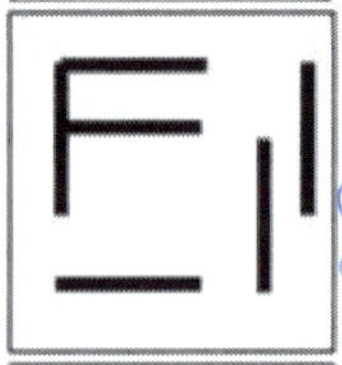
Set A
Set B
Neither

53
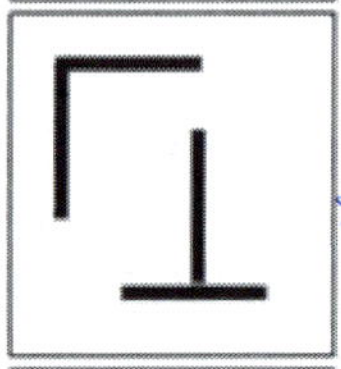
Set A
Set B
Neither

54
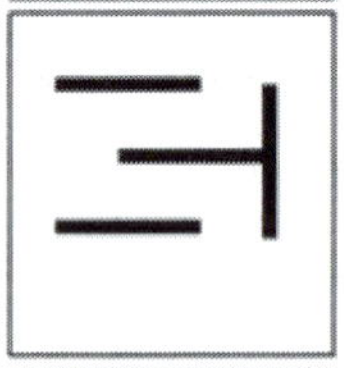
Set A
Set B
Neither

55
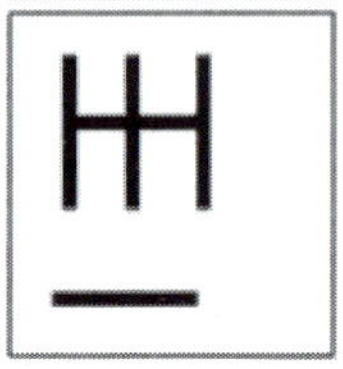
Set A
Set B
Neither

Full Mock Test 1 Situational Judgement (26 minutes for this section)

Hazel is working in a general surgery ward as part of her hospital placement. She has heard rumours that a fellow medical student, Sophia, is having a relationship with one of the surgical registrars. Hazel has noticed that Sophia always seems to get to observe operations that the registrar is involved with and feels that this will unfairly affect her end of placement report.

How appropriate are the following actions for Hazel?

1. Ask around on the ward whether the rumours are true

A. A very appropriate thing to do

B. Appropriate, but not ideal

C. Inappropriate, but not awful

D. A very inappropriate thing to do

2. Confront Sophia about the rumours

A. A very appropriate thing to do

B. Appropriate, but not ideal

C. Inappropriate, but not awful

D. A very inappropriate thing to do

3. Report her concerns to her clinical supervisor (the registrar's boss)

A. A very appropriate thing to do

B. Appropriate, but not ideal

C. Inappropriate, but not awful

D. A very inappropriate thing to do

4. Do nothing and hope she gets more opportunities on the next placement

A. A very appropriate thing to do

B. Appropriate, but not ideal

C. Inappropriate, but not awful

D. A very inappropriate thing to do

5. Speak to the registrar about getting more opportunities in surgery

A. A very appropriate thing to do

B. Appropriate, but not ideal

C. Inappropriate, but not awful

D. A very inappropriate thing to do

Christopher, a medical student, is working on an elderly care ward. He has been asked to carry out an audit on medical equipment used on the ward. Christopher finds that some equipment is missing. He is aware that a bank nurse, Imogen, has an elderly father who recently had a stroke and is almost certain that she has taken the equipment home to help him.

How appropriate are the following actions for Christopher?

6. Tell the senior nurse in charge that Imogen has taken the equipment.

A. A very appropriate thing to do

B. Appropriate, but not ideal

C. Inappropriate, but not awful

D. A very inappropriate thing to do

7. Cover up the fact that some equipment is missing in his report.

A. A very appropriate thing to do

B. Appropriate, but not ideal

C. Inappropriate, but not awful

D. A very inappropriate thing to do

8. Mention to the senior nurse in charge that Imogen should not be offered any more shifts.

A. A very appropriate thing to do

B. Appropriate, but not ideal

C. Inappropriate, but not awful

D. A very inappropriate thing to do

Amelia is in her first week helping on a ward. She notices that one of the doctors there appears to be neglecting minor health and safety rules.

How appropriate would the following courses of action be?

9. Assume the doctors involved know what they're doing better than she does and that she must have been mistaken.

A. A very appropriate thing to do

B. Appropriate, but not ideal

C. Inappropriate, but not awful

D. A very inappropriate thing to do

10. Assume that the rules being neglected must not be that important or may be optional.

A. A very appropriate thing to do

B. Appropriate, but not ideal

C. Inappropriate, but not awful

D. A very inappropriate thing to do

11. Mention her concerns to the doctor involved and ask why they didn't follow the rules.

A. A very appropriate thing to do

B. Appropriate, but not ideal

C. Inappropriate, but not awful

D. A very inappropriate thing to do

12. Mention her concerns to the head of the ward while keeping the doctor anonymous to check that she was correct in her concerns.

A. A very appropriate thing to do

B. Appropriate, but not ideal

C. Inappropriate, but not awful

D. A very inappropriate thing to do

13. Double check the health and safety rules she believes are being neglected after her placement to confirm that they have not been changed.

A. A very appropriate thing to do

B. Appropriate, but not ideal

C. Inappropriate, but not awful

D. A very inappropriate thing to do

14. Report the doctor involved for poor conduct.

A. A very appropriate thing to do

B. Appropriate, but not ideal

C. Inappropriate, but not awful

D. A very inappropriate thing to do

Nathan is on work experience shadowing a doctor around a ward. The doctor is called away and a distressed patient, mistaking Nathan for a doctor, approaches him to ask about their condition. Nathan believes he recognises the condition from reading he has been doing recently.

How appropriate would the following courses of action be?

15. Nathan uses the best of his medical knowledge to try to work out the patient's condition and tells them that

A. A very appropriate thing to do

B. Appropriate, but not ideal

C. Inappropriate, but not awful

D. A very inappropriate thing to do

16. Nathan explains that he is not qualified to help and leaves the patient.

A. A very appropriate thing to do

B. Appropriate, but not ideal

C. Inappropriate, but not awful

D. A very inappropriate thing to do

17. Nathan finds the doctor and asks them.

A. A very appropriate thing to do

B. Appropriate, but not ideal

C. Inappropriate, but not awful

D. A very inappropriate thing to do

18. Nathan explains that he is not qualified and so may not be accurate but reassures the patient that the doctor will answer their questions when they return.

A. A very appropriate thing to do

B. Appropriate, but not ideal

C. Inappropriate, but not awful

D. A very inappropriate thing to do

19. Nathan suggests that the patient sits down and wait for a doctor then find a nurse and points out that the patient appears to be distressed.

A. A very appropriate thing to do

B. Appropriate, but not ideal

C. Inappropriate, but not awful

D. A very inappropriate thing to do

20. Nathan pretends not to have heard the patient and avoids them.

A. A very appropriate thing to do

B. Appropriate, but not ideal

C. Inappropriate, but not awful

D. A very inappropriate thing to do

After a great deal of time and effort, Christos is struggling, to understand some of his course material and wants to find help.

How appropriate are the following methods for this situation?

21. Go online and find others' work to help him learn the course.

A. A very appropriate thing to do

B. Appropriate, but not ideal

C. Inappropriate, but not awful

D. A very inappropriate thing to do

22. Ask friends on the course for their notes so he can check for information he may have missed or find better ways of looking at things he doesn't understand.

A. A very appropriate thing to do

B. Appropriate, but not ideal

C. Inappropriate, but not awful

D. A very inappropriate thing to do

23. Ask his tutor to go through the sections he struggles with.

A. A very appropriate thing to do

B. Appropriate, but not ideal

C. Inappropriate, but not awful

D. A very inappropriate thing to do

24. Attempt to give himself more time to try to understand the material.

A. A very appropriate thing to do

B. Appropriate, but not ideal

C. Inappropriate, but not awful

D. A very inappropriate thing to do

25. Give up the course as he does not feel able to understand important information.

A. A very appropriate thing to do

B. Appropriate, but not ideal

C. Inappropriate, but not awful

D. A very inappropriate thing to do

Diya is worried about the health of one of his relatives. The relative frequently complains of blurred vision and other symptoms, asking to know what is wrong with them. Their GP however has informed them that it is not serious.

How appropriate are the following actions in the situation?

26. Recommend his relative sees their regular GP follows their advice.

A. A very appropriate thing to do

B. Appropriate, but not ideal

C. Inappropriate, but not awful

D. A very inappropriate thing to do

27. Recommend they see a different doctor at the same practice to get a second opinion.

A. A very appropriate thing to do

B. Appropriate, but not ideal

C. Inappropriate, but not awful

D. A very inappropriate thing to do

28. Attempt to use medical text books and the internet to help his relative diagnose what is wrong with them.

A. A very appropriate thing to do

B. Appropriate, but not ideal

C. Inappropriate, but not awful

D. A very inappropriate thing to do

29. Try to arrange a meeting with a doctor he trusts and knows to be an expert in eye conditions.

A. A very appropriate thing to do

B. Appropriate, but not ideal

C. Inappropriate, but not awful

D. A very inappropriate thing to do

30. Recommend his relative asks for a referral to the local hospital.

A. A very appropriate thing to do

B. Appropriate, but not ideal

C. Inappropriate, but not awful

D. A very inappropriate thing to do

Edward, a medical student, volunteers to help a family friend to move house. Later, his tutor suggests that, since he is struggling with his course, he attends a series of lectures and sessions designed to help with exam revision. Edward agrees, only to find that one of the sessions is on 'moving day'

How appropriate are the following actions in this situation?

31. Go to the session as Edward's medical course is more important than helping his friend.

A. A very appropriate thing to do

B. Appropriate, but not ideal

C. Inappropriate, but not awful

D. A very inappropriate thing to do

32. Help his friend, then catch up on what he missed from the session later with another student.

A. A very appropriate thing to do

B. Appropriate, but not ideal

C. Inappropriate, but not awful

D. A very inappropriate thing to do

33. Explain the problem to his friend and offer to help after the session.

A. A very appropriate thing to do

B. Appropriate, but not ideal

C. Inappropriate, but not awful

D. A very inappropriate thing to do

34. Persuade another student to go help his friend move while he goes to the support session.

A. A very appropriate thing to do

B. Appropriate, but not ideal

C. Inappropriate, but not awful

D. A very inappropriate thing to do

35. Explain the problem to his tutor and ask to see the notes for the session in advance so he can go over them in his own time.

A. A very appropriate thing to do

B. Appropriate, but not ideal

C. Inappropriate, but not awful

D. A very inappropriate thing to do

36. Pretend to forget one of the engagements and go to the other, then apologise later for forgetting.

A. A very appropriate thing to do

B. Appropriate, but not ideal

C. Inappropriate, but not awful

D. A very inappropriate thing to do

Freya, a medical student, does poorly in her exams and is informed that if she does not improve significantly she will have to drop out of the course. Due to complications that come up in her personal life, however, as she reaches her retake she feels even less prepared for her exam.

How appropriate are the following actions in this situation:

37. Give up, drop out of the course look for something else she can do that will help people without needing a medical degree.

A. A very appropriate thing to do

B. Appropriate, but not ideal

C. Inappropriate, but not awful

D. A very inappropriate thing to do

38. Explain her problems to her tutor and see if she can get the retake rescheduled, or at least get as much help as possible.

A. A very appropriate thing to do

B. Appropriate, but not ideal

C. Inappropriate, but not awful

D. A very inappropriate thing to do

39. Try regardless but prepare to apply for other courses as well as revising.

A. A very appropriate thing to do

B. Appropriate, but not ideal

C. Inappropriate, but not awful

D. A very inappropriate thing to do

40. Look into retaking her medical course again, maybe redoing a year at another university or the possibility of redoing the whole degree.

A. A very appropriate thing to do

B. Appropriate, but not ideal

C. Inappropriate, but not awful

D. A very inappropriate thing to do

41. Focus all her efforts on doing the exam and merely hope to score highly enough.

A. A very appropriate thing to do

B. Appropriate, but not ideal

C. Inappropriate, but not awful

D. A very inappropriate thing to do

Bernice does not feel prepared to take her end of year exams. She does not want to admit that she needs help at the risk of seeming incompetent and is consequently severely tempted to copy someone else's work for a presentation which will be assessed.

How important should the following criteria be in deciding what the Bernice should do?

42. How much time doing the work will take versus looking up someone else's work.

A. Very important

B. Important

C. Of minor importance

D. Not important at all

43. What is the 'right' thing to do.

A. Very important

B. Important

C. Of minor importance

D. Not important at all

44. How important the upcoming tests are to her future career.

A. Very important

B. Important

C. Of minor importance

D. Not important at all

45. Using someone else's material could be considered efficient revision.

A. Very important

B. Important

C. Of minor importance

D. Not important at all

46. How likely Bernice is to be caught.

A. Very important

B. Important

C. Of minor importance

D. Not important at all

47. The amount of spare time she is spending on things other than her course.

A. Very important

B. Important

C. Of minor importance

D. Not important at all

Olivia is studying dentistry. Her new best friend at university, Maggie, has just told her she is pregnant. She is considering having an abortion as she doesn't want her studies to be affected but she is unsure if she might regret it, either now or in the future, and wants Olivia's advice.

How important are the following to consider?

48. Olivia's own views on abortion.

A. Very important

B. Important

C. Of minor importance

D. Not important at all

49. How Maggie feels about motherhood.

A. Very important

B. Important

C. Of minor importance

D. Not important at all

50.Whether Maggie's family will be supportive of her.

A. Very important

B. Important

C. Of minor importance

D. Not important at all

51. The university is known to have not been supportive of other students in similar situations in the past.

A. Very important

B. Important

C. Of minor importance

D. Not important at all

52. The need to be supportive whatever Maggie's decision

A. Very important

B. Important

C. Of minor importance

D. Not important at all

Nigel, a junior doctor responds to an intercom request for medical assistance at a railway station. Upon arrival at the scene a very elderly doctor is already treating the patient. She says she hasn't practiced medicine in fifteen years.

How important is it for Nigel to consider the following?

53. Experience is very valuable in medicine so he should respect the older doctor's credentials

A. Very important

B. Important

C. Of minor importance

D. Not important at all

54. A newly qualified doctor may be more aware of current protocol and practice

A. Very important

B. Important

C. Of minor importance

D. Not important at all

55. Responding to an emergency call like this often causes unexpected challenges.

A. Very important

B. Important

C. Of minor importance

D. Not important at all

56. The patient would benefit from two doctors working together

A. Very important

B. Important

C. Of minor importance

D. Not important at all

57. An elderly doctor may have health issues connected to old age such as dementia or physical degeneration of some kind

A. Very important

B. Important

C. Of minor importance

D. Not important at all

Sam is studying dentistry. A new friend he has made at Uni, Tom, mentioned to him that he failed to disclose some motoring offences on background check. Sam feels uncomfortable about this and thinks he should tell someone, although he is not sure who.

How important are the following to consider?

58. If Sam reports Tom to the university, they may kick him off the course and this could end Tom's dreams of becoming a dentist.

A. Very important

B. Important

C. Of minor importance

D. Not important at all

59. If Sam reports Tom to the university and they don't kick him off the course, this will make things very awkward for the rest of Sam's studies as Tom will know it was Sam who reported him.

A. Very important

B. Important

C. Of minor importance

D. Not important at all

60. If Sam doesn't report Tom to the university, another student who may have got Tom's place has missed out on their opportunity to study there.

A. Very important

B. Important

C. Of minor importance

D. Not important at all

61. Motoring offences have nothing to do with Tom's ability to practice as a dentist.

A. Very important

B. Important

C. Of minor importance

D. Not important at all

Sharon is a final year medical student and is attending a family event. Two of her cousins have young babies and are discussing the MMR injection. One of the cousins is adamant that her son will not have the injection because it 'causes autism' whereas the other cousin says that the injection is perfectly safe and that it's not safe to leave your children unprotected. The discussion becomes quite heated and they invite Sharon to give her opinion.

How important is it for Sharon to consider the following?

62. The study that showed the MMR 'causes autism' has been thoroughly discredited

A. Very important

B. Important

C. Of minor importance

D. Not important at all

63. Parents have the right to make health care decisions for their children, as they see fit.

A. Very important

B. Important

C. Of minor importance

D. Not important at all

64. Sharon is not a qualified doctor so isn't in a position to offer an opinion

A. Very important

B. Important

C. Of minor importance

D. Not important at all

65. Once a discussion becomes 'heated' it's best to leave it in the interests of family harmony.

A. Very important

B. Important

C. Of minor importance

D. Not important at all

Pearl is a newly qualified doctor working on an elderly care ward. One of her patients, who has extensive and complex issues, has a procedure the following week about which she is very anxious. She asks if Pearl could go with her as she says she has never felt as at ease with any other doctor. Pearl is supposed to be on annual leave the following week but is considering coming into work just for that one day.

How important is it for Pearl to consider the following?

66. It is a great compliment that this patient feels so confident with her

A. Very important

B. Important

C. Of minor importance

D. Not important at all

67. Doctors have a special responsibility and should sometimes be prepared to sacrifice aspects of their own lives to help their patients

A. Very important

B. Important

C. Of minor importance

D. Not important at all

68. The patient will receive good care from any of the staff working on the ward

A. Very important

B. Important

C. Of minor importance

D. Not important at all

69. Annual leave is a crucial part of Pearl being the best doctor she can be

A. Very important

B. Important

C. Of minor importance

D. Not important at all

Full Mock Test 1 Answers

1. The correct answer is B. **A s**lower shutter speed gives a longer exposure
The slower shutter speed means the lens is open longer, therefore increasing the exposure of the film to the light. Paragraph 2 states that exposure is referred to as shutter speed, therefore the slower shutter speed means a longer exposure.

2. The correct answer is D. 16
Going up 'one stop' means using lower f-stop numbers. This doubles the amount of light reaching the film. This means to decrease the amount of light reaching the film you must increase the f-stop numbers. Therefore the answer is 16.

3. The correct answer is B. Slow shutter speed, short focal length, smaller f-number
A slow shutter speed allows more light into the lens (paragraph 2), as does a short focal length lens (paragraph 3) and smaller f-numbers increase the amount of light into the lens (paragraph 5)

4. The correct answer is C. Doubling the f-number halves the amount of light that reaches the film
Doubling the f-number does not half the amount of light reaching the film. Although moving up an f-number will halve the amount of light reaching the film, the f-number itself is not doubled to achieve this effect. The text states- 'If the f-number is decreased by a factor of the square-root of 2, the aperture diameter is increased by the same factor, and its area is increased by a factor of 2'

5. The correct answer is C. Cyclones form over land mass
The second paragraph states that 'they develop over large bodies of warm water', therefore they cannot form over land mass.

6. The correct answer is A. Tropical cyclones help to maintain a relatively stable and warm temperature worldwide
The final sentence states that 'they also carry heat energy away from the tropics making them an important part of global atmospheric circulation'.

7. The correct answer is B. Water from the ocean evaporates, when this saturated air reaches the colder atmosphere the water vapour condenses
As the first paragraph states cyclones form 'when water evaporated from the ocean is released as the saturated air rises, resulting in condensation of water vapor contained in the moist air'. The saturated air reaches a point where the temperature is cooler and the water in the air condenses.

8. The correct answer is C. Cyclones can cause devastation for many populations
It is not only coastal populations that are affected by cyclones, inland regions can be affected by flood waters (paragraph 2) and the second last sentence states that cyclones can relieve drought conditions so not all the effects of cyclones are negative.

9. The correct answer is A. True. Bob Dylan was born Robert Zimmerman and is a musician.

10. The correct answer is B. False. Robert Zimmerman was born in 1941.

11. The correct answer is C. Can't tell. Although Bob Dylan's most celebrated works date from the 1960s, it is unclear as to how popular he was prior to the 1960s.

12. The correct answer is A. True. Bob Dylan has been touring steadily since the late 1980s i.e. since his forties. There was no mention of the end of touring and therefore, according to the text, Bob Dylan toured in his fifties.

13. The correct answer is A. True. The B-17 is a four-engine heavy bomber aircraft.

14. The correct answer is C. Can't tell. Although the B-17s were developed by Boeing for the United States Army Air Corps, there is no mention of where the aircrafts were actually built.

15. The correct answer is C. Can't tell. There is no mention of World War I so it is not possible to state who bombed whom during that war.

16. The correct answer is A. True. The United States Eighth and Fifteenth Air Forces were based in England and Italy, respectively.

17. The correct answer is B. 50% of infections are fatal if left untreated
The passage describes how only about 1 in 10 (10%) of infections lead to active disease, of which 50% will kill if left untreated. Option A is incorrect mycobacterium tuberculosis is described as being the 'usual' culprit. Option C is incorrect as the text states that "In 2007, there were an estimated 13.7 million chronic active cases globally". Option D is incorrect as the need for blood tests to detect latent TB is described in the text.

18. The correct answer is C. Diagnosis of latent TB relies on the tuberculin skin test (TST) and/or blood tests
This statement is stated in the passage. Option A is incorrect as the spread of tuberculosis through human contact is discussed but not through contact with faeces. Option B is incorrect as the absolute number of tuberculosis cases has been decreasing since 2006. Option D is incorrect as one third of the world's population is thought to be infected with M. tuberculosis.

19. The correct answer is B. Treatment of TB will become more problematic due to antibiotic resistance
Antibiotic resistance is described in the text as a 'growing problem'. Option A is incorrect as the absolute numbers of TB are described as falling. Option C is incorrect as the information about the changing proportion

of infected people implies that it will rise given that new infections are equal to 1% population pa. Option D is incorrect as there is nothing in the text about increasing HIV prevalence, merely high rates.

20. The correct answer is A. More than half of the population of Asia and Africa test positive in tuberculin tests About 80% of the population in many Asian and African countries tests positive in tuberculin tests - not necessarily all of Africa and Asia. Option B is incorrect as "Infection of other organs causes a wide range of symptoms". Option C is incorrect as "Microscopic examination and microbiological culture of body fluids can also diagnose active tuberculosis" Option D is incorrect as the first paragraph states that tuberculosis used to be known as phthisis pulmonalis.

21. The correct answer is C. Can't tell. The reserve status of the Everglades is neither confirmed nor denied.

22. The correct answer is A. True. The geography (and the ecology) of the Everglades involves everything affecting its natural environment in southern Florida.

23. The correct answer is A True. Before drainage, the Everglades used to be an interwoven mesh of marshes and prairies.

24. The correct answer is C. Can't tell. Although Marjory Stoneman Douglas wrote her definitive description of the Everglades region in 1947 it does not necessarily follow that she lived in the region at that time.

25. The correct answer is D. The world population is more than 7 billion people
We know that the European population is up to 739 million and comprises 11% of the world population. This places the world population under 7 billion. Option A is incorrect as the passage states, "The Industrial Revolution, which began in Great Britain around the end of the 18th century, gave rise to radical economic" growth. Option B is true as we know from the text that the Mediterranean Sea is the southern border of Europe and hence Europe is to the north of it. Option C is incorrect as, "During the Cold War, Europe was divided along the Iron Curtain between NATO in the west and the Warsaw Pact in the east".

26. The correct answer is B. Europe is a not a continent in a physical geographical sense
This is inferred by the description of the continent and the 'general' acceptance of borders. The borders are described as 'arbitrary' and the incorporation of cultural and political elements, rather than strict geophysical factors, is stressed. Option A is incorrect as the EU is clearly distinct from the Schengen Area, where border controls have been abolished. Simple calculations make option C very unlikely given that Europe has 11% of the world's population but less than 7% of the land area. Option D cannot be shown and seems unlikely given that ancient Greece and ancient Rome are described as the birthplace of Western culture.

27. The correct answer is A Europe has growing influence
The text says that the EU has growing influence over its member states but also that since the mid-20th century the US and Soviet Union took prominence. Option B is true as described in the text - the Americas, most of Africa, Oceania and large portions of Asia constitute most of the world. The industrial revolution began in Great Britain which is part of Europe (option C). Option D can be shown by the description of the Iron Curtain dividing the continent.

28. The correct answer is C. Africa is home to more than 11% of the world's population
This must be true as we know Africa to have a larger population than Europe and Europe houses 11% of the world's population. Option A is incorrect as Asia is another continent discussed in the passage not a country in Europe. Option B is incorrect as Europe is described as divided from Asia by watershed divides. Option D is incorrect as Europe as a continent covers 2% of the Earth's surface, 6.8% of the land area.

29. The correct answer is B. Tolerance is associated with long term use of a drug
The last paragraph states that tolerance 'may occur with chronic administration of a drug'

30. The correct answer is B. Occasional or recreational users of illegal drugs would not be classified as drug misusers
The first paragraph states 'The term drug misuse is applied to any drug-taking which harms or threatens to harm the physical or mental health of an individual, or other individuals, or which is illegal'. Even taking a drug once that could cause harm means that the user could be classified into the category of 'drug misuser'

31. The correct answer is B. Some people are more likely to become dependent than others
Paragraph 3 states 'dependence depends on many factors, including the type of drug, the route of administration, the pattern of drug taking and the individual' implying that some individuals are more likely to become dependent than others.

32. The correct answer is C. Tolerance requires a decrease in the frequency or dose of the drug

33. The correct answer is C. Rescuing a kidnapped princess
The text states that episodes tend to feature the characters doing 'everyday activities'.

34. The correct answer is A. Riding bikes and travelling in cars
We know that the first two series showed the characters not wearing seatbelts and cycle helmets necessitating a reanimation. The other activities are cited or likely but we cannot know they occurred within the first two series.

35. The correct answer is C. All animals maintain some characteristics of their species
The continuation of some species behaviour (animal snorting, food choices) is described in the text. Options A and B are anthropomorphic qualities which are cited as not happening in the text. Option D seems true given that Peppa Pig is alliterative and Tiddles the Tortoise and Polly Parrot are also alliterative however Peppa's younger brother is called George which means that his name is not alliterative.

36. The correct answer is B. Peppa Pig was used to promote services for young children given her wide appeal. Although this is not expressly cited in the text, it is the most likely of all of the options. There is no suggestion that Peppa appeared in any political manifesto at any point and the event which she specifically did not attend was a launch. The political leanings of the makers of the programme cannot be assessed or guessed (option C). Similarly, there is no suggestion that Peppa 'switched allegiances' (option D)

37. The correct answer is C. The first use of radar was for marine life surveillance
The text states "The first use of radar was for military purposes: to locate air, ground and sea targets". Option A is incorrect as the passage states radar was used during World War II and that the term 'radar' was coined in 1940. Option B is incorrect as this statement can be found in the passage. Option D is incorrect as "Aircraft can land in fog at airports equipped with radar-assisted ground-controlled approach systems".

38. The correct answer is D. Satellite detection.
The modern uses stated in the passage are highly diverse, including air traffic control; ocean surveillance systems, and meteorological precipitation monitoring, but satellite detection is not included.

39. The correct answer is C. Both use the electromagnetic spectrum
Option C is the only option stated as a similarity within the text. Radar uses radio waves whilst lidar uses visible light (option A), There is no information about the uses of lidar so options B and D cannot be confirmed or otherwise.

40. The correct answer is A. Radio waves can travel through air, matter and vacuum
The passage doesn't directly state this but the use of radar in both the air, space (vacuum) and ground penetration are all cited. Option B is incorrect as radar is an objection-detection system. Option C is incorrect as the passage states that the position of an object can be known if its bearing and range are detected. Option

D is incorrect as the passage states radars is used to forecast and watch weather so the radio waves used must detect the different conditions.

41. The correct answer is A. True. Joseph Smith became chief designer after the death of R. J. Mitchell in 1937.

42. The correct answer is B. False. The Spitfire was produced in greater numbers than any other British aircraft, but during the Battle of Britain more Hurricanes were in use.

43. The correct answer is A. True. "It was built in many different variants with four different types of engine and several wing configurations."

44. The correct answer is C. Can't tell. It was used as a fighter over Germany but not necessarily as a bomber.

1.

This college has enough space to fully deliver this programme There are 8 classrooms which can hold 4 classes each day, so 20 per week. A total of 160 hours of potential lesson space. Each course needs 5 hours per week and there are 10 courses, so 50 hours a week.	Yes
The college could treble the number of courses they offer and still be able to schedule the classes	Yes
Each course has a daily class of 1 hour Each course needs 5 hours per week, not necessarily 1 per day	No
The college must employ at least 10 teachers It is possible that some teachers would be able to teach more than one course	No
The college could decommission half of their classrooms without making timetabling impossible Even with only 4 classrooms the college would have up to 80 hours of classroom space to accommodate 50 hours of lesson time	Yes

2.

Sue could empty all of the chocolates into 2 tubs She has 2.5 tubs worth of chocolate	No
All of the boxes of biscuits have been opened The chocolate biscuits from all three boxes have been eaten	Yes
Sue could put all of the biscuits in the biscuit tin We don't know how big the biscuit tin is nor how many biscuits the boxes still contain	No
There are at least three colours of flower on display after Sue finishes The carnations could have been pink and yellow meaning only pink and yellow flowers would be on display	No
More than one patient gave the nurses this loot The opening line described grateful patients - plural	Yes

3.

Soft fruit yields were 50% higher The information said 'up to' 50% higher	No
The rain in the winter had no impact on the crop yield of soft fruits We don't have information about the impact of winter rains	No

The relationship with above average rain and above average yields is directly proportional No

Any 'above average' rain can increase crop yields by up to 50%

In a dry year the crop yields will be below average No
A dry year may yield average crop yields

Average rainfall in spring will result in average crop yields Yes

4.

Some legal registration certificates for cars are issued electronically No
We know that not all legal registration certificates are for cars and only some are issued electronically.
No cars have legal registration certificates which cost £20 Yes
All cars have this certificate but no certificates cost £20

Legal registration certificates which are not for cars cost £20 No
No legal registration certificates cost £20

Electronically issued certificates make up a proportion of certificate issues Yes
Some are issued electronically, so others must be issued otherwise

Legal registration certificates are necessary for other vehicles as well as cars No
We don't know what the non-car certificates are for

5. The correct answer is C. Matthew worked the longest
We know that Psychology took the longest (2.5 hours) so Chemistry - taking an hour longer than History - must have taken 2 hours whilst History took 1 hour. Biology must therefore have taken 1.5 hours. Beatrice worked the second longest so must be doing Chemistry, meaning Benjamin must have worked 1.5 hours and Joel worked 1 hour. Therefore, Matthew must have worked on Psychology and worked the longest.

6. The correct answer is B. Grace has her activity on Wednesday
Grace must have her class on a Wednesday - we know it isn't Monday or Tuesday. Jacob has his activity on a Thursday, and the Friday activity is gymnastics and we know Grace does music.

7. The correct answer is C. The drinks arrived after the salad
We know the drinks didn't come first or last from points one or two. The rice came immediately after the drinks so must have arrived at 7.00 and the drinks must have arrived at 6.55. The chicken arrived at 7.05 so the salad must have arrived at 6.50.

8. The correct answer is C. Tom sits between Alex and Ellen
We know that seats d and e are taken by John and Vivienne, but we don't know which one is in which seat. When we place Alex in seat c, and we know Ben must have a centre side seat (b or g) as he is between two people - neither of whom is John or Vivienne - we know that Ellen and Lydia must have seats a and f and therefore Ben must be sitting in seat g. Ellen must be in seat a and Tom must be in seat b.

9. The correct answer is C. Carlisle University got a new facility thanks to Intergalactic
The information is insufficient to complete the table.
Andover, Edward and Farley, A multimedia suite OR a swimming pool
Bridlington, Harlon and Son, A multimedia suite OR a swimming pool
Carlisle, InterGalactic, theatre
Doncaster, General Engineering, research lab

10. The correct answer is B. The text states that there are links between the study of maths and music and the option suggests that even though the disciplines are seemingly unrelated there is scope for inspiration and broader horizons if both are studied together.
Option A adds a new factor - that of relaxation and refreshment - to the suggestion which is unwarranted based on the text. Option C dismisses music as merely creative and suggests it's a distraction rather than engaging with the point made in the text. Option D doesn't address any possible link between music and maths and dismisses the proposition without argument.

11. The correct answer is D. No - there is no way to make a fair judgement
The text shows that there is ambiguity in both the definition of intelligence and in the test process. Option D is the only response to the proposition which doesn't place too much confidence in the tests given.

12. The correct answer is B. Yes – but efforts must be made to minimise the risk to health and the environment
Option A introduces the notion of poor people which is not mentioned at all in the initial argument
Option C draws the unreasonable conclusion that if business owners and investors like it then it must be bad
Option D makes an invalid comparison between the problems solved vs the problems created.

13. The correct answer is C. No – foreign aid can do some good which is better than doing no good
The proposition is solely about how foreign aid is not a quick or complete solution for national and international problems and this is the only option that alludes to this.

14. The correct answer is D. Triangle
The second equation shows that a square is equal to a crescent plus a triangle. The third euqation shows that a triangle is half of a crescent.
The incomplete equation is like the first one, but we have three squares. As a square is worth more than a crescent the missing shape must be worth less than a crescent – hence a triangle.
15. The correct answer is C. No – nicotine itself may be a cancer-causing chemical so they are still dangerous
This is the only statement which directly addresses the issue in the original proposition.
Statement A – the antisocial or nasty smelling aspect of tobacco smoking is not part of the original proposition.
Statement B – there is no mention of the economics of the change
Statement D – introduces an entirely new point and doesn't engage with the proposition at all.

16. The correct answer is C. No – there are some products that people will always want to see before purchase so there will always be some high street shops
This is the only statement which addresses the proposition's assertion that there will be an eventual death of real shops.
Statement A – no reference is made to the levels of increase in online shopping and the statement is vague. It doesn't address the likely trends in real shops.
Statement B – introduces the idea that price is the main determinant rather than other factors such as convenience or choice
Statement D – introduces an entirely new concept.

17.

The family owned both rabbits at the same time	No
The description of the garden coop says it held rabbits (plural) but they may have lived there consecutively rather than concurrently.	
Two hamsters died of natural causes	No
We know that 2 of the hamsters died due to the family cat but don't know how the other 2 left the household.	
The chickens and the rabbits lived with the family at the same time	No
The text tells us that the rabbits lived in the garden coup before the chickens arrived.	
The most pets the Smiths could have owned at once is 11	Yes
The most animals which could have all lived in the household at the same time is	

3 chickens, 4 hamsters, 3 cats, 1 goldfish
The family owned 2 rabbits and a goldfish at one time No
There is no information about when the goldfish lived in the household and if it overlapped with any other pets

18. The correct answer is D. No – it is difficult to assess the needs of any household and these restrictions may cause unintended hardship
This statement addresses the proposition and the restrictions suggested within.
Statement A and B are somewhat judgemental
Statement C – introduces the idea of government tracking, which is not warranted by the proposition

19. The correct answer is C. There are a total of 147 non-insects represented in the chart
There is actually 57 + 56 + 34 + 15 = 162
A. There are 58 + 68 black insects represented in the chart
B. The tropical parasites rectangle does not overlap at all with the red bugs diamond
D. The oval shows us that there are 68 black ants, 39 red ants and 65 other ants

20. The correct answer is B. Out of all the novels that feature winged creatures, just over 10% also feature creatures which are deadly, malevolent and mythical.
A. All novels with malevolent creatures in also contain winged creatures. False
B. Out of all the novels that feature winged creatures, just over 10% also feature creatures which are deadly, malevolent and mythical. True – total winged – 66 and 7 is 10.60 % of 66
C. Novels with malevolent and mythical creatures (25) are equal to those that feature deadly creatures. False
D. Novels with mythical, deadly, and malevolent creatures (5) are equal to novels with mythical, deadly, malevolent and winged creatures (7). False

21. The correct answer is B. David doesn't work at the delivery company
David cannot earn the most. Eleanor works at the shop and can't earn the least. The factory pays £7.00 per hour but not to Georgina. Frank works at either the factory or the delivery company. The shop worker must earn £8.00 as we know the factory worker earns £7.00.
Eleanor works at the shop for £8.00 per hour
David earns £7.50 per hour so can't work at the factory or the delivery firm. Therefore, he must work at cinema

22. The correct answer is C. 21
The text tells us that 14 tables were selling bric-a-brac so we can surmise that the question mark in the diamond shape should be a 3.
There are 30 tables in all; therefore, the other question mark represents a 4.

23. The correct answer is C.
Venn diagram A does not add up to 40 and 60.
Venn diagram B does not add up to 40 and 60.
Venn diagram D has ten too few cats.

24. The correct answer is C. 67
Chemistry and Biology – 15
Chemistry and Physics – 14
Chemistry and Maths – 7
Biology and Physics – 4
Biology and Maths – 7
Physics and Maths – 20

25. The correct answer is B. Mona Patel 0776955555, monapatel456@hotmail.com
    The triangle is email and the circle a mobile phone number. Adam Bird (option D) also has a landline number.

26. The correct answer is D. No, choosing a blue pair both times is less likely than 0.07
The correct probability is 0.02 or 1/49. As the chosen pair of socks is replaced before the next draw the events are independent. The probability of choosing a blue pair the first time is 1/7; the probability of choosing a blue pair the second time is also 1/7. The probability of choosing a blue pair both times is 1/7 x 1/7 = 1/49 = 0.02

27. The correct answer is C. No - because two babies have already been born
Two of the babies have already been born meaning that the 'odds' of all five being boys are dramatically slashed from the 1/32 which would have been the case at the outset. Whilst A and B (and D) are all technically correct none of them consider that the unknowns in this scenario are only 3/5 cases.

28. The correct answer is A. Yes, this group and the group that own both are mutually exclusive
It is not possible for a child to simultaneously own both a laptop and a phone and own only a laptop or a phone. To calculate the probability of owning either, add the probability of owning a laptop to the probability of owning a phone and subtract the probability of owning both.
0.28 + 0.76 – 0.21 = 0.83

29. The correct answer is D. No, their chance of winning or drawing is more than 70%
The previous form statistics would look like this:
United win 50/80 or 62.5%
City win 20/80 or 25% (10% increase of this takes it to 27.5%)
Draw 10/80 or 12.5%

If the illnesses in the United side increase their chances of a loss by 10% then the statistics would look like this:
United win 65%
(City win) United loss 27.5%
Draw 12.5%

1. The correct answer is C. £3814.56
Mrs Singh got 20% off so she paid 80% of £4768.20 which is 4768.20 × 0.8 = 3,814.56

2. The correct answer is E. £12.78
Total takings were £1764.23 138 customers were served. Average spend is £1764.23/138 = 12.784 or £12.78

3. The correct answer is A. £1058.54 - £1,764.23 × 0.6 = 1058.538 or £1058.54

4. The correct answer is B. £44102.20
Loan £125,000 - costs + takings
Costs were a total of £82,662.03. (£78,458.47 + £3,814.56 +£389)
Takings were £1,764.23
£125,000 - £82,662.03 + £1,764.23

5. The correct answer is D. Event C (motorbike) - A = 0.073; B = 0.020; C = 0.7; D = 0.271; E = 0.003

6. The correct answer is A. 0.020 - 0.073 × 0.271 = 0.019783 = 0.020

7. The correct answer is C. 353/490 - 1/49 + 7/10 = 10/490 + 343/490 = 353/490

8. The correct answer is C. 0.204
Event C AND (Event D OR Event B) = 0.7 AND (0.271 OR 0.020) = 0.7 × (0.271 + 0.020) = 0.2037 = 0.204

9. The correct answer is D. £43.81
The total weekly income for the household is £99.15 + £150.00 + £33.70 +£20.96 + £14.27 = £318.08. The total weekly expenditure for the household is £150.00 + £14.27 + £70.00 + £40.00 = £274.27. The disposable income is the total income less the total expenditure = £318.08 - £274.27 = £43.81

10. The correct answer is B. 12/25
A 14% reduction in their housing benefit equals a reduction of £150 * 0.14 = £21. The family's disposable income is £43.81. The reduction in income is £21 / £43.81 = 0.47934. The fraction closest to this is 12 / 25 = 0.48

11. The correct answer is D. £40.43
Because the child leaves, the household income drops by £13.40 + £10.48 = £23.88. However, the household expenditure also drops by (£70.00 * 0.15) + (£40.00 * 0.25) = £20.50. This means the weekly disposable income is now (£318.08 - £23.88) – (£274.27 - £20.50) = £40.43

12. The correct answer is E. 60 weeks
12% of the household disposable income of £43.81 = 43.81 * 0.12 = £5.26. To save up £315 will take 315 / 5.26 = 59.92 weeks = 60 weeks of saving

13. The correct answer is B. 3.06 AU - 457 743 646/149 597 870.69 = 3.059 = 3.06

14. The correct answer is A. 1 light year
This calculation can be done approximately, as we are dealing with such large numbers: 1 light year is easily larger than 998,867,654,567 miles (1 light year = 5,874,601,673,400 miles) and 567 km. 23 AU approximately equals 150,000,000 km = 93 225 606 miles. Therefore, the light year is the largest.

15. The correct answer is E. (5 874 601 673 400 x 8)/12
(Distance/12 months) × 8 months = (Distance × 8 months)/12 months

16. The correct answer is B. 326.3% - (3.263/1)×100 = 326.3 %

17. The correct answer is C. 15% - ((35+84+26)/(35+84+26+118+30+675)) × 100 = (145/968) × 100 = 14.979 = 15%

18. The correct answer is E. £161 - (35+84+26+118+30+675)/6 = 968/6 = 161.33 = £161

19. The correct answer is A. 64.9%
Bill percentage = ((35+84+26+118+30+675)/1492) × 100
Bill percentage = (968/1492) × 100
Bill percentage = 64.879 or 64.9% to 1 decimal place.

20. The correct answer is C. 12.32%
Normal monthly bills = 35+84+26+118+30+675 = 968;
This month's adjustments = + (2×2.99) - 15.82 = 5.98 - 15.82 = -9.84;
This month's bill = 968 - 9.84 = 958.16;
Council tax percentage = (118/958.16) × 100 = 12.315 = 12.32 %

21. The correct answer is D. 53,000
Mean = (39754+56753+24787+64665+87664+45876)/6
Mean = 319499/6
Mean = 53,250 or 53,000 to 2 significant figures.

22. The correct answer is A. 62,877 - Range = highest – lowest, Range = 87664-24787, Range = 62877

23. The correct answer is B. 51,315
The median score is the middle-ranked value.

With an even number of scores there will be two middle values, in which case they are added together and divided by two. The ranked scores are: 24787, 39754, 45876, 56753, 64665, 87664; the middle two values are 45876 and 56753; median = (45876+56753)/2 therefore median = 51,314.5 or 51,315 as a whole number.

24. The correct answer is C. 48,158
New total = previous leader board + increase in DaveP's score + new player's score so new total = (39754+56753+24787+64665+87664+45876) + 5842 + 11765
New Total = 319499 + 5842 + 11765 therefore New Total = 337106
New mean = 337,106/7 (1 additional player)
New mean = 48,158

25. The correct answer is C. 0.429 - 3 out of 7 = 3/7 = 0.42857 = 0.429

26. The correct answer is A. 220.15g - 370 × 0.595 = 220.15 g

27. The correct answer is D. £2.36
Good Price = Farm Fresh /5
Good Price = £5.90/5
Good Price = £1.18
Speciality brand = Good Price x 2
Speciality brand = £1.18 × 2
Speciality brand = £2.36

28. The correct answer is A. £0.03
280g × 0.969% = 271.32 g of meat;
Price per gram = £9.45/271.32
Price per gram = £0.03483 or £0.03 to the nearest penny

29. The correct answer is C. 14 - 70/5 = 14

30. The correct answer is C. 18.37%
% space on G = 90/(70+100+90+230)) × 100
% space on G = (90/490) × 100
% space on G = 18.36734 or 18.37% to 2 decimal places

31. The correct answer is D. 159 MB
Extra disk space = 69% of 230 MB
Extra disk space = 230 × 0.69 = 158.7 or 159 MB

32. The correct answer is A. 40%
Unused space = 70 – (6×7)
Unused space = 70 – 42 = 28
% original drive space still available = (28/70) × 100 = 40%

33. The correct answer is C. 1802
Personal trainers are 27% of 6674
Personal trainers = 6674 × 0.27
Personal trainers = 1801.98 or 1802 to the nearest whole number

34. The correct answer is C. 1001
24% - 9% = 15%.
15% of 6675 = 6674 × 0.15

15% = 1001.1 = 1001 to the nearest whole number.

35. The correct answer is B. 272
Dance teachers = 24% of 6674
Dance teachers = 1601.76
Yoga qualified = 17% of 1601.76 =
Yoga qualified = 272.29 or 272 to the nearest whole number

36. The correct answer is E. 9.7%
Current lifeguards = 6674 × 0.09
New total lifeguards = 600.66 +50
New percentage = (656.66 /6724)× 100
New percentage = 9.68 or 9.7% to 1 decimal place

Question Set 1 (questions 1-5)
Set A: has 1 black and 1 grey shape that contains right angles. Set B: has 2 white shapes that contain right angles

1. Neither
2. Set B
3. Neither
4. Set A
5. Set B

Question Set 2 (questions 6-10)
Set A: central star, the same number of big and small arrows but pointing in opposite directions.
Set B: central star, two small arrows pointing towards star from different directions

6. Set A
7. Set B
8. Set A
9. Neither
10. Set A

11. The correct answer is C. - The second picture is a 90 degree right hand rotation of the first

12. The correct answer is D. - The characters on the top row in the first picture have only straight lines, the middle row contains a mixture of straight and curved lines and the bottom row has characters with only curved lines. In the second picture these rules are reversed.

Question Set 3 (questions 13-17)
Set A always contains a single triangle and Set B always contains a single circle

13. Set B
14. Set A
15. Set A
16. Neither
17. Set B

Question Set 4 (questions 18-22)
Set A always contains arrows pointing up, left and right in a 3:3:3 ratio. Set B always contains them in a 4:3:2 ratio.

18. Set B
19. Set A
20. Set A
21. Neither

22. Neither

Question Set 5 (questions 23-27)
Set A always contains two circles. Set B contains two triangles, at least one of which is made of dashed lines.

23. Set A
24. Set A
25. Set B
26. Neither
27. Set B

Question Set 6 (questions 28-32)
Set A: at least one intersection in each shape, circles of the same size do not intersect with each other
Set B: at least one intersection in each box - all intersections are between circles of the same size

28. Set A
29. Set A
30. Set B
31. Set A
32. Neither

33. The correct answer is C. The pictures have an increasing number of lines that point directly upwards. In picture A no lines point up, in picture B there is one and so on. Picture C has four upward pointing lines.

34. The correct answer C. The oval shape is moving clockwise around the large square, the small square is moving anti-clockwise around the large square but only half a length at a time, the triangle is moving anti-clockwise around the large square.

35. The correct answer is B. The shapes move in regular sequence from one picture to the next.

Question Set 7 (questions 36-40)
Set A always has two shapes of the same colour and always contains at least one shape with a straight edge.
Set B always has 3 shapes of the same colour.

36. Set A
37. Set B
38. Neither
39. Neither
40. Set B

Question Set 8 (questions 41-45)
Set A always contains three horizontal and three vertical arrows.
Set B always contains four horizontal and four vertical arrows.

41. Set B
42. Neither
43. Neither
44. Neither
45. Set A

Question Set 9 (questions 46-50)
Set A always contains a set of three shapes with the same number of sides, two white and one black.
Set B always contains a set of two shapes with the same number of sides, both are white.

46. Set A
47. Set A
48. Set B
49. Neither
50. Set A

Question Set 10 (questions 51-55)
Set A always contains two parallel lines. (Two lines of the same length in line with each other with no other line of the same orientation between them). Set B always contains three parallel lines. (Three lines of the same length in line with each other with no other line of the same orientation between them)

51. Set A
52. Set B
53. Neither
54. Neither
55. Set B

1. The correct answer is D. A very inappropriate thing to do – 2 marks (1 mark for C. Inappropriate but not awful)
This action will just add to the rumours which may not be true, in which case damaging Sophia's professional reputation

2. The correct answer is D. A very inappropriate thing to do – 2 marks (1 mark for C. Inappropriate but not awful)
Although it might be a good idea to speak to Sophia (who may not be aware of the rumours) the use of the word 'confront' makes it inappropriate as it suggests Hazel has already made up her mind that the rumours are true and is jealous of the extra opportunities Sophia appears to receive as a result. Whether the rumours are true or not, this action will likely impact on the relationship between Sophia and Hazel.

3. The correct answer is B. Appropriate but not ideal – 2 marks (1 mark for A. A very appropriate thing to do or C. Inappropriate but not awful)
It would be better to speak to Sophia first and give her the opportunity to clarify whether there is any truth to the rumours. If the rumours are not true, Hazel could offer to go with Sophia to speak to the clinical supervisor about the situation.

4. The correct answer is C. Inappropriate but not awful – 2 marks (1 mark for B. Appropriate but not ideal or D. A very inappropriate thing to do)
This action suggests Hazel is not that interested in seeking more opportunities to expand her experience and is not proactive in creating opportunities to learn.

5. The correct answer is A. A very appropriate thing to do – 2 marks (1 mark for B. Appropriate but not ideal)
This action shows that Hazel is willing to create more learning opportunities for herself. It may be that the reason Sophia is getting in on more surgeries is because she asked to be involved and not because she is having a relationship with the registrar.

6. The correct answer is B. Appropriate but not ideal – 2 marks (1 mark for A. A very appropriate thing to do or C. Inappropriate but not awful)
It is always best to speak to the person concerned before going to their manager. Although this will resolve the issue, it's not the most sensitive way of dealing with the situation.

7. The correct answer is D. A very inappropriate thing to do – 2 marks (1 mark for C. Inappropriate but not awful)
This action shows that Christopher has no regard for honesty, even if his intentions are good, part of being a medical professional is writing accurate and honest reports. It also could put patients on the ward at risk if they need the equipment and it is not available.

8. The correct answer is C. Inappropriate but not awful – 2 marks (1 mark for B. Appropriate but not ideal or D. A very inappropriate thing to do)
This is inappropriate because a medical student should not be telling the senior nurse in charge who to employ. It's not awful because Christopher's advice will be ignored for this very reason.

9. The correct answer is C. Inappropriate but not awful – 2 marks (1 mark for B. Appropriate but not ideal or D. A very inappropriate thing to do) While it is probable that the doctor has a reason for their actions simply assuming that a professional is correct because they out rank you could lead to mistakes in later practice.

10. The correct answer is D. A very inappropriate thing to do – 2 marks (1 mark for C. Inappropriate but not awful) Disregarding a rule simply because some professionals do not follow it is very poor practice.

11. The correct answer is A. A very appropriate thing to do – 2 marks (1 mark for B. Appropriate but not ideal) While it is most likely that the doctor merely forgot the rule there may be an actual reason that it does not appear to be being followed. Asking the doctor involved allows the problem to be solved as well as potentially allowing the student to learn more about being a doctor on a ward.

12. The correct answer is A. A very appropriate thing to do – 2 marks (1 mark for B. Appropriate but not ideal) This means that any problem with a doctor's practice on the ward can be rectified while ensuring that any reports that need to go do so through the proper channels instead of just leaving it up to the student.

13. The correct answer is B. Appropriate but not ideal – 2 marks (1 mark for A. A very appropriate thing to do or C. Inappropriate but not awful) The student should make sure she is certain of whether a rule is definitely being broken before she acts to prevent wasting everyone's time or appearing incapable. However - doing it after her placement means that, should she be correct, no improvement to practice will happen.

14. The correct answer is C. Inappropriate but not awful – 2 marks (1 mark for B. Appropriate but not ideal or D. A very inappropriate thing to do) This ensures something is done about the neglecting of the rule but is likely an overreaction to an issue that could be dealt with faster and more effectively by other means.

15. The correct answer is D. A very inappropriate thing to do – 2 marks (1 mark for C. Inappropriate but not awful) Nathan's diagnosis may not be accurate but it still might prejudice the patient's opinion on their condition.

16. The correct answer is B. Appropriate but not ideal – 2 marks (1 mark for A. A very appropriate thing to do or C. Inappropriate but not awful) While this avoids causing any problems it does nothing on its own to deal with the patients distress about their condition.

17. The correct answer is C. Inappropriate but not awful – 2 marks (1 mark for B. Appropriate but not ideal or D. A very inappropriate thing to do) Given the doctor has been called away they are likely to be busy with another patient or job that Nathan will be distracting them from. Still if Nathan is tactful or waits this does reassure the patient that something is being done and helps them to be seen quickly.

18. The correct answer is A. A very appropriate thing to do – 2 marks (1 mark for B. Appropriate but not ideal) This helps reassure the patient as well as informing them that he is not qualified to judge.

19. The correct answer is B. Appropriate but not ideal – 2 marks (1 mark for A. A very appropriate thing to do or C. Inappropriate but not awful) While the ward's staff may well have already noticed the patient, pointing them out allows them to be helped as quickly as possible and also ensures that any additional problems that may have led to their distress can be spotted. However - the nurses have their own work to do and may not appreciate a med student asking them to do something else.

20. The correct answer is C. Inappropriate but not awful – 2 marks (1 mark for B. Appropriate but not ideal or D. A very inappropriate thing to do) Functionally this works but it demonstrates a poor ability to relate to patients and does nothing to help the distressed patient.

21. The correct answer is B. Appropriate but not ideal – 2 marks (1 mark for A. A very appropriate thing to do or C. Inappropriate but not awful) While this may help the student understand the material better it may also lead them to unknowingly (or even consciously) copy parts from others' work which could cause problems. 'Online' is also unregulated and accuracy is far from certain.

22. The correct answer is B. Appropriate but not ideal – 2 marks (1 mark for A. A very appropriate thing to do or C. Inappropriate but not awful) This could help the student who is struggling but also could take time away from other students who may need it to work as well as possibly resulting in the student just copying work from their friends. Also - there is a risk of swapping one set of misunderstandings for another.

23. The correct answer is A. A very appropriate thing to do – 2 marks (1 mark for B. Appropriate but not ideal) While the tutor may not have time to help the student go through every section letting their tutor know that they are struggling with parts of the course allows the tutor to help find ways to aid the student in understanding the material and handling the workload.

24. The correct answer is C. Inappropriate but not awful – 2 marks (1 mark for B. Appropriate but not ideal or D. A very inappropriate thing to do) This has limited use if the student is struggling due to a lack of insight or poor notes. The student has already invested a lot of time fruitlessly and there is no reason why further effort should be more useful. While memorising material could be of some use it is probably better to ask for help.

25. The correct answer is D. A very inappropriate thing to do – 2 marks (1 mark for C. Inappropriate but not awful) While this may be the outcome of failing to understand the course, simply giving up means the student will not improve. This is something to consider only after all other options have been exhausted.

26. The correct answer is B. Appropriate but not ideal – 2 marks (1 mark for A. A very appropriate thing to do or C. Inappropriate but not awful) The relative has already seen their GP but clearly doesn't quite trust, or understand, their diagnosis. Doing this may reassure them though. The GP does have a history with the patient so is in a good place to identify anything out of the ordinary with their condition.

27. The correct answer is A. A very appropriate thing to do – 2 marks (1 mark for B. Appropriate but not ideal) A second opinion from a doctor with full access to all of the notes made by the first doctor enables the patient to be reassured about the care they are receiving.

28. The correct answer is D. A very inappropriate thing to do – 2 marks (1 mark for C. Inappropriate but not awful) Mistakes can be made even by trained doctors so it is unlikely that a medical student will be able to accurately diagnose a patient especially given that they may be biased in their findings given that they are dealing with a member of their family. This therefore is fairly useless except to reassure the patient.

29. The correct answer is C. Inappropriate but not awful – 2 marks (1 mark for B. Appropriate but not ideal or D. A very inappropriate thing to do) While it is understandable that the student would want their relative seen by an expert, many of the ways they could make this happen could be seen as an abuse of power.

30. The correct answer is B. Appropriate but not ideal – 2 marks (1 mark for A. A very appropriate thing to do or C. Inappropriate but not awful) This allows the patient assurance that they have been checked over by an expert as opposed to a GP (who while skilled may not have the exact knowledge of certain conditions). However - if the GP thought this was necessary they should have made the referral.

31. The correct answer is B. Appropriate but not ideal – 2 marks (1 mark for A. A very appropriate thing to do or C. Inappropriate but not awful) While it could be argued that the medical course is more important doing nothing to help a friend you committed to helping is obviously far from perfect.

32. The correct answer is B. Appropriate but not ideal – 2 marks (1 mark for A. A very appropriate thing to do or C. Inappropriate but not awful) Since this is a prior commitment helping one's friend then catching up on the revision later makes sense but may come at the cost of success in the course.

33. The correct answer is A. A very appropriate thing to do – 2 marks (1 mark for B. Appropriate but not ideal) While rescheduling may be impossible this at least makes an attempt to solve both problems.

34. The correct answer is C. Inappropriate but not awful – 2 marks (1 mark for B. Appropriate but not ideal or D. A very inappropriate thing to do) While this solves both problems it is essentially using a friend's time to solve a problem that the student himself created. The friend may not appreciate a stranger coming to help either.

35. The correct answer is A. A very appropriate thing to do – 2 marks (1 mark for B. Appropriate but not ideal) While getting notes in advance may not be possible, at least trying is a very good idea before he makes a decision

36. The correct answer is D. A very inappropriate thing to do – 2 marks (1 mark for C. Inappropriate but not awful) This is essentially dishonesty which a doctor should not be in the habit of practising.

37. The correct answer is C. Inappropriate but not awful – 2 marks (1 mark for B. Appropriate but not ideal or D. A very inappropriate thing to do) This would mean the end of the students' medical aspirations. However it is at least plan a backup plan where the student can still help others and shows some planning.

38. The correct answer is A. A very appropriate thing to do – 2 marks (1 mark for B. Appropriate but not ideal) This ensures that the student's reasons for their lack of preparation are taken into account and helps their tutors to help them succeed.

39. The correct answer is A. A very appropriate thing to do – 2 marks (1 mark for B. Appropriate but not ideal) This attempts to plan for all scenarios ensuring that should she fail again she will have something to do while still doing her best to succeed.

40. The correct answer is B. Appropriate but not ideal – 2 marks (1 mark for A. A very appropriate thing to do or C. Inappropriate but not awful) While her dedication here is commendable it may be wise to consider whether the medicine course is right for her if she has to redo the entire thing, especially given that medicine is so difficult to get into as a course.

41. The correct answer is B. Appropriate but not ideal – 2 marks (1 mark for A. A very appropriate thing to do or C. Inappropriate but not awful) This may help to do well in the exams but it makes no allowances in case everything goes wrong.

42. The correct answer is B. Important – 2 marks (1 mark for A. Very important or C. Of minor importance) Aside from the moral implications there is very little point wasting time with dishonest practice that could simply be used to ask someone about your work or get help understanding it.

43. The correct answer is A. Very important – 2 marks (1 mark for B. Important) Patients and colleagues should be able to expect that a doctor will work morally and so in any decision what the right thing to do is an important consideration.

44. The correct answer is B. Important – 2 marks (1 mark for A. Very important or C. Of minor importance) It is more tempting to cheat on a more important test but is in turn arguably more immoral as the student will need to know the information well to be a doctor anyway.

45. The correct answer is B. Important – 2 marks (1 mark for A. Very important or C. Of minor importance) Almost everything we learn comes from the original work of someone else. It is, of course, important to attribute this where appropriate.

46. The correct answer is D. Not important at all – 2 marks (1 mark for C. Of minor importance) While this will most likely be a consideration in the student's mind it should not be. The sort of mindset that says it is important is ultimately unfit for medical practice.

47. The correct answer is A. Very important – 2 marks (1 mark for B. Important) If Bernice has a large amount of time dedicated to leisure, she may want to reschedule to place more time on her studies at least until exams are over.

48. The correct answer is D. Not important at all – 2 marks (1 mark for C. Of minor importance) Maggie has not asked Olivia what her views on abortion are, nor has she asked what Olivia would do in this situation. Olivia's role here is to give advice and help Maggie explore the various options open to her and her feelings about them. This is good practice for Olivia to be caring yet impartial.

49. The correct answer is A. Very important – 2 marks (1 mark for B. Important) This is very important as it has a direct impact on what action she chooses to take and how she will feel about her decision.

50. The correct answer is B. Important – 2 marks (1 mark for A. Very important or C. Of minor importance) This is important to take into consideration as she may well need their support whatever she chooses to do. However, the final decision should be hers.

51. The correct answer is B. Important – 2 marks (1 mark for A. Very important or C. Of minor importance) If Maggie's university does not have a policy in place or any support to help should she choose to have the baby, this does not mean that she should be prevented from having the baby and continuing her studies when appropriate. If she speaks to the relevant staff, a policy could be drawn up which would help her and the students who come after her. Alternatively, she could look into other childcare options.

52. The correct answer is A. Very important – 2 marks (1 mark for B. Important) Olivia may disagree with Maggie's choice; however, it is very important that she support her as a friend. Doctors need to learn where they have strong views on ethical issues that they cannot expect patients to behave as they might wish them to and even though Maggie is not her patient, Olivia should bear this in mind.

53. The correct answer is B. Important – 2 marks (1 mark for A. Very important or C. Of minor importance) A newly qualified doctor still has a lot to learn, and while they still have much to offer there is no substitute for experience in medicine. However - in this scenario the older doctor hasn't practiced for many years and their skills may be out of date or rusty.

54. The correct answer is B. Important – 2 marks (1 mark for A. Very important or C. Of minor importance) Ideas and policies change all the time in medicine and a much older doctor, especially one who hasn't practiced in some time, may be less aware of new methods and policies

55. The correct answer is D. Not important at all – 2 marks (1 mark for C. Of minor importance) Whilst it is often true that these types of alerts can seem like a 'headache' to a doctor, part of their professional responsibility is to use their knowledge and skills to help people who need them whenever and wherever the need arises.

56. The correct answer is A. Very important – 2 marks (1 mark for B. Important) This patient potentially has the chance of excellent care if the two doctors are able to work together. Mutual respect within the profession benefits everyone.

57. The correct answer is D. Not important at all – 2 marks (1 mark for C. Of minor importance) Age will eventually render some people incapable of performing professionally. However - unless Nigel sees signs of this he should not assume it.

58. The correct answer is B. Important – 2 marks (1 mark for A. Very important or C. Of minor importance) The ramifications of Sam reporting Tom to the university may be very significant and action shouldn't be taken lightly.

59. The correct answer is C. Of minor importance – 2 marks (1 mark for B. Important or D. Not important at all) If Sam did choose to report Tom and the university chose not to pursue it then it could be awkward. This may be a problem as the course is long and team work is likely to be a big part of the course. However - personal awkwardness, however uncomfortable, should not prevent Sam from choosing to do the right thing

60. The correct answer is C. Of minor importance – 2 marks (1 mark for B. Important or D. Not important at all) This is speculative. It is possible that the university wouldn't have taken motoring offences into account. It is not certain that the next student on 'the list' hasn't secured a place anywhere else.

61. The correct answer is C. Of minor importance – 2 marks (1 mark for B. Important or D. Not important at all) This may seem to be the intuitive conclusion, but honesty and integrity are important in all professional careers.

62. The correct answer is A. Very important – 2 marks (1 mark for B. Important)
This discussion is not between two shades of opinion. The study that suggested a link between MMR and autism has been comprehensively discredited and no reliable evidence of a link has ever been found.

63. The correct answer is A. Very important – 2 marks (1 mark for B. Important)
Parents make health decisions for their children. Although health care professionals can offer advice, they can only intercede and supersede those decisions in very specific circumstances

64. The correct answer is D. Not important at all – 2 marks (1 mark for C. Of minor importance) An opinion can be offered by anyone. An informed opinion can be offered by someone with information. As Sharon has been asked for her opinion, she is in a position to offer it.

65. The correct answer is C. Of minor importance – 2 marks (1 mark for B. Important or D. Not important at all)
This really would depend on lots of factors. However - sometimes discretion is the better part of valour and 'being right' is not as important as keeping the peace.

66. The correct answer is B. Important – 2 marks (1 mark for A. Very important or C. Of minor importance)
Pearl should be proud that a patient with a lot of medical history (who has seen a lot of different doctors) has been so positive about her.

67. The correct answer is C. Of minor importance – 2 marks (1 mark for B. Important or D. Not important at all)
Doctors deal with life and death situations and cannot 'work to rule' in exactly the same way some other people can. However - doctors are people too and need rest and relaxation and an opportunity to step back from their professional responsibilities.

68. The correct answer is B. Important – 2 marks (1 mark for A. Very important or C. Of minor importance)
While the patient may like Pearl the most it isn't reasonable to assume that she, and only she, can provide this patient with good care. If Pearl has confidence in her colleagues then she can rest assured that her absence will have no impact on the quality of care.

69. The correct answer is A. Very important – 2 marks (1 mark for B. Important)
Everyone, doctor or not, needs to have adequate rest, relaxation and recreation. Pearl could work during her holiday time but this would limit these restorative features and mean she may be less able to continue her placement and continue to learn and improve at the same level.

26/44

Full Mock Test 2 Verbal Reasoning (21 minutes for this section)

Influenza, commonly known as 'the flu', is an infectious disease of birds and mammals caused by RNA viruses of the family Orthomyxoviridae, the influenza viruses. The most common symptoms are chills, fever, runny nose, sore throat, muscle pains, headache (often severe), coughing, weakness/fatigue and general discomfort. Although it is often confused with other influenza-like illnesses, especially the common cold, influenza is a more severe disease caused by a different type of virus. Influenza may produce nausea and vomiting, particularly in children, but these symptoms are more common in the unrelated gastroenteritis, which is sometimes inaccurately referred to as 'stomach flu' or '24-hour flu'.

Typically, influenza is transmitted through the air by coughs or sneezes, creating aerosols containing the virus. Influenza can also be transmitted by direct contact with bird droppings or nasal secretions, or through contact with contaminated surfaces. Airborne aerosols have been thought to cause most infections, although which means of transmission is most important is not absolutely clear. Influenza viruses can be inactivated by sunlight, disinfectants and detergents. As the virus can be inactivated by soap, frequent hand washing reduces the risk of infection. Flu can occasionally lead to pneumonia, either direct viral pneumonia or secondary bacterial pneumonia, even in people who are usually healthy. In particular it is a warning sign if a child (or presumably an adult) seems to be getting better and then relapses with a high fever as this relapse may be bacterial pneumonia. Another warning sign is if the person starts to have trouble breathing.

Vaccinations against influenza are usually made available to people in developed countries. Farmed poultry is often vaccinated to avoid decimation of the flocks. The most common human vaccine is the trivalent influenza vaccine (TIV) that contains purified and inactivated antigens from three viral strains. Typically, this vaccine includes material from two influenza A virus subtypes and one influenza B virus strain. The TIV carries no risk of transmitting the disease. A vaccine formulated for one year may be ineffective in the following year, since the influenza virus evolves rapidly, and new strains quickly replace the older ones. Antiviral drugs such as the neuraminidase inhibitors oseltamivir among others have been used to treat influenza. Their benefits in those who are otherwise healthy do not appear to be greater than their risks. No benefit has been found in those with other health problems.

1. Which of the following statements is true?

A. TIV contains one strain from influenza type A and two strains from influenza type B
B. Influenza can only be inactivated by good hygiene practices
C. TIV puts you at risk of transmitting the disease
D. Flu can lead to bacterial pneumonia in healthy adults ✓

2. Which of the following statements is most likely to be true?

A. Influenza strains are constantly evolving
B. Influenza is sometimes known as 'stomach flu' or '24-hour flu' ✓
C. Antiviral drugs are best used for people with existing health problems
D. Vaccines are available in developed countries as they are expensive

3. Which of the following people is most likely to genuinely have influenza?

A. A child at school with a runny nose, headache and sore throat for five days ✓
B. An adult who had severe symptoms and vomiting for one day
C. A child who was recovering but now is feverish and struggling to breath
D. An adult who has been bed bound for four days with aches, fever and fatigue

4. Which of the following statements is most likely to be true?

A. Birds are likely to die if infected with flu
B. Washing your hands will be ineffective prevention as most infections are airborne X
C. The influenza virus infects animals, birds and people
D. An influenza vaccination will protect you for two years

Banana is the common name for herbaceous plants of the genus Musa and for the fruit they produce, which may be yellow, purple or red when ripe. In commerce 'banana' usually refers to soft, sweet 'dessert' bananas. Bananas are native to tropical Southeast Asia and were probably first domesticated in Papua New Guinea. Today, they are cultivated throughout the tropics in at least 107 countries, primarily for their fruit but also to make fibre. 'Cavendish' bananas are the main commercial cultivar.

Wild species have large, hard seeds but virtually all culinary bananas have tiny seeds. Fruit are classified either as dessert bananas or for cooking. Most export bananas are of the dessert types; about 10-15% of production is for export. The USA and EU are the dominant importers.

The banana plant is the largest herbaceous flowering plant; often mistaken for a tree, their main pseudostem grows from 6 to 7.6 metres tall, producing a single bunch of bananas before dying.

Banana fruit grow in hanging clusters, with up to 20 fruit to a tier. The assemblage of hanging clusters is known as a bunch, comprising 3-20 tiers, or commercially as a "banana stem", and can weigh from 30-50 kilograms. Individual fruits average 125g, of which approximately 75% is water and 25% dry matter.

Each stem normally produces a single, sterile, male banana flower. The female flowers appear further up the stem and produce the actual fruit without fertilisation. Due to having stiff stems bananas grow pointing up, not hanging down.

5. The USA imports 10% of all dessert bananas grown.

A. True
B. False
C. Can't tell

6. 'Cavendish' bananas have small seeds.

A. True
B. False
C. Can't tell

7. Bananas are 50% water.

A. True
B. False
C. Can't tell

8. Bananas are cultivated in more than 100 countries.

A. True
B. False
C. Can't tell

Although sawgrass and sloughs are the enduring geographical icons of the Everglades, other ecological features and systems are just as vital, and the borders marking them are subtle or non-existent. Pinelands and tropical hardwood hammocks are located throughout the sloughs; the trees, rooted in soil inches above the peat, marl, or water, support a variety of wildlife. The oldest and tallest trees are cypresses, whose roots are specially adapted to grow underwater for months at a time. The Big Cypress Swamp is well-known for its 500-year-old cypresses, though cypress domes can appear throughout the Everglades. As the fresh water from Lake Okeechobee makes its way to Florida Bay, it meets salt water from the Gulf of Mexico; mangrove forests grow in this transitional zone, providing nursery and nesting conditions for many species of birds, fish, and invertebrates. The marine environment of Florida Bay is also considered part of the Everglades because its sea grasses and aquatic life are attracted to the constant discharge of fresh water.

These ecological systems are always changing due to environmental factors. Geographic features such as the Western Flatwoods, Eastern Flatwoods, and the Atlantic Coastal Ridge affect drainage patterns. Geologic elements, climate, and the frequency of storms and fire are formative processes for the Everglades. They help to sustain and transform the ecosystems in the Shark River Valley, Big Cypress Swamp, coastal areas and mangrove forests. The Everglade ecosystems have been described as both fragile and resilient. Minor fluctuations in water levels have far-reaching consequences for many plant and animal species, and the system cycles and pulses with each change.

9. Sawgrass and sloughs are the most important ecological features of the Everglades.

A. True
B. False
C. Can't tell

10. There is wildlife living in the trees in the Everglades.

A. True
B. False
C. Can't tell

11. Cypress trees have a maximum life span of 100 years.

A. True
B. False
C. Can't tell

12. Unseasonal heavy rains that result in flooding would have a great impact on the Everglade ecosystems.

A. True
B. False
C. Can't tell

The geology of the Isle of Wight is dominated by sedimentary rocks of Cretaceous and Paleogene age. This sequence was affected by the late stages of the Alpine Orogeny, forming the Isle of Wight monocline, the cause of the steeply-dipping outcrops of the Chalk Group and overlying Paleogene strata seen at The Needles, Alum Bay and Whitecliff Bay.
Rocks of Devonian, Triassic and Jurassic age are known to be present in the subsurface of the island from boreholes and interpreted seismic reflection profiles. Up to 389 metres of presumed Devonian sedimentary rocks been proved by 6 boreholes drilled on the island, consisting of claystone, siltstone, sandstone and quartzite, similar in type to other dated Devonian sequences. A nearly full Triassic succession has been drilled, reaching a maximum thickness of 450 metres. Sandstones of the Sherwood Sandstone Group are overlain by claystones and siltstones of the Mercia Mudstone Group and limestones of the Penarth Group. A complete Jurassic succession is shown by the boreholes at Arreton, reaching more than 1400 metres in thickness, comprising mainly mudstones of the Lias Group, oolitic limestones of the Inferior and Great Oolite Group, claystones of the Kellaways and Oxford Clay Formations, bioclastic limestones of the Corallian Group, organic-rich mudstones of the Kimmeridge Clay Formation, limestones of the Portland Group and the lower part of the Purbeck Group. The entire sequence presents sedimentation in a shallow water environment.

13. Which of the following is definitely a place on the Isle of Wight?

A. Purbeck
B. Arreton
C. Sherwood
D. Penarth

14. Which of the following statements is most likely to be true based on the text?

A. All or part of the Isle of Wight was once covered by shallow water
B. There were once dinosaurs on the Isle of Wight
C. The Jurassic era rocks are 1400m under the surface
D. There is a lot of clay on the Isle of Wight

15. What can we know for certain about the 'Isle of Wight' based on the text?

A. It is an island
B. There are a total of six boreholes on it
C. There are visible strata of sedimentary rock
D. There are chalk formations

16. Which of the following statements is listed in the correct order (top to bottom)?

A. Mercia Mudstone, Sherwood Sandstone
B. Devonian, Triassic, Jurassic
C. Lias Group, Great Oolite Group, Kellaways
D. Kimmeridge Clay, Limestone of Portland Group

People with ESFJ (Extrovert, Sensing, Feeling, Judging) preferences radiate sympathy and fellowship. They concern themselves chiefly with the people around them and place a high value on harmonious human contacts. They are friendly, tactful and sympathetic. They are persevering, conscientious, orderly even in small matters, and inclined to expect others to be the same. They are particularly warmed by approval and sensitive to indifference. Much of their pleasure and satisfaction comes from the warmth of feeling of people around them. ESFJs tend to concentrate on the admirable qualities of other people and are loyal to respected persons, institutions, or causes, sometimes to the point of idealising whatever they admire.
They have the gift of finding value in other people's opinions. Even when these opinions are in conflict, they have faith that harmony can somehow be achieved and they often manage to bring it about. To achieve harmony, they are ready to agree with others' opinions, within reasonable limits. They need to be careful, however, that they don't concentrate so much on the viewpoints of others that they lose sight of their own. They are mainly interested in the realities perceived by their five senses, so become practical, realistic and down-to-earth. They take great interest in the unique difference in each experience. ESFJs appreciate and enjoy their possessions. They enjoy variety but can adapt well to routine.

17. Which of the following series of adjectives best describes an ESFJ personality preference:

A. Compassionate, realistic, theoretical
B. Reliable, amiable, careful
C. Cooperative, thorough, thoughtless
D. Conscientious, practical, opinionated

18. All of the following statements are true except:

A. ESFJs value other people's opinions
B. ESFJs do not like it when people do not have an opinion
C. ESFJs can try so hard to keep everyone happy that they can lose their own viewpoint
D. ESFJs prefer routine

19. Which of the following statements would not describe an ESFJs preferred work environment?

A. Organised
B. Friendly
C. Includes people who are appreciative
D. Includes people who are not oriented to helping others

20. On encountering a problem, an ESFJ would be unlikely to:

A. Examine the logical consequences
B. Respond quickly to resolve without considering the consequences
C. Gather all the evidence and relevant opinions
D. Consider the impact on others

Synonyms are different words with identical or very similar meanings. Words that are synonyms are said to be synonymous, and the state of being a synonym is called synonymy.
Synonyms can be any part of speech (e.g. nouns, adjectives, adverbs), as long as both members of the pair are the same part of speech. Some examples of English synonyms are:

- student and pupil (noun)
- buy and purchase (verb)
- sick and ill (adjective)
- quickly and speedily (adverb)

Note that synonyms are defined with respect to certain senses of words; for instance, pupil as the "aperture in the iris of the eye" is not synonymous with student, a long arm is not the same as an extended arm. In English, many synonyms evolved from the parallel use, in the early medieval period, of Norman French (from Latin) and Old English (Anglo-Saxon) words, often with some words being used principally by the Saxon peasantry ("freedom", "bowman") and their synonyms by the Norman nobility ("liberty", "archer").
Some lexicographers claim that no synonyms have exactly the same meaning (in all contexts) because etymology, orthography, phonic qualities, ambiguous meanings etc. make them unique. Different words that are similar in meaning usually differ for a reason: feline is more formal than cat; long and extended are only synonyms in one usage and not in others. The purpose of a thesaurus is to offer the user a listing of similar or related words; these are often, but not always, synonyms.

21. Mean (average) and mean (unkind) are synonymous.

A. True
B. False
C. Can't tell

22. Synonymy is dependent upon context.

A. True
B. False
C. Can't tell

23. Verbs may be synonymous.

A. True
B. False
C. Can't tell

24. The medieval French army contained archers.

A. True
B. False
C. Can't tell

The Penny Blue is frequently mistaken for a postage stamp of Britain. It is from a series of proof impressions that were made at the time Rowland Hill was looking at the new colours that were to be used for the stamps that would replace the Penny Black and the original 1840 issue of the Two Pence Blue.
The decision to change the black stamp to red had already been made, and at the same time the colour of the ink used for the cancellations was to be changed from red to black.
Although it had been decided that the two pence value stamp would remain blue, it would be printed using a different ink from that used on the original. (Thus when the stamp was printed it had the addition of white lines added above and below the inscription so that the new printings could be distinguished at a glance.)
For the printing of the three proof sheets, plate 8 - constructed for the production of the Penny Black - was used.
Rowland Hill chose the full deep blue colour for the two pence stamp.

Examples printed in the red-brown shade, if they made it onto postage, would be indistinguishable from later printings, printed in this colour as part of the general issue in 1841.
Die, plate, and paper proofs have been a common step in the process of stamp pre-production since the first stamps. These proofs are never usable as postage, and as a result do not constitute a 'postage stamp', rather they are a representation, frequently to test the type or colour of ink, how it will react on certain papers, as well as validating the image itself. This was more critical in the early days of stamp production where metal (and sometimes stone or even wooden plates) were used to make the stamp impression, and some inks caused undue wear on the plates.

25. Which of these statements is most likely to be true?

A. The 'Penny Blue' stamp was issued in 1840
B. 'Deep blue' was chosen in preference to 'Prussian blue'
C. The plate used to print the Penny Blue was later used for the Penny Black
D. The red-brown prototypes were readily distinguished from the 1841 general issue

26. Which of these statements is true?

A. The ink for cancellation was changed from blue to black at the same time as the new stamps were issued
B. The 'Penny Black' was replaced in 1841 by the 'Penny Red'
C. The ink for the 'two penny' blue did not need to be changed
D. The 1841 version of the two pence stamp was unchanged

27. All of the following statements are true except:

A. Three sheets of samples were provided for Rowland Hill to examine
B. Paper proofs are not true postage stamps
C. Proofs are used to test the colour, check the reaction of the paper, evaluate the image quality and examine the possibility of forgery
D. The 'Penny Red' was exactly like the 'Penny Black' apart from the change of ink

28. Which of these statements is least likely to be true?

A. Penny Red proof impressions were edited before stamp production
B. There was no 'Penny Blue' stamp
C. Stamps were printed from metal, stone or wood plates
D. Plates reacted badly to some types of ink

The London *Gazette* is one of the official journals of record of the British government, in which certain statutory notices are required to be published. It claims to be the oldest surviving, continuously published English newspaper, having been first published on 7 November 1665 as the Oxford *Gazette* for members of the Royal Court who had moved to Oxford and were unwilling to touch London newspapers during the Great Plague of London. Its first publication is noted by Samuel Pepys in his diary. It does not have a large circulation. When the King returned to London, the *Gazette* moved too, with the first issue of the London *Gazette* being published on 5 February 1666. The *Gazette* was not a newspaper in the modern sense: it was not printed for sale to the general public. In 1812 an officer of the London *Gazette* named George Reynell established the first advertising agency.
The Edinburgh and Belfast *Gazettes* reproduce certain materials of nationwide interest published in the London *Gazette* and also contain publications specific to Scotland and Northern Ireland, respectively. In turn, the London *Gazette* not only carries notices of UK-wide interest, but also those relating specifically to England. However, certain notices that are only of specific interest to Scotland or Northern Ireland are also required to be published in the London *Gazette*.
The London *Gazette* is published each weekday. Notices for the following, among others, are published:

- granting of Royal Assent to bills of the United Kingdom and Scottish parliaments
- corporate and personal bankruptcies
- granting of honours and military medals
- changes of coats of arms

29. Bankruptcies are reported in the *Gazette*.

A. True
B. False
C. Can't tell

30. The *Gazette* has a small readership.

A. True
B. False
C. Can't tell

31. The first printed advertisements appeared in the London *Gazette*.

A. True
B. False
C. Can't tell

32. Samuel Pepys wrote a diary.

A. True
B. False
C. Can't tell

Opponents Auto-Tune have argued that the plug-in has a negative effect on society's perception and consumption of music. In 2004, the UK's *The Telegraph* music critic Neil McCormick called Auto-Tune a 'particularly sinister invention that has been putting extra shine on pop vocals since the 1990s' by taking 'a poorly sung note and transpos[ing] it, placing it dead centre of where it was meant to be'.

In 2009, Time magazine quoted an unnamed Grammy-winning recording engineer as saying, "Let's just say I've had Auto-Tune save vocals on everything from Britney Spears to Bollywood cast albums. And every singer now presumes that you'll just run their voice through the box." The same article expressed "hope that pop's fetish for uniform perfect pitch will fade', speculating that pop-music songs have become harder to differentiate from one another, as 'track after track has perfect pitch.' According to Tom Lord-Alge Auto-Tune is used on nearly every contemporary record.

In 2010, the British television reality TV show *The X Factor* admitted to using Auto-Tune to improve the voices of contestants. Simon Cowell, one of the show's bosses, ordered a ban on Auto-Tune for future episodes. Also - in 2010 - *Time* magazine included Auto-Tune in their list of 'The 50 Worst Inventions'.

In a 2006 interview with Pitchfork Media, US singer-songwriter Neko Case gave an example of how prevalent pitch correction is in the industry:

'I'm not a perfect note hitter either but I'm not going to cover it up with Auto-Tune. Everybody uses it, too. I once asked a studio guy in Toronto, "How many people don't use Auto-Tune?" and he said, "You and Nelly Furtado are the only two people who've never used it in here." Even though I'm not into Nelly Furtado, it kind of made me respect her. It's cool that she has some integrity.'

Electropop recording artist Kesha has been widely recognised as using excessive Auto-Tune in her songs, putting her vocal talent under scrutiny. Music producer Rick Rubin wrote that 'Right now, if you listen to pop, everything is in perfect pitch, perfect time and perfect tune. That's how ubiquitous Auto-Tune is.' Time journalist Josh Tyrangiel called Auto-Tune 'Photoshop for the human voice.' Big band singer Michael Bublé criticised Auto-Tune as making everyone sound the same – 'like robots' - but admits he uses it when he records pop-oriented music.

33. According to the text, which of the following recording artists has definitely used Auto-Tune technology?

A. Britney Spears
B. Nelly Furtado
C. Michael Bublé
D. Kesha

34. All of the following criticisms of Auto-Tune were issued by *Time* magazine except:

A. 'Right now, if you listen to pop, everything is in perfect pitch, perfect time and perfect tune'
B. One of 'The 50 Worst Inventions'
C. 'Photo shop for the human voice'
D. 'A particularly sinister invention'

35. What is the most likely benefit of Auto-Tune based on the information in this text?

A. Singers will be able to spend less time recording thus freeing up studio time
B. It enables authentic singers to advertise their distinctiveness
C. It means there will be more pop stars
D. It makes the tone of people's voices sound better

36. Which of the following statements seems likely to be true?

A. *The X-Factor* would have had fewer viewers if it hadn't used Auto-Tune
B. Modern music buyers demand perfection and, thus, Auto-Tune
C. Auto-Tune makes everything sound better
D. Singers don't necessarily have much control over whether Auto-Tune is used in the production of their work

Clinical features of varicella-zoster infections

Chickenpox is a systemic viral infection caused by varicella-zoster virus (VZV), a herpes virus. Its public health importance lies in the risk of complications in immunosuppressed and pregnant patients. Herpes zoster (shingles) is caused by reactivation of latent VZV whose genomes persist in sensory root ganglia of the brain stem and spinal cord.

There is sometimes a prodromal illness of fever, headache and myalgia. The diagnostic feature is the vesicular rash, which usually appears first on the trunk. The rash starts as small papules, develops into clear vesicles, becomes pustules and then dries to crusts. There are successive crops of vesicles over several days. The hands and feet are relatively spared.

A more fulminant illness including pneumonia, hepatitis or disseminated intravascular coagulation may affect the immunocompromised, neonates and occasionally healthy adults, particularly smokers. Congenital varicella syndrome occurs following infections in the first 5 months of pregnancy, although most risk appears to be in weeks 13-20.

Shingles begins with pain in the dermatome supplied by the affected sensory root ganglion. The trunk is a common site. The rash appears in the affected area and is vesicular and rapidly coalesces. It is very painful and persists for several days and even weeks in the elderly.

The incubation period for chickenpox is 11-21 days, usually 15-18 days. Cases are infectious for up to 5 days before the onset of rash (usually 1-2 days) until 5 days after the first crop of vesicles. Infectivity may last longer in immunocompromised patients. Patients with herpes zoster are usually infectious only if the lesions are exposed or disseminated.

37. All of the following statements are true except:

A. The vesicular rash is the sign that usually provides a diagnosis
B. There can be an early stage of the disease which involves fever, headaches and myalgia
C. The rash usually appears on the hands and feet first before spreading
D. The rash lasts for 5 days

38. All of the following statements are true of chickenpox except:

A. The incubation period is usually 11-21 days
B. The host is infectious for up to 10 days
C. The incubation period for chickenpox can be as high as 3 weeks
D. Immunocompromised hosts may be infectious longer

39. According to the text, which of the following sets of symptoms cannot be caused by the zoster virus?

A. Temperature, myalgia, pneumonia
B. Pneumonia, liver complications, skin pustules
C. Skin pustules, renal complications, headaches
D. Painful rash, fever, myalgia

40. According to the text which of the following statements is true?

A. Once the rash appears, infected people are no longer infectious
B. People who are immunocompromised tend to have more severe and persisting disease
C. People who have had shingles may develop chickenpox later in life
D. Herpes zoster is not infectious

The House of Stuart is a European royal house founded in the late 14th century. By the 17th century its territory covered the entire British Isles. In total, nine Stuart monarchs ruled just Scotland from 1371 until 1603. After this there was a Union of the Crowns under James VI & I who had become the senior claimant to the holdings of the extinct House of Tudor.
The Stuarts ruled during a time of transition from the Middle Ages to the Renaissance. Monarchs such as James IV were known for sponsoring exponents of the Northern Renaissance. Shakespeare's best-known plays were authored during the Jacobean era, while the Royal Society and Royal Mail were established under Charles II.
James IV married King Henry VII's daughter, Margaret Tudor. The birth of their son, later James V, brought the House of Stuart into the line of descent of the House of Tudor, and the English throne. Margaret Tudor later married Archibald Douglas and their daughter Margaret was the mother of Lord Darnley who married Mary, Queen of Scots, the daughter of James V.
The couple's only child James VI & I became King of Scotland and England in 1603. The two Kingdoms shared a monarch but had separate governments and institutions. Conflict arising from this marked the reign of Charles I culminating in the English Civil War. The execution of Charles I by the English Parliament in 1649 began the English Interregnum. The younger Charles returned to Britain to assume his thrones in 1660 as Charles II of England and Scotland.

41. Robert II of Scotland was the first of nine Stuart kings of Scotland.

A. True
B. False
C. Can't tell

42. James VI & I was King James VI of Scotland and James I of England.

A. True
B. False
C. Can't tell

43. Charles II of England and Scotland was the son of Charles I.

A. True
B. False
C. Can't tell

44. James IV of Scotland was the grandfather of James VI & I.

A. True
B. False
C. Can't tell

Full Mock Test 2 Decision Making (31 minutes for this section)

1. The park has two lakes, one of which is used for boating. Both lakes have many ducks, geese and other waterfowl. There are three play areas aimed at different age groups and lots of open lawn area for ball games etc. There are many flower beds and lots of mature trees and shrubs. There is one large bandstand and also a cricket club. Within the park there is a leisure centre, a café and a church. The park is divided into two sections by a railway line over which there are two bridges. On one side there is the larger lake, café and church. The other side has the cricket club, leisure centre and play areas.

Select the words 'Yes' or 'No' if the conclusion does or doesn't follow

The side of the park with the larger lake is the larger side	Yes / No
All three play areas can be accessed without crossing the railway bridge	Yes / No
There are ducks in both halves of the park	Yes / No
The smaller lake is not used for boating	Yes / No
The café is closer to the church than the cricket club	Yes / No

2. A group of friends went out for dinner. Some of them ordered three courses but most of them only had a starter or a dessert along with a main course. They all ordered a single cold drink. Some people stayed on for a coffee but some of them left after dessert.

Select the words 'Yes' or 'No' if the conclusion does or doesn't follow

Some people had a starter, a main course and coffee	Yes / No
Some people left before dessert	Yes / No
Everyone had a main course	Yes / No
The number of cold drinks sold was equal to the number of main courses	Yes / No
Fewer people had coffee than had a starter	Yes / No

3. The Elephant and Castle shopping centre, once a symbol of hope and regeneration, could be on its last legs. Built on a site that was heavily bombed in World War Two, the precinct opened in 1965 and was praised for its design and ambition. But in six months' time, the centre - which is home to a vibrant Latin American community - could be demolished as part of a wider redevelopment project for the area.

Select the words 'Yes' or 'No' if the conclusion does or doesn't follow

World War Two ended before 1965	Yes / No
There is a wide redevelopment project planned for the area	Yes / No
The Latin American community is the dominant group in the area	Yes / No
The shopping centre is faded and depreciating in value	Yes / No
The Elephant and Castle shopping centre will be demolished	Yes / No

4. Select the words 'Yes' or 'No' if the conclusion does or doesn't follow

Over half of all social media users as shown are aged under 35	Yes / No
Of the social media platforms shown, Facebook has the most representative age distribution	Yes / No
On average around a quarter of people aged 25-34 use social media	Yes / No
If people continue to use the same social media platforms as they get older then these proportions will shift in the coming years	Yes / No
Less than 10% of all social media use is from people aged over 65	Yes / No

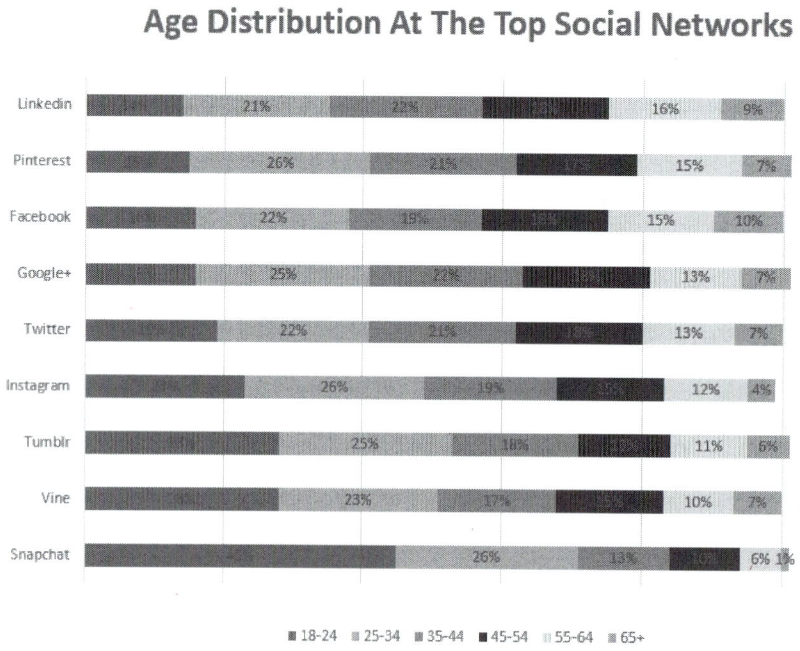

5. Gareth is buying a car and is doing research as to which one offers the best fuel efficiency. There are four cars he is considering. The cars are blue, red, silver and black. They mpg ratings on offer are 25mpg (miles per gallon of fuel), 27mpg, 29mpg and 31mpg. The cars cost £1500, £1600, £1700 and £1800.

- The most expensive car is the silver car; it is not the most fuel efficient
- The least fuel-efficient car is also the cheapest
- The red car is more fuel efficient than the blue car and more expensive than the black car
- The car which gets 27mpg costs £1700 (it's not blue)

Which of the following statements is true?

A. The most fuel-efficient car is the most expensive
B. The least fuel-efficient car is the cheapest
C. The car which costs £1600 gets 29mpg
D. The silver car is more efficient than the black car

6. Nicola owns a fudge shop in a seaside town. She wraps the different flavours of fudge she makes in different coloured paper. One day she assesses how much of each type of fudge she has sold to discover her four top selling flavours.

Top four flavours – cherry, chocolate, coffee, vanilla

Wrapping colour – gold, green, pink, silver

- Nicola's most popular fudge comes in a silver wrapper
- Cherry fudge comes in a pink wrapper
- Chocolate fudge is the third most popular
- The green wrapped fudge was placed one place below the gold wrapped fudge and two places below the cherry flavour

Which of the following must be true?

A. Nicola's most popular fudge is vanilla
B. Coffee fudge comes in a green wrapper
C. Gold wrapped fudge is chocolate flavour
D. Cherry fudge is the third most popular

7. Four runners join up for a 5km run. Each of them wears a different coloured running outfit and registers a slightly different time.

Runners – Andy, Francesca, George, and Rachel

Outfits – blue, pink, red, and white

Times – 24 minutes, 26 minutes, 28 minutes, and 29 minutes

- Rachel always wears red when she runs
- The runner is white was the fastest
- The runner in blue took four minutes longer to complete the circuit than Andy
- Rachel ran the circuit 2 minutes faster than George

Which of the following statements is true?

A. Andy wore blue
B. George took 26 minutes to run the course
C. The 29-minute run was by a person wearing blue
D. Francesca wore pink

	A	B	C	D	E
1	a				
2			b		c
3			City Park		
4		d			
5				e	

8. The five buildings marked on this map are a hotel, a business centre, a shopping mall, a leisure centre and a housing unit.

The two most distant units from each other are the business centre and the shopping mall

The hotel has direct park views

The leisure centre has diagonal park views

The closest two units are the hotel and the housing unit

Which of these statements is true?

A. Unit A is a business centre
B. Unit B is a hotel
C. Unit C is a leisure centre
D. Unit D is a housing unit
E. Unit E is a shopping mall

9. Three friends (Martha, Norman and Olive) are playing lawn bowls. The small black circle is the 'Jack' (target ball).

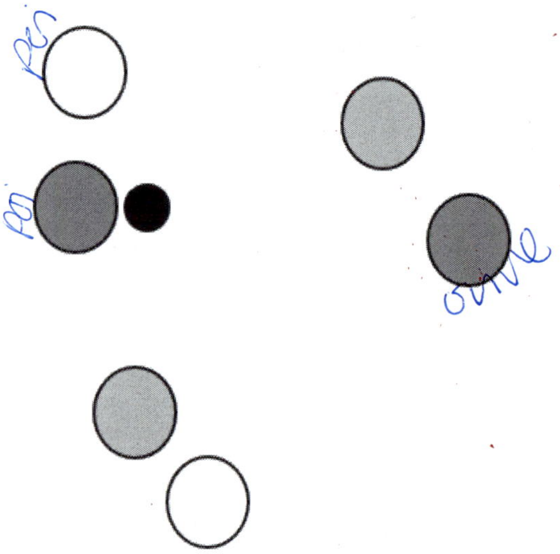

- Norman didn't get a bowl in the closest two
- Olive's first throw is the furthest away from the Jack
- Only the two closest bowls to the Jack receive any points
- If a player gets the first and second closest then they get double points

Which statement is not true?

A. Martha threw the white bowls
B. Norman was awarded some points in this round
C. Olive threw the winning bowl
D. Martha and Olive shared the points

10. The minimum wage should be set at a rate that ensures any full-time worker earning it will be able to afford a basic standard of living

Select the strongest argument from the options below:

A. Yes – if workers don't earn enough to live then the welfare system has to top up their income
B. Yes – it is important for personal dignity that workers are paid a fair amount
C. No – most people earning minimum wage are young people earning pocket money
D. No – a 'basic standard of living' varies so rates should reflect the economy more generally

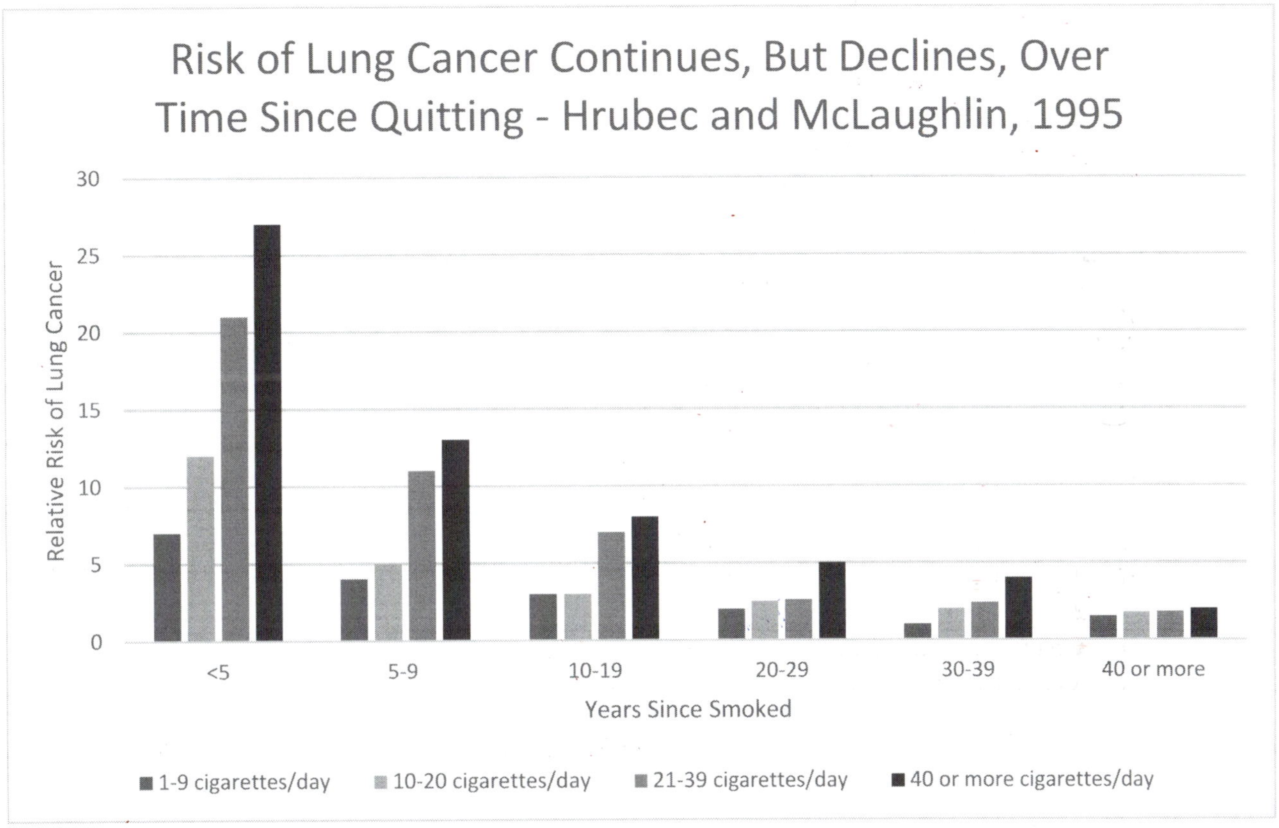

11. Which of the following statements is true based on the shown data?

A. Smoking fewer cigarettes leads to a much lower risk
B. 40 years after quitting smoking the risk of lung cancer equalises with a non-smoker
C. 25 years after quitting smoking, the difference between 10 or 35 cigarettes per day makes negligible difference
D. Anyone who quits a 5 per day habit will have their lung cancer risk steadily decline

12. Students who go academically poor schools and still get excellent exam results should be given preferential treatment by universities

A. Yes – achieving well at a poor school is a greater achievement than achieving well at a good school and universities should take into account the character and work ethic of the student, who overcame their circumstances

B. Yes – universities should actively work to increase the diversity of their students to contribute to social mobility which will create a more equitable and merit-based society

C. No – universities should only consider academic rigour and not the advantages or disadvantages a student has enjoyed or suffered

D. No – it is not fair to discriminate against students who have had the privilege to have gone to academically good schools

13. Despite the convenience and advantages associated with e-readers – such as being able to carry many books in one device, being able to read in the dark and being able to purchase many more books than the average bookstore can stock – many people refuse to use them. Those who want to continue to read printed books cite a love of the sensory experience of reading; the weight of a book, the action of turning a page, the smell of the paper. It is suggested that digitalising some of the more pleasurable things in life can unintentionally take away some of the previously unnoticed joys of a simpler time.

Which of the following can be concluded from the passage?

A. Simple times were more joyful times

B. Typically, bookstores only stock a very limited selection of texts

C. Technological progress can have unintended, detrimental consequences

D. People who continue to read books aren't concerned by inconveniences

Region	Average Asking Price			Grade 3 to 1 Premium		Grade 2 to 1 Premium	
	Grade 1	Grade 2	Grade 3	(£)	(%)	(£)	(%)
West Midlands	£218,903	£187,317	£165,984	£52,919	32%	£31,586	17%
North West	£184,659	£164,205	£145,269	£39,390	27%	£20,454	12%
Yorks & Humber	£181,821	£164,654	£148,934	£32,886	22%	£17,166	10%
South East	£408,201	£367,986	£336,222	£71,979	21%	£40,215	11%
East of England	£353,496	£322,547	£293,673	£59,823	20%	£30,949	10%
South West	£300,862	£284,000	£253,791	£47,071	19%	£16,862	6%
London	£678,595	£659,397	£598,054	£80,542	13%	£19,198	3%
North East	£144,192	£134,322	£127,102	£17,090	13%	£9,870	7%
East Midlands	£201,874	£190,208	£178,549	£23,325	13%	£11,666	6%
National Average	**£350,339**	**£313,450**	**£297,967**	**£52,372**	**18%**	**£36,889**	**12%**

14. The table shows the average house price in different regions for homes which are close to an 'outstanding' primary school (grade 1), a 'good' primary school (grade 2) or a primary school which has been rated by Ofsted as 'requires improvement' (grade 3).

Select the words 'Yes' or 'No' if the conclusion does or doesn't follow

Only 3 regions have a below average percentage premium for a grade 3 home over a grade 1 home	Yes / No
The average given here is the median	Yes / No
The premium is less in areas with generally higher house prices as people there can take their children out of the state school system and use private education instead.	Yes / No
The cheapest homes in England can be found in the North East	Yes / No
Those who pay the most to live near a Grade 1 school, rather than a Grade 3 school, live in London	Yes / No

15. A commitment to organic farming and organic produce may seem very admirable and does ensure that the consumers of such produce have fewer chemicals associated with agriculture in their bodies. However – it is naïve to think that such farming can be sustainable on a global scale. The labour-intensive nature of organic farming and correspondingly lower yields mean it is not economic to farm this way, nor could the method effectively feed all the people on the planet.

Which of the following can be concluded from the passage?

A. Agricultural chemicals are very bad for your health
B. Wider adoption of organic farming would help tackle unemployment
C. Intensive agriculture on differs from organic farming due to chemical use
D. Organic produce will inevitably cost more to the consumer

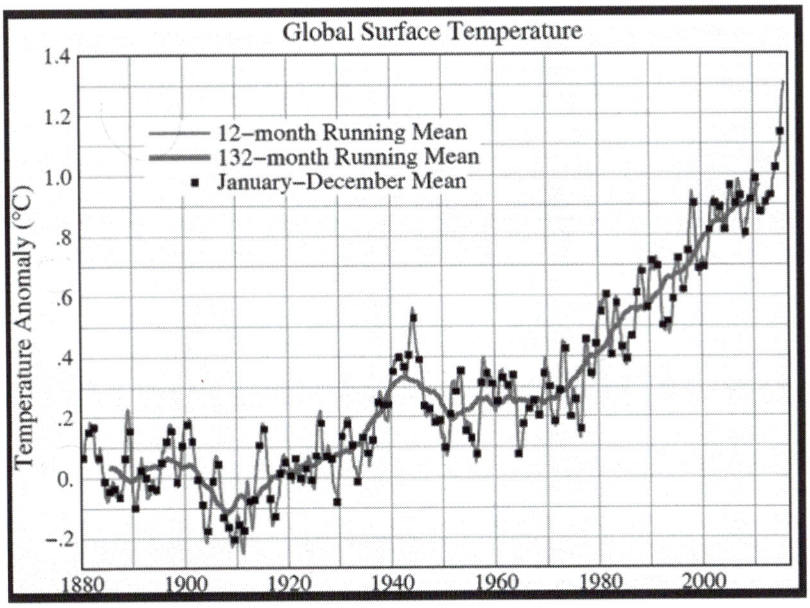

16. Select the conclusion that can be drawn from the graph:

A. The overall picture is one of fluctuation
B. There are natural variations in the global climate
C. The annual mean shows a steady increase in global temperatures
D. The long-term trend cannot be observed using short term measurements

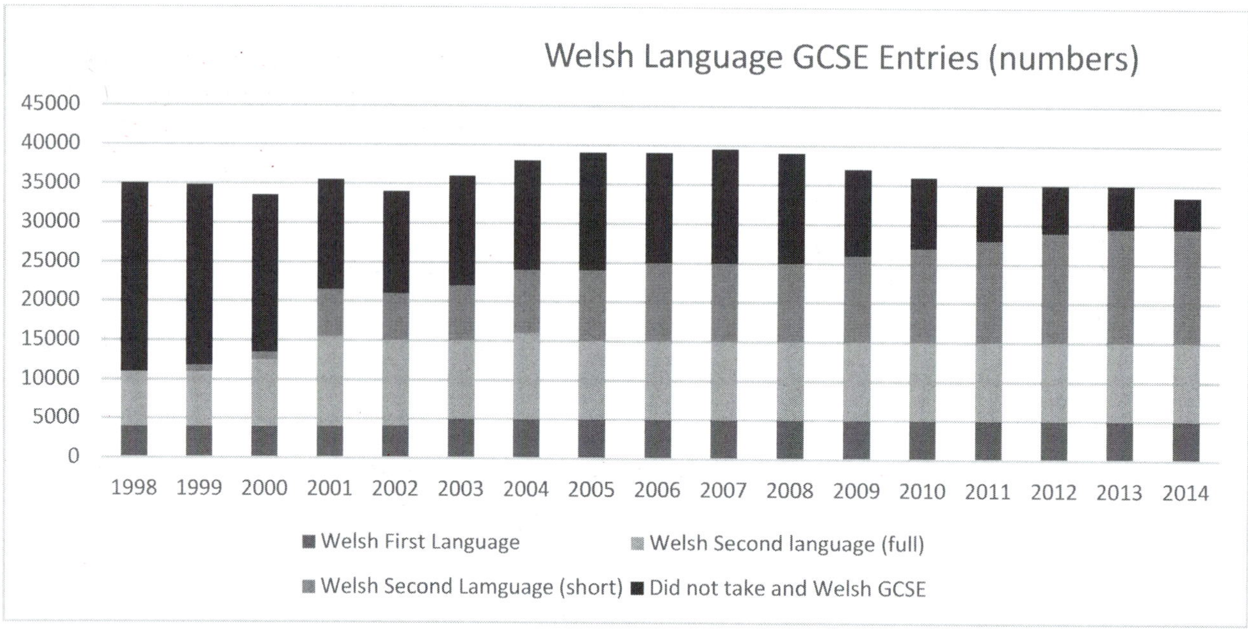

17. Select the words 'Yes' or 'No' if the conclusion does or doesn't follow

A higher percentage of students took some sort of Welsh GCSE in 2002 than 2001	Yes / No
The Welsh Second Language (short) was introduced in 1999	Yes / No
There have been between 35,000 and 40,000 Welsh GCSE students throughout the period shown	Yes / No
The number of Welsh first language pupils has remained quite static at between 4,000 and 5,500	Yes / No
The largest change over this period was that more students took Welsh Second Language (short) as opposed to not taking any Welsh GCSE	Yes / No

18. People who travel widely have a much greater appreciation of the diversity of culture and lifestyle in different places in the world

A. Yes – nothing quite compares to seeing other places with your own eyes
B. Yes – people who travel widely have fully experienced a range of other cultures
C. No – it is possible to read far more widely than most people will ever travel
D. No – most travellers only go to tourist places and don't see the 'real' country

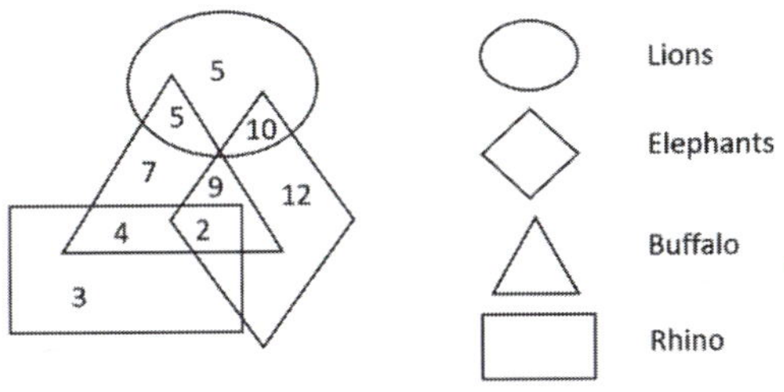

19. This diagram represents the animal sightings of various groups who went on safari while on holiday in Africa. Which statement is true?

A. 15 groups saw lions
B. The rarest animal to see was the rhino
C. Many groups saw three of the four animals
D. More groups saw just one animal than multiple animals

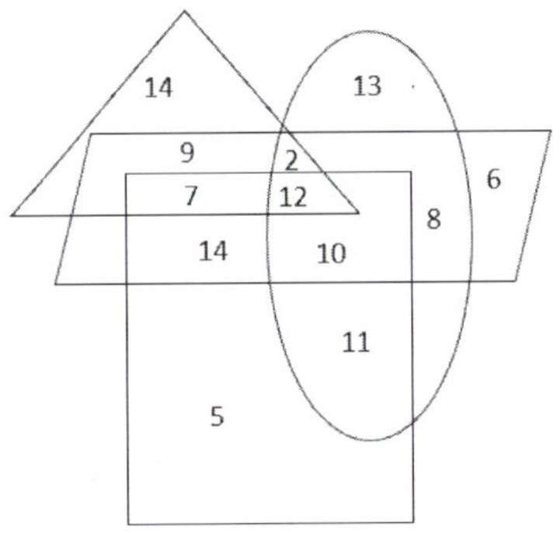

20. This Venn diagram shows the number of students taking various classes at a school of dance and drama.

The oval represents ballet
The parallelogram represents tap dance
The triangle represents speech and drama
The square represents freestyle

Which of the following statements is true?

A. The most commonly taken subject overall is freestyle
B. Fewer students take both ballet and freestyle than take speech and tap
C. Fewer than 20 students in total take three out of the four classes offered
D. More than a third of speech students only study speech

21. Five people (Howard, Justin, Kevin, Ian and Luca) are comparing their commute distances and trying to rank them from shortest to longest.

- Howard travels a shorter distance than Justin
- Kevin travels further than Ian
- Justin travels further than Kevin or Ian
- Ian travels further than Howard but not as far as Kevin

Who travels the shortest distance and longest distance of this group?

A. Ian (shortest) and Luca (longest)
B. Howard (shortest) and Justin (longest)
C. Kevin (shortest) and Howard (longest)
D. Luca (shortest) and Kevin (longest)

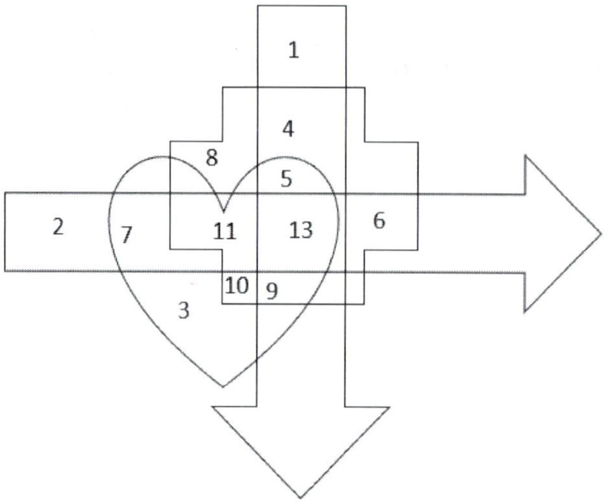

22. This diagram shows some information about a number of football teams.

The heart represents teams having a stadium of more than 10,000 capacity
The cross represents teams having won a trophy in the last 50 years
The right pointing arrow represents teams playing in red
The down pointing arrow represents teams never having been relegated

Which of the following statements is true?

A. No teams have won a trophy and have never been relegated
B. 12 teams in the sample have not won a trophy in the last 50 years
C. Playing in red makes you more likely to win a trophy based on this information
D. Most teams in this sample have a 10,000+ capacity stadium

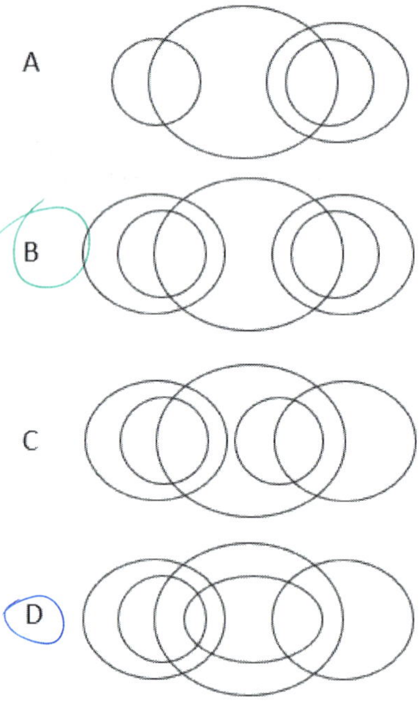

23. All cars have wheels. Some cars run on diesel. Some trains run on diesel. All trains run on tracks.

Which of the diagrams best describes the information given?

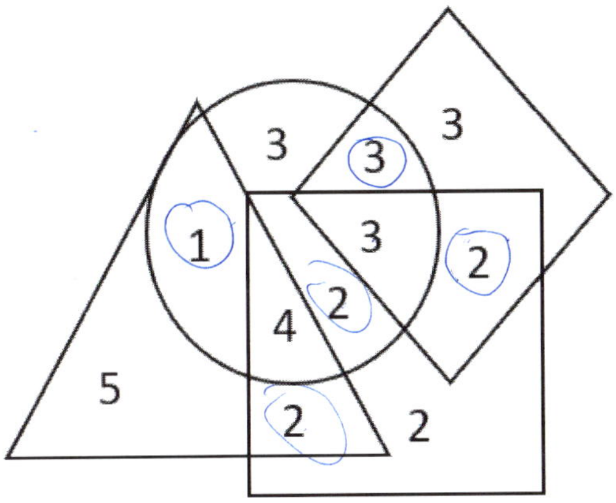

24. Miss Cooper took her class on an overnight field trip. Every single child forgot at least one vital thing.

Triangle – toothbrush
Circle – pyjamas
Square – phone charger
Diamond – spare underwear

What proportion of children forgot exactly two items?

A. A quarter
B. A third
C. Half
D. Two thirds

25. Kevin and Lucy are twins in the class. Their mum delivered the pyjamas and underwear they both forgot. How many children in total now have no pyjamas?

A. 16
B. 15
C. 14
D. 13

26. Isabel and Jonathan have gone into a travel agent to book a holiday. They are undecided as to whether to stay in a hotel, a villa, an apartment or a glamping tent. They countries they are considering are France, Spain, Portugal, Italy, and Greece. All combinations of accommodation and country are possible.

Which of the following is the most likely possible outcome?

A. Isabel and Jonathan choose to stay in a hotel
B. Isabel and Jonathan decide against Portugal and Spain
C. Isabel and Jonathan choose Italy
D. Isabel and Jonathan decide against a villa or an apartment

27. There are 29 children in Class 5. Their teacher monitored their attendance for one week (Monday – Friday).

- 22 children were there everyday
- The only day all 29 children were at school was Wednesday
- A group of five were absent on Friday due to a football match at another school
- The total number of 'attendances' for the week was 137.

How many children were at school on Monday?

A. 27
B. 28
C. 29
D. Can't tell

28. Someone is throwing two dice. They believe there is a 50% chance that the total score thrown will be 8 or above.

A. Yes – there is a 50% chance that each dice thrown will land on 4, 5 or 6 so the total score would be above 8
B. Yes – there are many combinations equally 8 or above that don't require a number above 3 to be thrown
C. No – as both dice must show 4 or above, there is only a 25% chance of throwing 8 or above
D. No – there are fewer dice combinations which add up to 8 or more than those which add up to 7 or less.

29. Rachel has a bag with six colours of wool in it. There are 3 balls of blue wool, 2 balls of purple wool and 1 ball of pink wool. She randomly picks the first ball – blue – and knits half of a blanket. She needs another ball of wool to complete the blanket. She thinks the chance of knitting the whole blanket blue is 50%. Is she right?

A. Yes - she has a greater than 50% chance of taking another blue ball of wool out to complete the first blanket
B. Yes – as there are only three colours the chances of two identical colour balls coming out consecutively is very high.
C. No – there is less than a 50% chance of Rachel picking a blue ball to complete the blanket
D. No – there is a 1 in 3 chance she will pull out a purple ball of wool next time

Full Mock Test 2 Quantitative Reasoning (24 minutes for this section)

27/37

Recipe for vegetable soup

Chop a medium onion of around 150g along with 675g potatoes, 150g carrots and 150g of parsnips. Using 2 tablespoons of vegetable oil, fry the onions for 6 minutes and gradually add half of the chopped vegetables.

Once the vegetables begin to brown, add the remaining vegetables along with 75g of peas. Next, put two 200g tins of chopped tomatoes into the pan with 100g of kidney beans and half a pint of stock.

Cover the pan and simmer for about half an hour until the vegetables have softened. Season the mixture and remove from the heat. Place the mixture into a liquidiser and once the desired consistency is achieved, pour into a bowl and serve immediately.

1. Not including the vegetable oil and stock, what will be the weight of the soup?

A. 1625g
B. 1500g
C. 1850g
D. 1550g
E. 1700g

2. Not including the vegetable oil and stock, what percentage of the soup will consist of tinned ingredients? Give the answer to the nearest whole number.

A. 36%
B. 20%
C. 32%
D. 31%
E. 29%

3. If Mrs Cook was to increase the amount of potatoes used by 27%, what would be the mass of potatoes used in the soup? Give the answer to the nearest gram.

A. 182 g
B. 857 g
C. 25 g
D. 787 g
E. 935 g

4. If Mrs Cook increases the simmering time by 85 %, what would be the new boiling time?

A. 0.56 hours
B. 3563 seconds
C. 0.26 hours
D. 3330 seconds
E. 26 minutes

Chemical	Amount
Rixypolydon	1/7
Bincom	34/82
Granular Silycom	3/13
Yernyphosotride	2/19
Polytomi	1/50

Chemicals used in a shampoo
Amounts are shown as fractions by weight

5. Which chemical will be the heaviest?

A. Rixypolydon
B. Bincom
C. Granular Silycom
D. Yernyphosotride
E. Polytomi

6. One of the chemicals has been left off the list, what fraction of the weight will this chemical be? Give the answer to 3 decimal places.

A. 0.239
B. 0.062
C. 0.240
D. 0.086
E. Cannot tell

7. If the bottle of shampoo weighs 1200g, with 30% of the weight being packaging, what is the weight of the Granular Silycom?

A. 840 g
B. 194 g
C. 360 g
D. 83 g
E. 277 g

8. The price of the shampoo is £2.30, but the company would like to sell the product in Europe for 3.99 euros. If the current exchange rate is £1 = 1.07 euros, how much more money will they make per unit in Europe?

A. £1.43
B. £2.46
C. £1.69
D. £1.07
E. £1.97

A group of men decides to do a parachute jump for charity. During the jump, the C-182 aircraft will leave the Meadows airfield at 14:00 and climb to 13,000 feet. There will be 6 people participating in the jump and they will be in tandem with 6 professional parachutists. They will all exit the aircraft in pairs once it has reached altitude, free falling at an average speed of 120mph for 1 minute, after which they will have to release their parachute.
1000 feet = 0.189 miles
1 mile = 1,609 metres

9. After leaving the airfield the aircraft ascends at 800 feet per minute. At what time will it reach its intended altitude?

A. 14:11
B. 14:06
C. 14:24
D. 14:16
E. 14:18

10. At what average speed will the parachute jumpers fall, in metres per second?

A. 0.07 m/s
B. 193,080 m/s
C. 53.6 m/s
D. 0.03 m/s
E. 13.4 m/s

11. If the mean weight of each person jumping is 70 kg, and the take-off weight of the aircraft is 10,000 kg, approximately what percentage of the take-off weight is made up by the people jumping?

A. 0.7 %
B. 4.2 %
C. 70 %
D. 84 %
E. 8.4 %

12. At what altitude must the jumpers release their parachutes?

A. 10,582 feet
B. 13,000 feet
C. 87 feet
D. 2,418 feet
E. 4,572 feet

The graph shows the response of a valve on a pressure vessel, where Max Chamber Pressure (Pc) equals 9.18 bar. The valve is switched on at Time = ON and switched off at Time = OFF

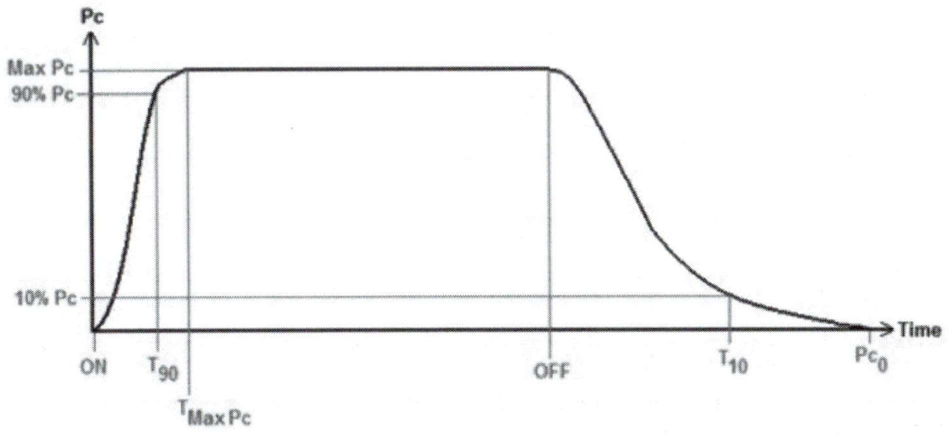

13. What is the chamber pressure at T90?

A. 9.18 bar
B. 8.262 bar
C. 0.102 bar
D. 862.18 bar
E. 826.2 bar

14. What is the chamber pressure at T10?

A. 91.8 bar
B. 918 bar
C. 0.092 bar
D. 0.009 bar
E. 0.918 bar

15. How would you calculate the duration of the VALVE ON time?

A. OFF – ON
B. ON – OFF
C. ON
D. Pc0 – ON
E. OFF - T90

16. A valve gives a pressure reading of 2 bar at T10. What is Max Pc?

A. 2 bar
B. 10 bar
C. 20 bar
D. 200 bar
E. 0.2 bar

Flight information

Options selected	Details and costs
Return ticket (flight only)	£219.50 per person (including charges)
Choose seat number	£10 per person
Seats together	£20 per person
Early booking reduction	£15 per person
Baggage allowance	22kg per person £7 per kilo excess
Cancellation	Non-refundable <3 months before travel

17. What is the total flight cost for a family of 4 booking early and choosing to sit together?

A. £1,058
B. £878
C. £921
D. £959
E. £938

Accomodation details

Villa cost p/wk	£899
Cancellation	More than 70 days - less deposit
	70-50 days - 50% cost of accommodation
	49-29 days - 70% cost of accommodation
	28-11 days - 90% cost of accommodation
	10 days or fewer - 100 %

Assume 1 mile = 1.609 km

18. Due to unforeseen circumstances it might be necessary to cancel the holiday. It is now 5 weeks before the departure date. What is the potential financial loss?

A. £1,837.00
B. £1,567.30
C. £1,747.10
D. £899.00
E. £1,387.50

19. Fortunately it was not necessary to cancel the holiday. During the course of the flight the pilot announced that the average speed of the plane was 500 mph. If the total flight time is 4 hours 10 minutes, how far in km had they travelled after 1.5 hrs?

A. 3,352.35 km
B. 750 km
C. 1,589.65 km
D. 1,206.75 km
E. 804.50 km

20. The family converted £850 into euros. During the holiday they spent 831.71 euros. What amount in pounds sterling did they return with? (Buy rate 1.137, sell rate 0.879)

A. £153.50
B. £89.75
C. £118.44
D. £20.80
E. £16.08

School	Seats on Bus	Pupils using Bus
North Hills	30	18
East Coast	28	27
Westwoods	35	32
Southlake	30	29

21. What percentage of seats is used on the North Hills bus?

A. 80%
B. 40%
C. 60%
D. 70%
E. 50%

22. What percentage of seats is empty on all the buses? Give the answer to the nearest whole number.

A. 14%
B. 16%
C. 86%
D. 13%
E. 17%

23. One more pupil decides to use the bus to East Coast School. By what percentage does the proportion of seats used change? Give the answer to 2 decimal places.

A. 3.58%
B. 1.00%
C. 100%
D. 2.48%
E. 3.57%

24. Southlake School decide to get a new 32-seater bus to replace the old one. What is the difference in the percentage of empty seats on the new bus compared with the old bus?

A. 6%
B. 2%
C. 1%
D. 9%
E. 4%

House	Distribution of Pupils
St George's	37%
St Andrew's	14%
St Patrick's	8%
St David's	23%
St Thomas's	18%

A school decided to divide the pupils into groups called Houses. They let the pupil's decide what House they wanted to be in, and the table shows the distribution of pupils per House.

Number of pupils = 482

25. How many pupils are in St Thomas's House? Give the answer to the nearest whole number.

A. 26
B. 18
C. 87
D. 27
E. 83

26. If 60 % of the pupils in St Andrew's House are male, how many female pupils are in St Andrew's House? Give the answer to the nearest whole number.

A. 26
B. 40
C. 193
D. 27
E. 67

27. If three pupils leave St George's to join St Thomas's House, how many pupils are now in St Thomas's House? Give the answer to the nearest whole number.

A. 89
B. 90
C. 88
D. 87
E. 86

28. If 40 new students join the school and are divided equally between the Houses, how many pupils are now in St Patrick's House? Give the answer to the nearest whole number.

A. 46
B. 41
C. 47
D. 42
E. 39

Marge decides to invest in some shares on the stock market. She has £1,500 that she would like to invest, buying one share per chosen company. She will only put two-thirds of the investment into high-risk shares, whilst the rest will go into low-risk, low-return shares. The high risk shares she has decided to invest in includes £600 for Global Bank, £250 for Greencoz and the remaining high-risk amount in Pollo Investments. The low risk shares she has decided to invest in are for SaveShare. High-risk investments typically see a 60% increase in value after one year, but this is not guaranteed. In addition, high-risk investments can see a loss of up to 30% in value. Low risk investments see a guaranteed increased in value of 5% after one year.

29. How much money will Marge be investing in Pollo Investments?

A. £650
B. £500
C. £200
D. £50
E. £150

30. What will Marge's SaveShare shares be worth after 1 year?

A. £525
B. £25
C. £476
D. £505
E. £1,575

31. What is the best possible share price for Greencoz after 1 year?

A. £250
B. £325
C. £175
D. £150
E. £400

32. If the markets perform badly and Marge sells her shares after 1 year, what is the worst-case amount she will be left with?

A. £0
B. £525
C. £500
D. £1225
E. £700

The newly generous Scrooge has promised to pay for Bob Cratchit and his family to go on holiday for 5 days (six nights). He now has to make arrangements

Bob's Family	**1 wife, 4 children including Tiny Tim**
Boarding house rates in Brighton	10 shillings per night for adults, 5 for children
Boarding house rates in Southsea	8 shillings per night for adults, 4 for children
Boarding house rates in Harwich	6 shillings per night for adults, 3 for children
Return train fare to Brighton	6 shillings for adults, 3 for children (Tiny Tim has a disabled badge and travels free)
Return train fare to Southsea	8 shillings for adults, 4 for children (Tiny Tim has a disabled badge and travels free)
Return stage coach to Harwich (no train available)	10 shillings for adults and 5 for children (no disablity concession)

12 pennies in each shilling and 20 shillings in each pound
Currency expressed £1/1/1 (one pound, one shilling, one pence)

33. How much will it cost Scrooge for the Brighton holiday?

A. £12/ - / -
B. £12/ 1 / -
C. £12/ 4 / -
D. £13/ - / -
E. £13/ 1 / -

34. How much will it cost Scrooge for the Southsea holiday?

A. £9/ 12 / -
B. £10/ 20 / -
C. £11/ - / -
D. £11/ 4 / -
E. £12/ - / -

35. How much will it cost Scrooge for the Harwich holiday?

A. £8/ 4 / -
B. £8/ 12 / -
C. £8/ 12 / -
D. £8/ 16 / -
E. £9/ 4 / -

36. The parsimonious old Scrooge would buy the cheapest offer.
How much more will the generous hearted version have to pay choosing the most expensive holiday? (in old money)

A. £1/ 16 / -
B. £2/ 1 / -
C. £3/ 17 / -
D. £8/ 16 / -
E. £11/ - / -

Full Mock Test 2 Abstract Reasoning (13 minutes for this section)

Set A | Set B

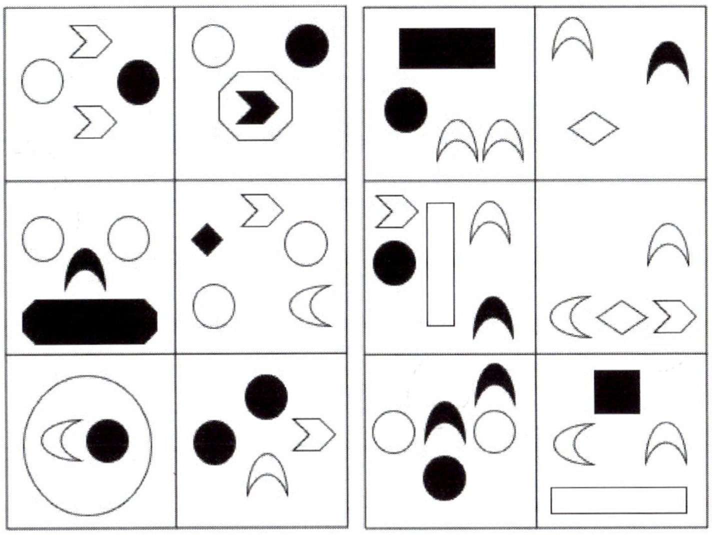

1 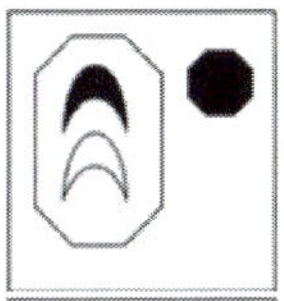
Set A
Set B
Neither

2 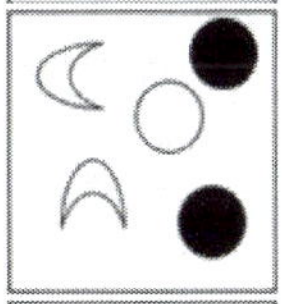
Set A
Set B
Neither

3 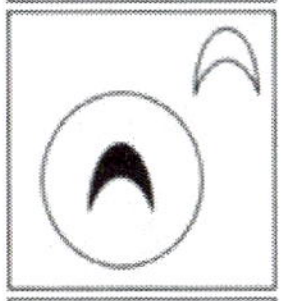
Set A
Set B
Neither

4 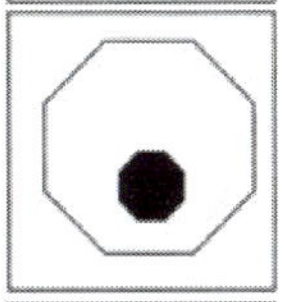
Set A
Set B
Neither

5 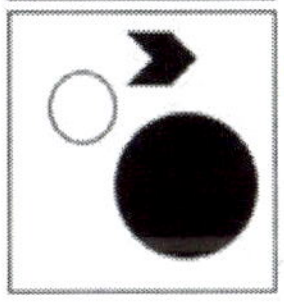
Set A
Set B
Neither

To which of the two sets do the following shapes belong?

Set A | Set B

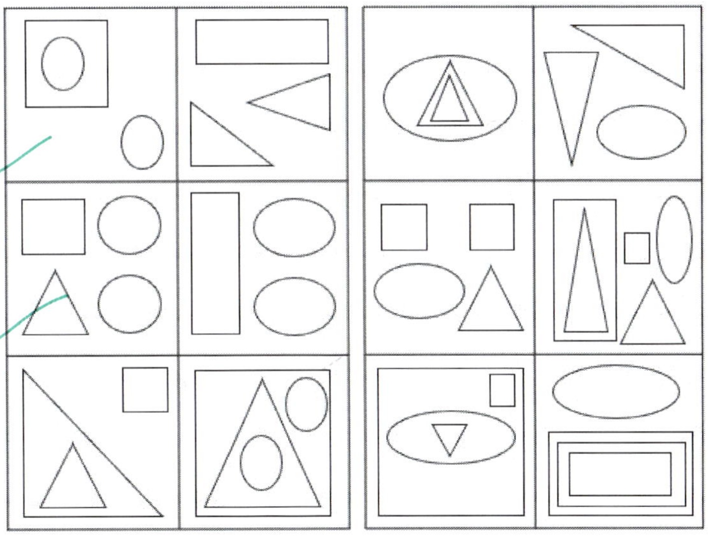

6 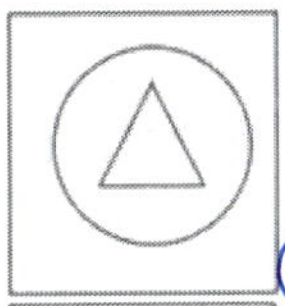
Set A
Set B
Neither

7 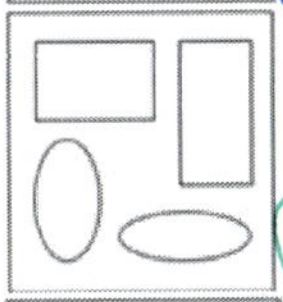
Set A
Set B
Neither

8 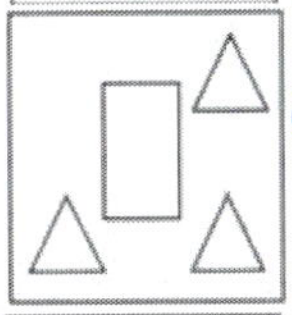
Set A
Set B
Neither

9 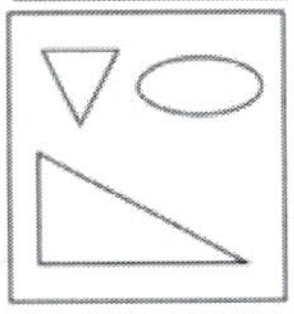
Set A
Set B
Neither

10 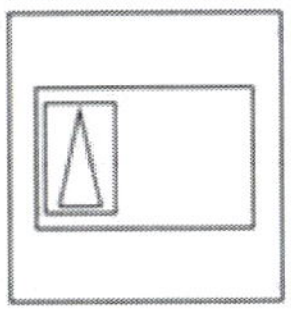
Set A
Set B
Neither

Set A

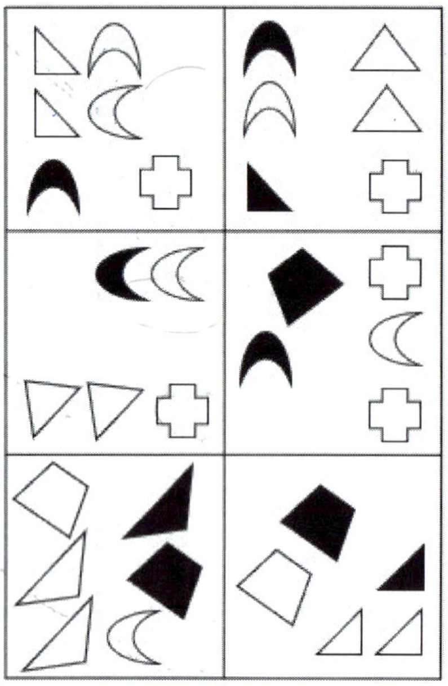

Set B

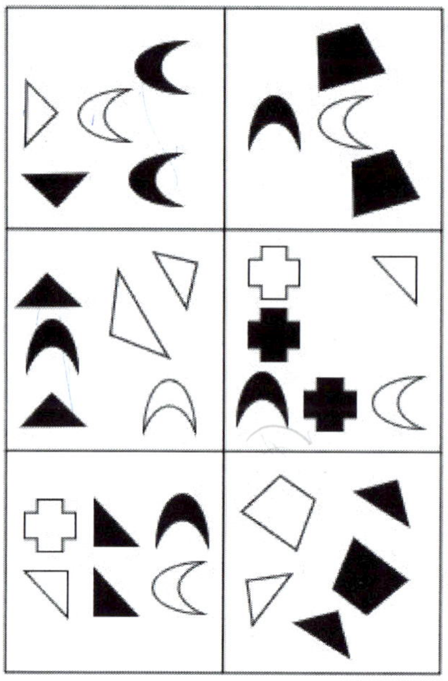

11 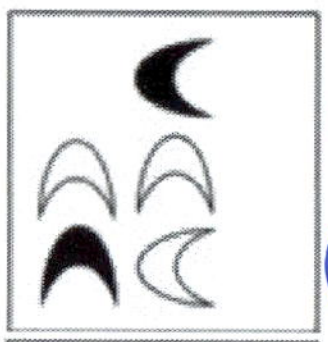

Set A
Set B
Neither

12 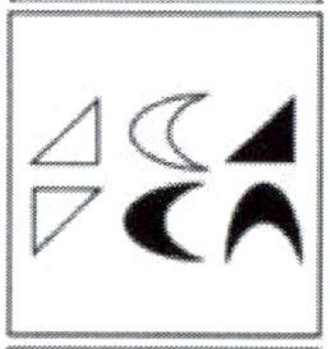

Set A
Set B
Neither

13 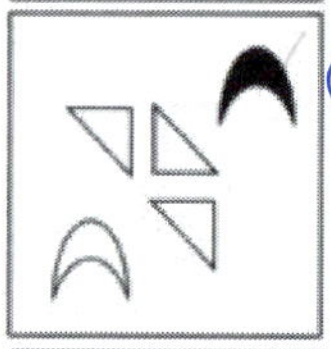

Set A
Set B
Neither

14 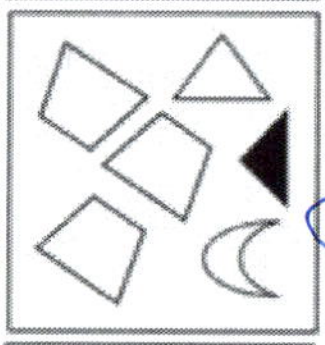

Set A
Set B
Neither

15 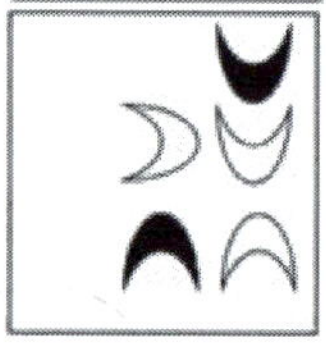

Set A
Set B
Neither

To which of the two sets do the following shapes belong?

Set A

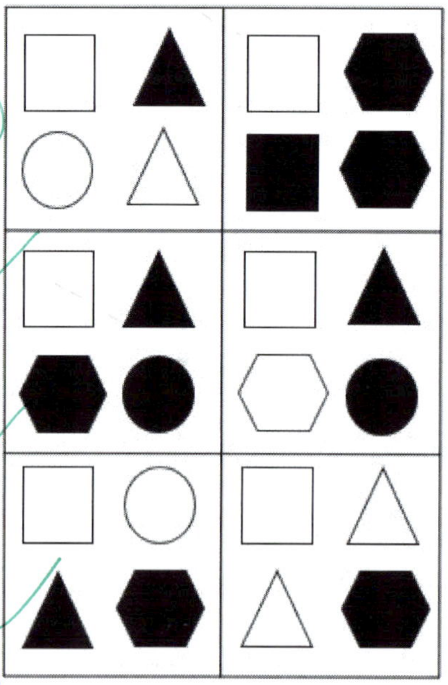

Set B

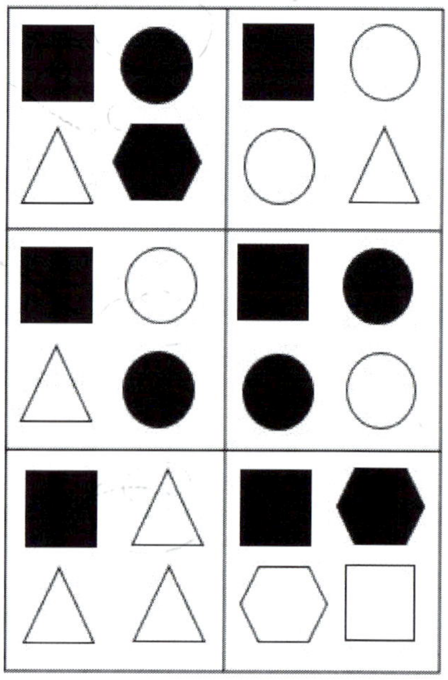

16 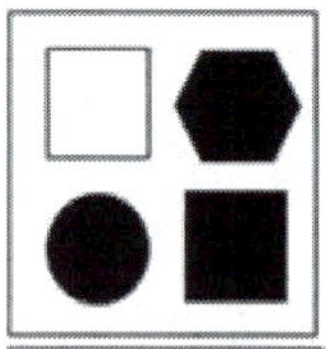

Set A
Set B
Neither

17 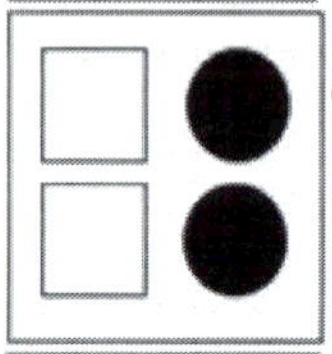

Set A
Set B
Neither

18 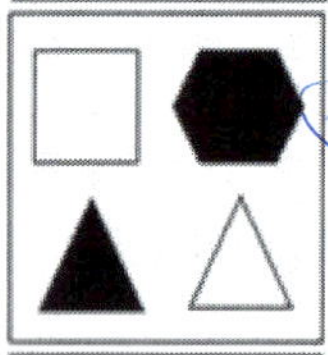

Set A
Set B
Neither

19 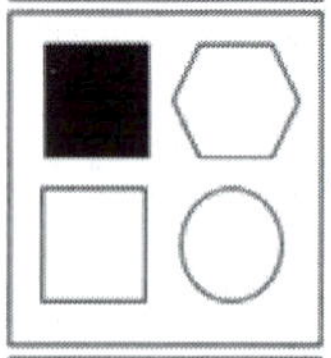

Set A
Set B
Neither

20 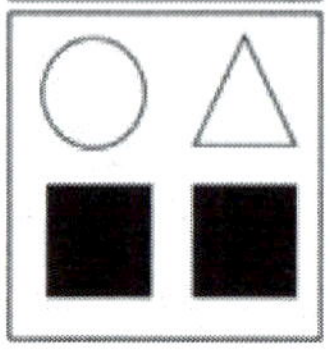

Set A
Set B
Neither

Set A | Set B

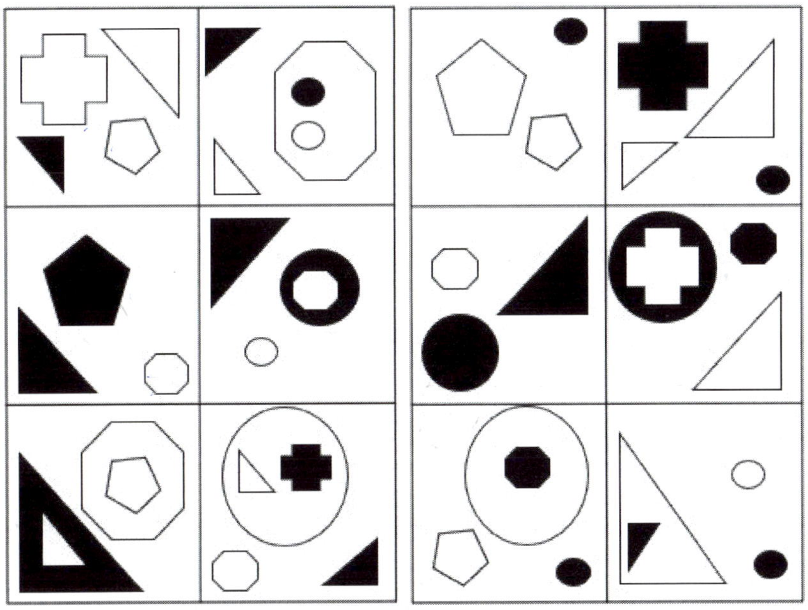

21 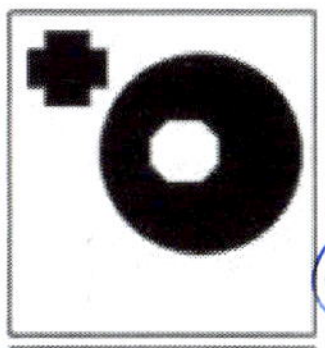
Set A
Set B
Neither

22 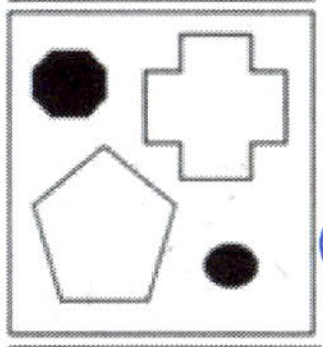
Set A
Set B
Neither

23 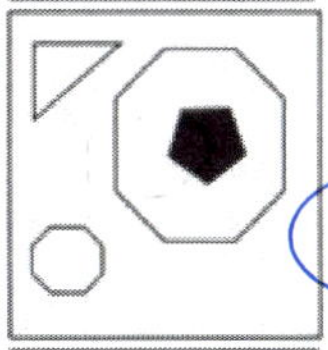
Set A
Set B
Neither

24 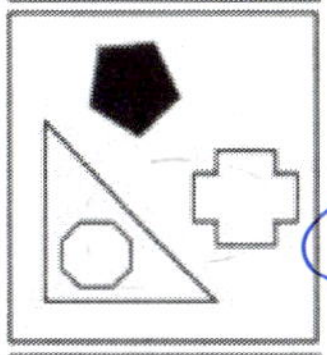
Set A
Set B
Neither

25 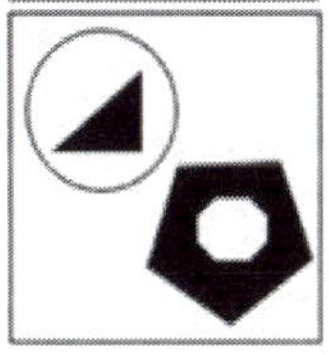
Set A
Set B
Neither

To which of the two sets do the following shapes belong?

Set A | Set B

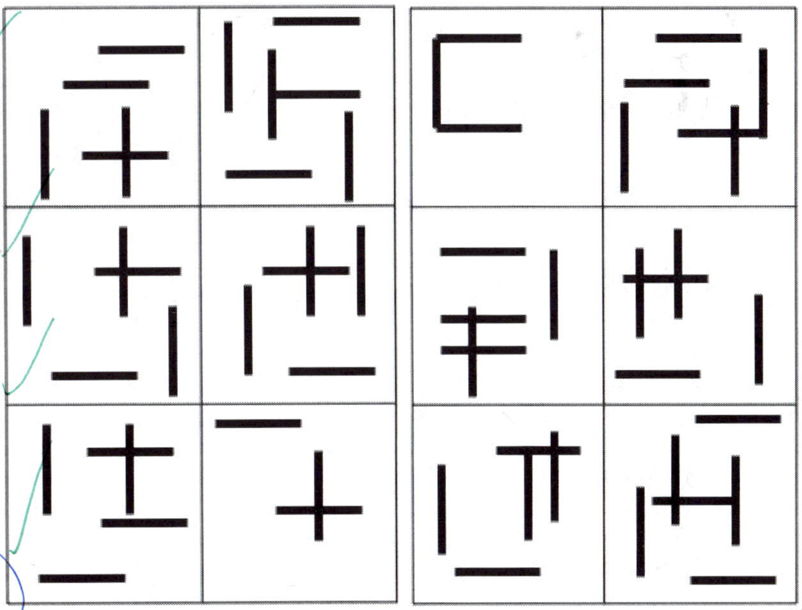

26 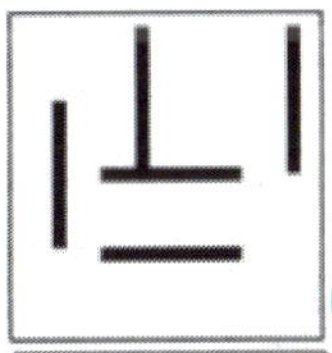
Set A
Set B
Neither

27 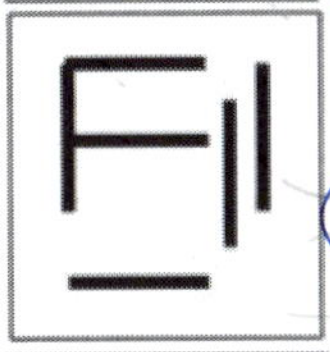
Set A
Set B
Neither

28 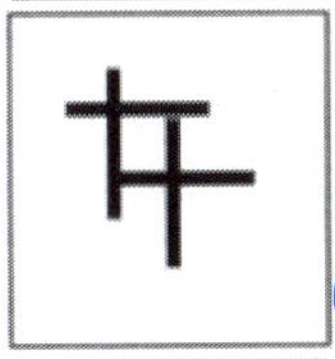
Set A
Set B
Neither

29 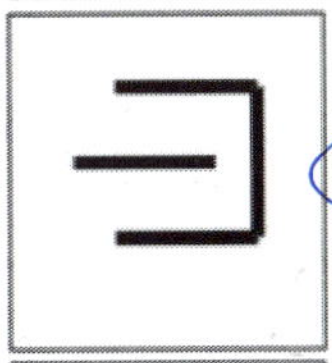
Set A
Set B
Neither

30 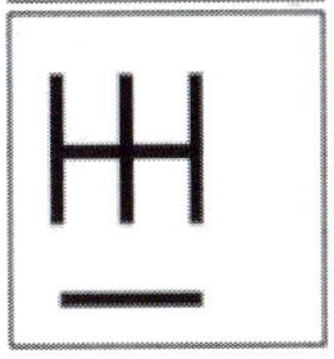
Set A
Set B
Neither

31

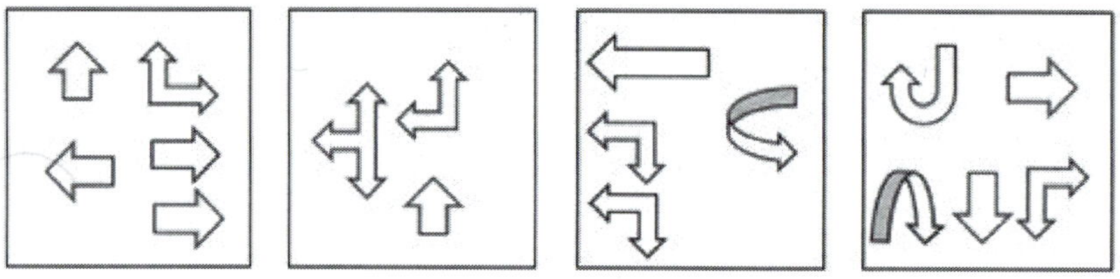

Which figure completes the series?

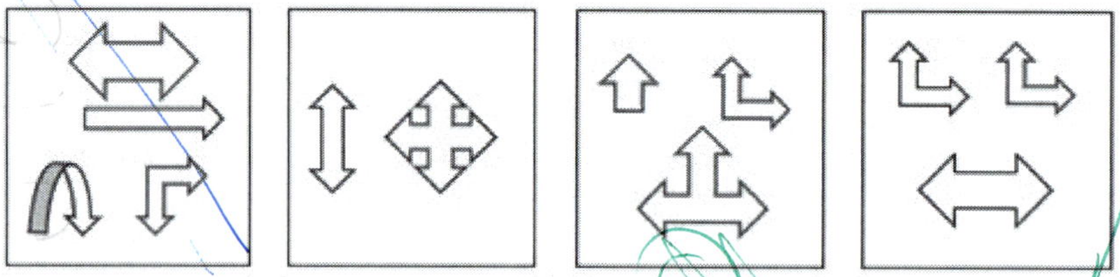

A B C D

32

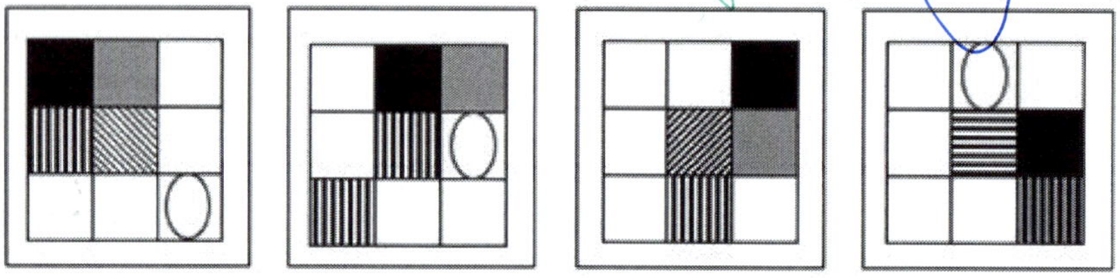

Which figure completes the series?

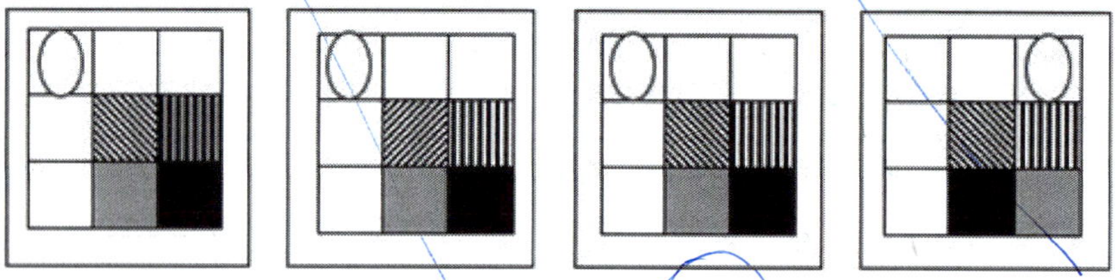

A B C D

33

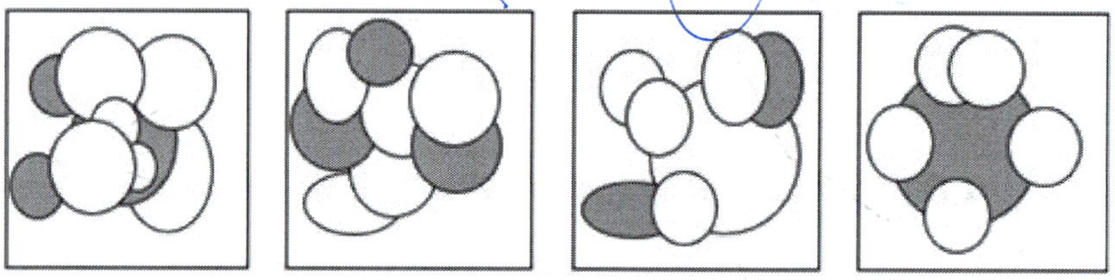

Which figure completes the series?

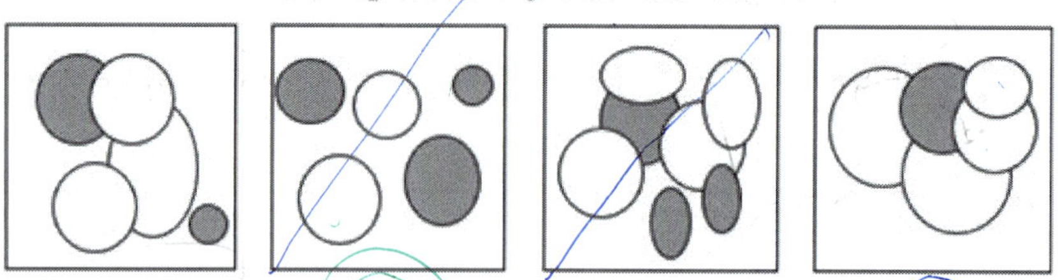

A B C D

Set A

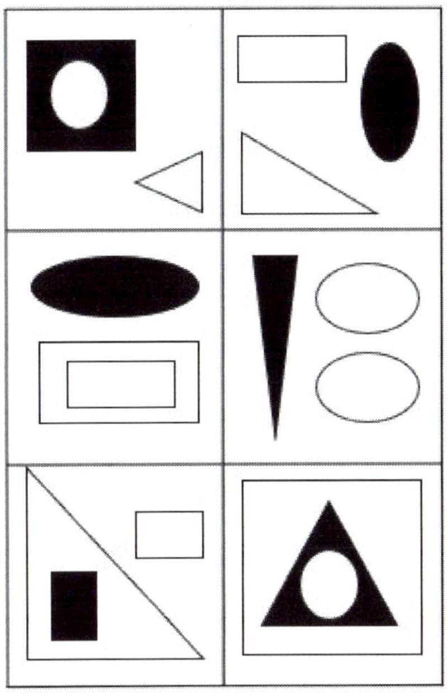

Set B

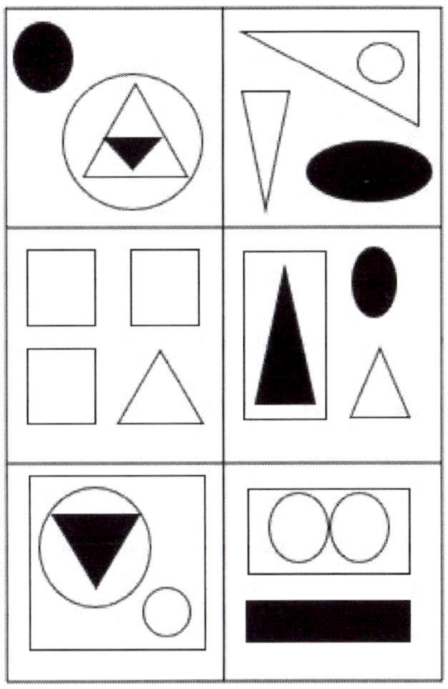

34 

Set A
Set B
Neither

35 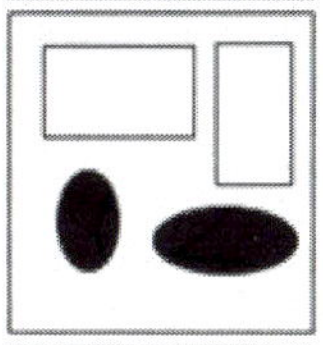

Set A
Set B
Neither

36 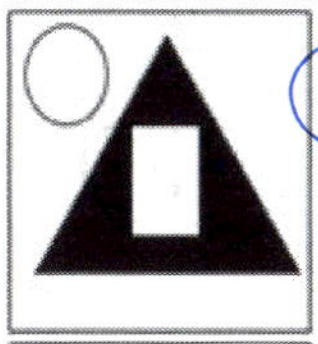

Set A
Set B
Neither

37 

Set A
Set B
Neither

38 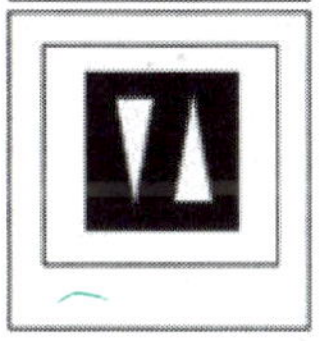

Set A
Set B
Neither

To which of the two sets do the following shapes belong?

39 

Set A
Set B
Neither

40 

Set A
Set B
Neither

41 

Set A
Set B
Neither

42 

Set A
Set B
Neither

43 

Set A
Set B
Neither

Set A

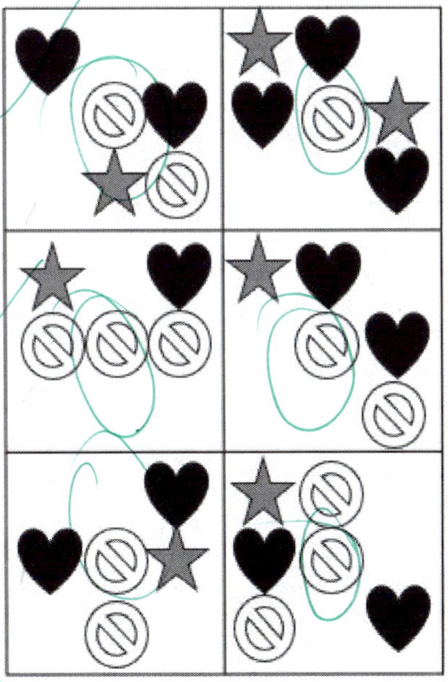

Set B

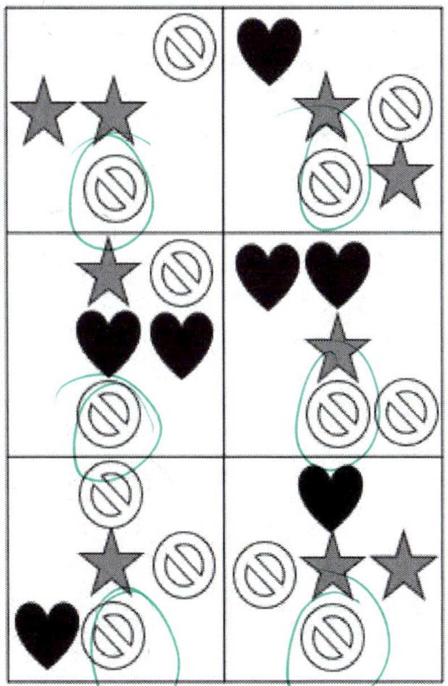

Set A

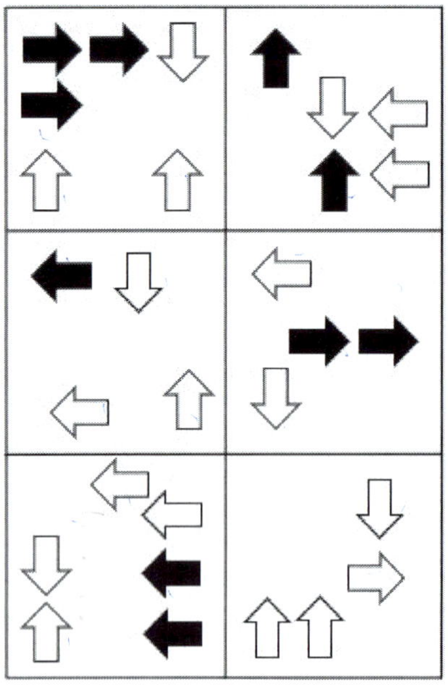

Set B

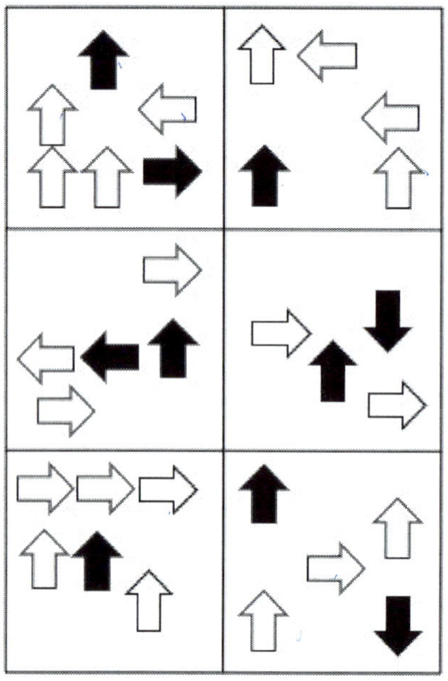

44 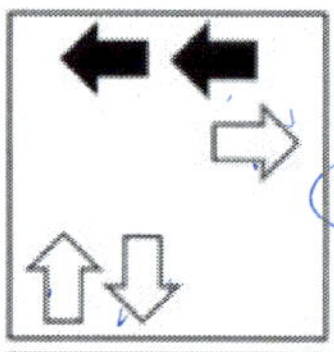
Set A
Set B
Neither

45 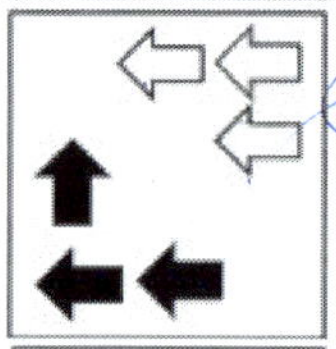
Set A
Set B
Neither

46 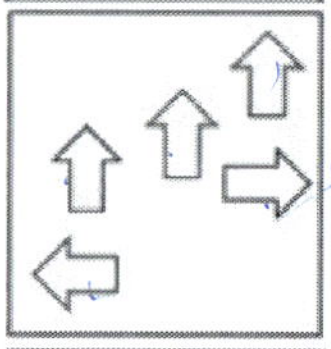
Set A
Set B
Neither

47 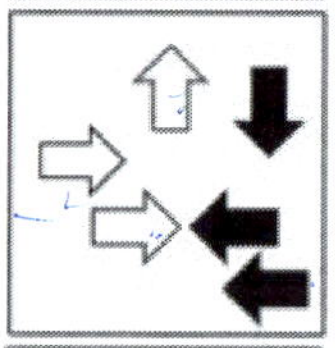
Set A
Set B
Neither

48 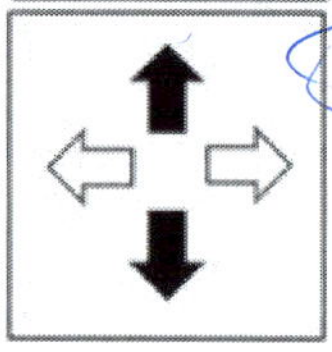
Set A
Set B
Neither

To which of the two sets do the following shapes belong?

Set A

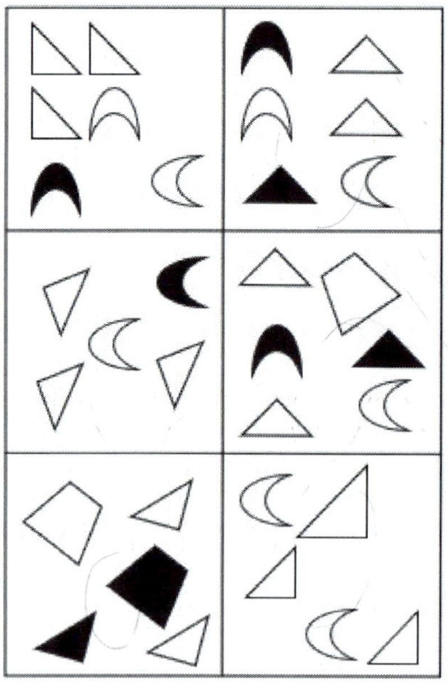

Set B

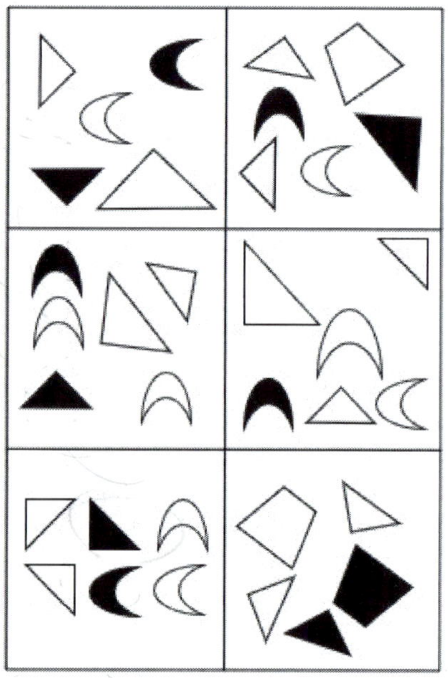

49 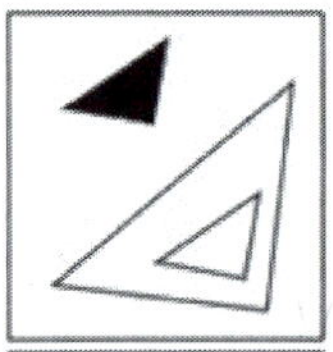
Set A
Set B
Neither

50 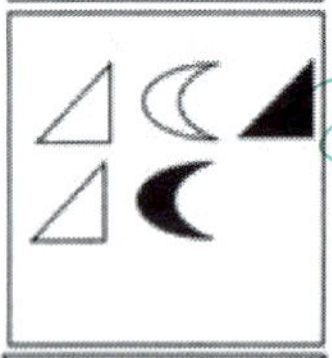
Set A
Set B
Neither

51 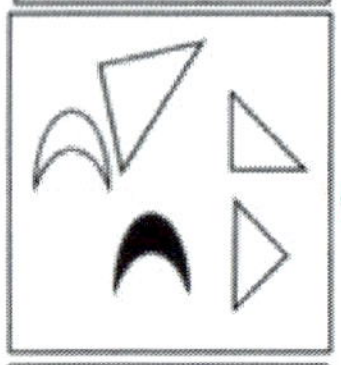
Set A
Set B
Neither

52 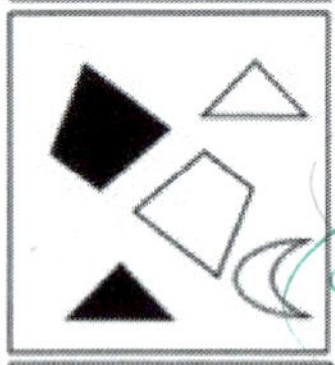
Set A
Set B
Neither

53 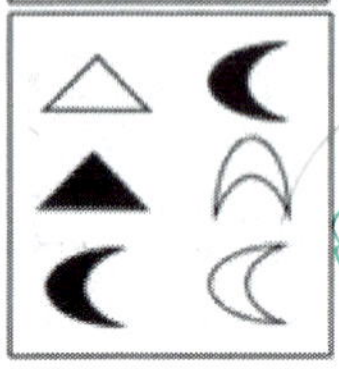
Set A
Set B
Neither

54

 is to 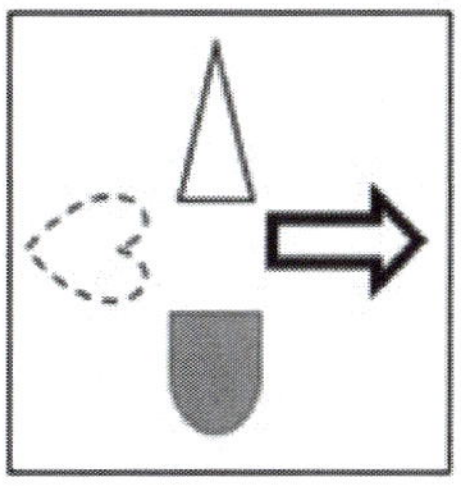

as

 is to 

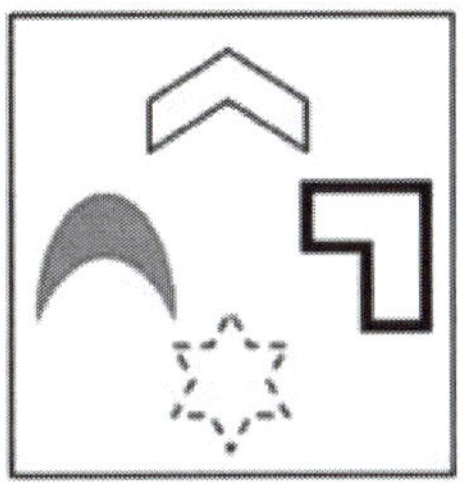
A

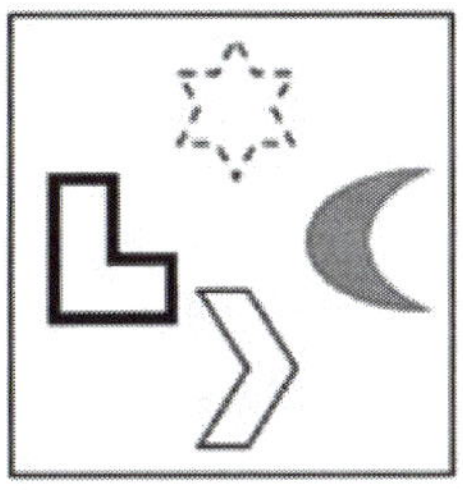
B

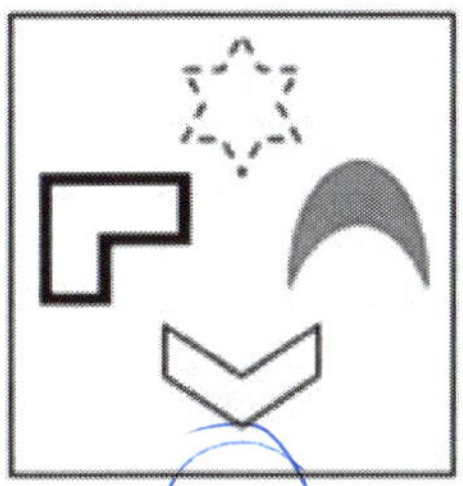
C

D

55

 is to 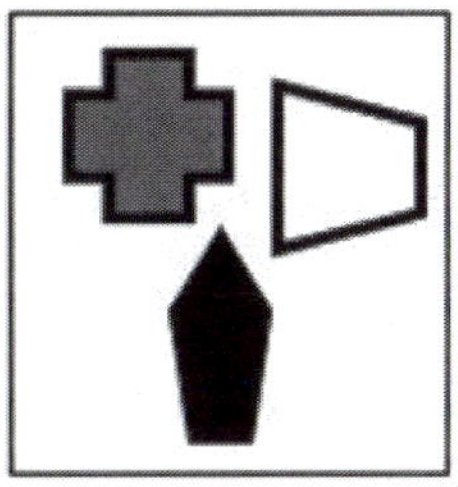

as

 is to 

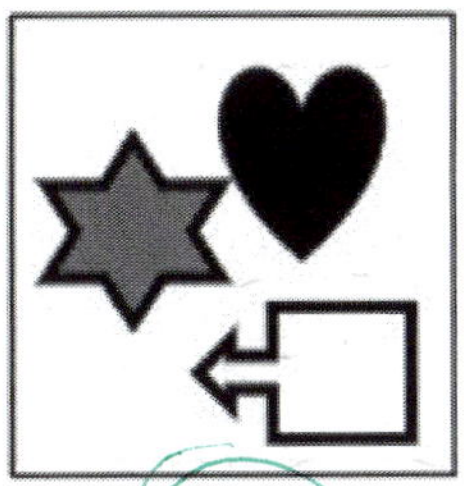
A

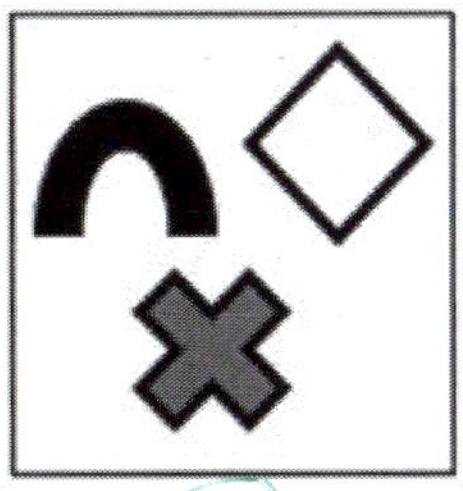
B

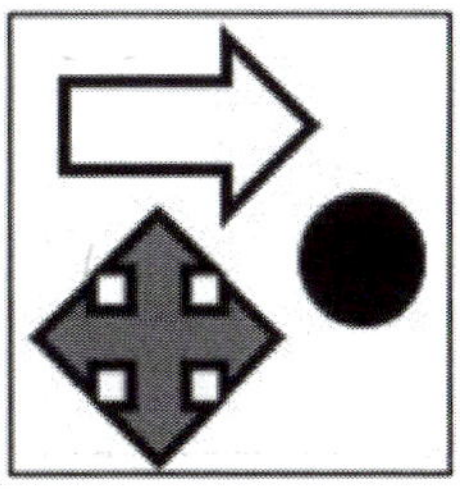
C

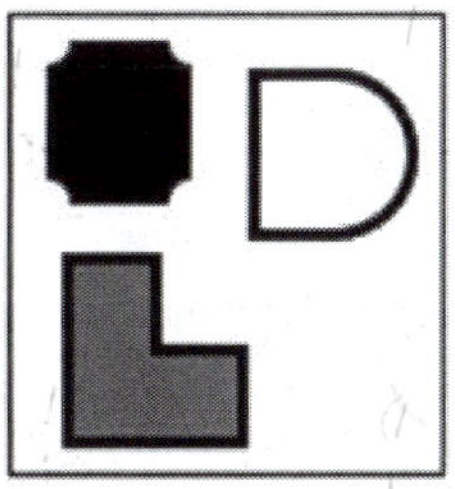
D

Full Mock Test 2 Situational Judgement (26 minutes for this section)

32/69

A woman frequently comes into A&E for drink related injuries. One of the doctors thinks that the woman may have children and is worried about their safety.

How appropriate would each action be in the circumstances:

1. Contact social services expressing concern about the patient's possible children and leave them to act.

A. A very appropriate thing to do
B. Appropriate, but not ideal
C. Inappropriate, but not awful
D. A very inappropriate thing to do

2. Ask the patient whether they have children and if so where they are and who is taking care of them.

A. A very appropriate thing to do
B. Appropriate, but not ideal
C. Inappropriate, but not awful
D. A very inappropriate thing to do

3. Ignore the misgivings on the grounds that they are not relevant to treating the current patient.

A. A very appropriate thing to do
B. Appropriate, but not ideal
C. Inappropriate, but not awful
D. A very inappropriate thing to do

4. Check the patient's records to see if they have children and the health of those children.

A. A very appropriate thing to do
B. Appropriate, but not ideal
C. Inappropriate, but not awful
D. A very inappropriate thing to do

5. Make an appointment for the patient for the next week.

A. A very appropriate thing to do
B. Appropriate, but not ideal
C. Inappropriate, but not awful
D. A very inappropriate thing to do

Tai is doing a work experience placement in a GP surgery. His duties are mainly restricted to filing and answering the telephone but when there is a clinic for elderly patients, he is enlisted to help them get in and out of the minibus and help them move around the surgery. One gentleman presses a £10 note into his hands as he leaves saying, "Thanks for your help."

How appropriate are the following courses of action by Tai?

6. Insist to the gentleman that he cannot take the money.

A. A very appropriate thing to do
B. Appropriate, but not ideal
C. Inappropriate, but not awful
D. A very inappropriate thing to do

7. Thank the gentleman and accept the money.

A. A very appropriate thing to do
B. Appropriate, but not ideal
C. Inappropriate, but not awful
D. A very inappropriate thing to do

8. Thank the gentleman and tell him he'll buy chocolates for the whole team.

A. A very appropriate thing to do
B. Appropriate, but not ideal
C. Inappropriate, but not awful
D. A very inappropriate thing to do

9. Ask the practice manager for advice.

A. A very appropriate thing to do
B. Appropriate, but not ideal
C. Inappropriate, but not awful
D. A very inappropriate thing to do

Petra is struggling with a specific part of her coursework for one of her A-levels. She has previously asked her teacher for help, but he was dismissive and irritated with her and now she is afraid to ask again.

How appropriate are the following actions by Petra?

10. Go and see the teacher again and politely ask him to help her.

A. A very appropriate thing to do
B. Appropriate, but not ideal
C. Inappropriate, but not awful
D. A very inappropriate thing to do

11. Ask her friends if they can try to explain it.

A. A very appropriate thing to do
B. Appropriate, but not ideal
C. Inappropriate, but not awful
D. A very inappropriate thing to do

12. Go and see another teacher who teaches a similar subject but a different class.

A. A very appropriate thing to do
B. Appropriate, but not ideal
C. Inappropriate, but not awful
D. A very inappropriate thing to do

13. Do the best she can but not worry too much as the coursework won't count towards her final grade.

A. A very appropriate thing to do
B. Appropriate, but not ideal
C. Inappropriate, but not awful
D. A very inappropriate thing to do

Oscar is applying to medical school. For the last two years he has had a Saturday job at a local chemist. His job almost entirely consists of selling non-pharmacy products such as toiletries but on occasion he helps the pharmacist sort out prescriptions. He is now filling in his UCAS form.

How appropriate are the following actions by Oscar?

14. Include the information about his Saturday job in his general work experience.

A. A very appropriate thing to do
B. Appropriate, but not ideal
C. Inappropriate, but not awful
D. A very inappropriate thing to do

15. Include information about his Saturday job as evidence that he has some understanding of working in the medical field.

A. A very appropriate thing to do
B. Appropriate, but not ideal
C. Inappropriate, but not awful
D. A very inappropriate thing to do

16. Ask the pharmacist if he can volunteer some extra time and observe, and possibly help, with the pharmaceutical side of the business.

A. A very appropriate thing to do
B. Appropriate, but not ideal
C. Inappropriate, but not awful
D. A very inappropriate thing to do

17. Try to deal with customers who visit the chemist to collect their prescriptions by asking the questions and following the procedures that he has seen his colleagues doing.

A. A very appropriate thing to do
B. Appropriate, but not ideal
C. Inappropriate, but not awful
D. A very inappropriate thing to do

A group of 5 final year students must do a group presentation on diabetes management that will be 25% of each person's mark for this module. They have been meeting twice a week to generate ideas and plan work sharing. Laura has not been as interactive with the group as the others and has not offered any ideas during brainstorming sessions. Richard who has been leading the task feels that Laura's lack of contribution is worrying and unfair.

How appropriate are each of the following responses by Richard in this situation?

18. In the next group meeting, ask Laura specifically for ideas.

A. A very appropriate thing to do
B. Appropriate, but not ideal
C. Inappropriate, but not awful
D. A very inappropriate thing to do

19. Speak to Laura privately about noticing she is quiet in the group and ask if she is okay or needs help.

A. A very appropriate thing to do
B. Appropriate, but not ideal
C. Inappropriate, but not awful
D. A very inappropriate thing to do

20. Speak to other group members about Laura's lack of contribution

A. A very appropriate thing to do
B. Appropriate, but not ideal
C. Inappropriate, but not awful
D. A very inappropriate thing to do

21. Offer an option for the group to contribute ideas by email or in writing

A. A very appropriate thing to do
B. Appropriate, but not ideal
C. Inappropriate, but not awful
D. A very inappropriate thing to do

Ben, an 8-year-old boy who suffers from asthma, had a very bad night where his mum noticed he was wheezing heavily. The following morning, she booked him for an emergency appointment with a locum doctor. During the consultation, as soon as the stethoscope was placed on Ben's chest, he pulled away and started crying. The crying started to exacerbate his wheezing.

How appropriate are each of the following responses by the locum doctor in this situation?

22. Suggest the mother books another appointment at a later date.

A. A very appropriate thing to do
B. Appropriate, but not ideal
C. Inappropriate, but not awful
D. A very inappropriate thing to do

23. Carry on with the check up

A. A very appropriate thing to do
B. Appropriate, but not ideal
C. Inappropriate, but not awful
D. A very inappropriate thing to do

24. Take a detailed history with Ben's mother while Ben calms down

A. A very appropriate thing to do
B. Appropriate, but not ideal
C. Inappropriate, but not awful
D. A very inappropriate thing to do

25. Pause the consultation and speak kindly to Ben explaining exactly what he is doing and why

A. A very appropriate thing to do
B. Appropriate, but not ideal
C. Inappropriate, but not awful
D. A very inappropriate thing to do

Leanne, a medical student attends the pain clinic weekly as part of her hospital placement. Already late for her morning session, she cannot find her student identification badge and then recalls she left it at her friend's house. The student ID has her photograph, name, course and year of study, and must be worn at all times during placement sessions.

How appropriate are each of the following responses by Leanne

26. Head straight to the clinic without her identification badge

A. A very appropriate thing to do
B. Appropriate, but not ideal
C. Inappropriate, but not awful
D. A very inappropriate thing to do

27. Collect her badge and call the hospital to make them aware she will be running late

A. A very appropriate thing to do
B. Appropriate, but not ideal
C. Inappropriate, but not awful
D. A very inappropriate thing to do

28. Ask her friend to detour to the hospital on his way to work and deliver the badge to her

A. A very appropriate thing to do
B. Appropriate, but not ideal
C. Inappropriate, but not awful
D. A very inappropriate thing to do

A GP receptionist is called by a patient looking to make an appointment which they say is urgent. However, it has been a particularly busy day and as a result all the urgent appointments for that day are booked, as are all the regular appointments for that week.

How appropriate would it be for the receptionist to take the following action in this situation:

29. Tell the patient to call back tomorrow and make an appointment in one of that day's urgent slots.

A. A very appropriate thing to do
B. Appropriate, but not ideal
C. Inappropriate, but not awful
D. A very inappropriate thing to do

30. Take information on the problem from the patient to try to decide how urgent the problem is before acting.

A. A very appropriate thing to do
B. Appropriate, but not ideal
C. Inappropriate, but not awful
D. A very inappropriate thing to do

31. Look through the appointments made in that day to find a routine check-up, cancel it to make space for the 'emergency' patient and offer them that appointment.

A. A very appropriate thing to do
B. Appropriate, but not ideal
C. Inappropriate, but not awful
D. A very inappropriate thing to do

Laura, a medical student, is on a placement at the hospital. She has been given the opportunity to draw blood under the supervision of junior doctors. She has learnt this in lectures, however, she is still not confident in her blood drawing skills. It is a couple of days before Laura's clinical skills exam and she wants to practise drawing blood.

How appropriate are each of the following responses by Laura in this situation?

32. Discuss her concerns about this procedure with one of the doctors

A. A very appropriate thing to do
B. Appropriate, but not ideal
C. Inappropriate, but not awful
D. A very inappropriate thing to do

33. Search online for clinical skills information and videos

A. A very appropriate thing to do
B. Appropriate, but not ideal
C. Inappropriate, but not awful
D. A very inappropriate thing to do

34. Practise on her course mates who are also medical students

A. A very appropriate thing to do
B. Appropriate, but not ideal
C. Inappropriate, but not awful
D. A very inappropriate thing to do

35. Review her lecture notes and text books for information

A. A very appropriate thing to do
B. Appropriate, but not ideal
C. Inappropriate, but not awful
D. A very inappropriate thing to do

36. Go ahead with the clinical skills test, trusting her knowledge and learning thus far

A. A very appropriate thing to do
B. Appropriate, but not ideal
C. Inappropriate, but not awful
D. A very inappropriate thing to do

Jake and Calvin, two medical students, are walking to the anatomy room to attend their first dissection lesson. These lessons are compulsory for all medical students to attend to progress their studies. Jake tells Calvin that he was feels nauseous whenever he thinks about seeing human flesh. Jake becomes very pale and refuses to enter the anatomy room.

How appropriate are each of the following responses by Calvin in this situation?

37. Tell Jake to come to class as it will affect his academic progress if he doesn't attend

A. A very appropriate thing to do
B. Appropriate, but not ideal
C. Inappropriate, but not awful
D. A very inappropriate thing to do

38. Try to reassure Jake and calm him down

A. A very appropriate thing to do
B. Appropriate, but not ideal
C. Inappropriate, but not awful
D. A very inappropriate thing to do

39. Let Jake calm down on his own

A. A very appropriate thing to do
B. Appropriate, but not ideal
C. Inappropriate, but not awful
D. A very inappropriate thing to do

40. Ask Jake to speak to the anatomy lecturer and let him know how he is feeling about the class

A. A very appropriate thing to do
B. Appropriate, but not ideal
C. Inappropriate, but not awful
D. A very inappropriate thing to do

A group of three students have been given an assignment to work on together. The group has one week to choose a topic from a list and prepare a presentation. At their first group study session, one of the students, Charlotte, decides on a topic and delegates tasks to the other two students, Mark and Susie. Mark is unhappy that Charlotte has taken charge and also feels like she has delegated most of the work and is not doing much herself.

How appropriate are each of the following responses in this situation?

41. Refuse to accept the tasks Charlotte has delegated

A. A very appropriate thing to do
B. Appropriate, but not ideal
C. Inappropriate, but not awful
D. A very inappropriate thing to do

42. Talk to Susie about the situation and make a plan

A. A very appropriate thing to do
B. Appropriate, but not ideal
C. Inappropriate, but not awful
D. A very inappropriate thing to do

During a lecture, two students, Ava and Lucas, are constantly interrupting the lecturer to ask questions unrelated to the class. Some of the students find this amusing and start to laugh and talk to each other whilst the lecturer is trying to continue with the lecture. Oliver is sitting on the table in front of Ava and Lucas and is finding it increasingly difficult to concentrate on what the lecturer is saying.

How important are the following considerations for Oliver when deciding how to respond to the situation?

43. How his actions may affect future marks he receives from this lecturer

A. Very important
B. Important
C. Of minor importance
D. Not important at all

44. The fact that he may miss out on important information he needs to progress in his studies

A. Very important
B. Important
C. Of minor importance
D. Not important at all

45. The other students are laughing and enjoying the 'banter'

A. Very important
B. Important
C. Of minor importance
D. Not important at all

46. It is the lecturer's responsibility to maintain a good learning atmosphere in his class

A. Very important
B. Important
C. Of minor importance
D. Not important at all

Heidi, a student nurse, has been given a major role in a sketch for the annual hospital charity dinner. She has been asked to play a senior doctor, Dr Sharma, who works at the hospital. Upon reading the script, she feels that the jokes are more offensive than funny and make her feel uncomfortable. She mentions this to the director but is told she is being overly sensitive.

How important are the following considerations for Heidi when deciding how to respond to the situation?

47. Dr Sharma will be attending the charity dinner

A. Very important
B. Important
C. Of minor importance
D. Not important at all

48. The director does not find the script offensive

A. Very important
B. Important
C. Of minor importance
D. Not important at all

49. Heidi has a major role in the skit

A. Very important
B. Important
C. Of minor importance
D. Not important at all

50. Heidi is not comfortable with playing the role with the current script

A. Very important
B. Important
C. Of minor importance
D. Not important at all

A patient tells a student nurse, Karen, that she had an interesting conversation with a final year medical student, Harry. The patient tells Karen that Harry was boasting about the fact that he had submitted his brother's work as his own during his last assignment. Harry has never had any reports of plagiarism in the past and comes from a family of doctors. The patient has previously made several complaints about members of staff at the hospital.

How important are the following considerations for Karen when deciding how to respond to the situation?

51. Harry comes from a family of doctors

A. Very important
B. Important
C. Of minor importance
D. Not important at all

52. Harry hasn't had any previous reports of plagiarism

A. Very important
B. Important
C. Of minor importance
D. Not important at all

53. Karen is also a student

A. Very important
B. Important
C. Of minor importance
D. Not important at all

54. The patient is known to be someone who likes to complain about staff

A. Very important
B. Important
C. Of minor importance
D. Not important at all

A medical student realises that the information given by one of his lecturers is out of date when he compares it both to his up-to-date textbook and online resources. The old information has been shown to be harmful to patients in some instances.

How important is it to consider the following?

55. Even up-to-date advice becomes obsolete eventually.

A. Very important
B. Important
C. Of minor importance
D. Not important at all

56. The lecturer may not have practiced medicine for many years but should make an effort to stay current.

A. Very important
B. Important
C. Of minor importance
D. Not important at all

57. The lecturer's errors should be brought to their attention.

A. Very important
B. Important
C. Of minor importance
D. Not important at all

Ria is a very capable student and is predicted 4 grade A* in her A levels. Ria has, for as long as she can remember, wanted to be a midwife. However - her parents and teachers are keen for her to apply for a medical degree and suggest that she could specialise in Obstetrics eventually. Ria has done a few work experience placements and still strongly wants to be a midwife, but her parents and teachers say it would be a 'waste' for her not to aim 'higher'.

How important are the following considerations?

58. Being happy in your chosen career is more important than money or status.

A. Very important
B. Important
C. Of minor importance
D. Not important at all

59. Very capable students should make the most of their natural abilities and pursue more difficult academic pathways.

A. Very important
B. Important
C. Of minor importance
D. Not important at all

60. Ria's parents and teachers will be disappointed if she doesn't apply for medicine.

A. Very important
B. Important
C. Of minor importance
D. Not important at all

61. Midwifery offers opportunities for a fulfilling career and the chance to 'make a difference'.

A. Very important
B. Important
C. Of minor importance
D. Not important at all

Shaun is nearing his medical finals. He is on a long-haul flight when there is a request for 'a doctor or medically trained person' to make themselves known to the cabin crew.

How important are the following considerations?

62. Shaun is not a qualified doctor.

A. Very important
B. Important
C. Of minor importance
D. Not important at all

63. Shaun may be the closest thing to a doctor on the flight.

A. Very important
B. Important
C. Of minor importance
D. Not important at all

64. If Shaun makes an error he may be liable for damages.

A. Very important
B. Important
C. Of minor importance
D. Not important at all

65. Shaun's knowledge at this stage of his training is not very different to what his knowledge will be in a few months' time.

A. Very important
B. Important
C. Of minor importance
D. Not important at all

Vivienne is very good at maths and prior to some mock exams she tutors a small group of her friends. In the examination itself she realises that she has taught them a key formula incorrectly meaning they cannot arrive at the correct answer using it.

How important are the following considerations?

66. Vivienne made an honest mistake whilst trying to help.

A. Very important
B. Important
C. Of minor importance
D. Not important at all

67. Vivienne's friends took a risk when accepting tutoring from a peer, rather than a teacher.

A. Very important
B. Important
C. Of minor importance
D. Not important at all

68. The extra tutoring from Vivienne helped her friends with most of the exam even accounting for this mistake.

A. Very important
B. Important
C. Of minor importance
D. Not important at all

69. The exams affected are mocks.

A. Very important
B. Important
C. Of minor importance
D. Not important at all

Full Mock Test 2 Answers

1. The correct answer is D. Flu can lead to bacterial pneumonia in healthy adults
This can be seen in the passage. Option A is incorrect as TIV contains two strains of influenza type A and one strain from influenza type B. Option B is incorrect as influenza can also be inactivated by sunlight. Option C is incorrect as the vaccine is safe as it does not put you at risk of transmitting the disease.

2. The correct answer is A. The influenza strains are constantly evolving
This can be seen in the last paragraph where the passage describes how vaccines have to be constantly changed as the strains of influenza change. Option B is incorrect as the passage stresses that these naming protocols are inaccurate and unrelated to actual influenza. Option C is incorrect as the passage states that there has been no benefit found in using antiviral for people with other health problems. Option D is incorrect as while the passage states that vaccines are available in developed countries it does not say why.

3. The correct answer is D. An adult who has been bed bound for four days with aches, fever and fatigue
The symptoms of 'true influenza' are described as being severe (work or school not an option), lasting longer than 24 hours, and less likely to produce nausea and vomiting in adults. Based on the information in the text it is likely that option A is a common cold, option B gastroenteritis, and option C may be a child who had influenza but who is now developing pneumonia.

4. The correct answer is A. Birds are likely to die if infected with flu
Farmed birds are routinely vaccinated to prevent 'decimation' of the flocks which strongly suggests that fatalities are significant. Option B is incorrect as handwashing is described as reducing the risk of infection; additionally it is stated that the most important or common means of transmission is not confidently known. Option C is incorrect as there is a family of influenza viruses, not a single one. Option D is incorrect as the passage states that the vaccination may be ineffective within a year because the virus evolves so quickly.

5. The correct answer is C. Can't tell. Only 10-15% of dessert bananas are exported, and the USA is one of two major importers, but quantities imported are not defined.

6. The correct answer is C. Can't tell. 'Cavendish' bananas are a commercial variety and the passage only states that wild species have large seeds while most culinary bananas have tiny seeds.

7. The correct answer is B. False. 'Individual fruits average 125g (0.28 lb), of which approximately 75% is water and 25% dry matter'.

8. The correct answer is A. True. Bananas are 'cultivated throughout the tropics in at least 107 countries'.

9. The correct answer is B. False. Sawgrass and sloughs are the enduring geographical icons of the Everglades, but other ecological features are described as 'just as vital'. If other features are just as important, they cannot be the MOST important.

10. The correct answer is A. True. The trees, rooted in soil inches above the peat, marl, or water, support a variety of wildlife.

11. The correct answer is B. False. The Big Cypress Swamp is well-known for its 500-year-old cypresses.

12. The correct answer is A. True. As minor fluctuations in water levels have far-reaching consequences for many plant and animal species, flooding would have a great impact on those plant and animal species.

13. The correct answer is. B. Arreton
Arreton is described as the location of one or some of the boreholes. The other places are mentioned as being part of a 'group' but we cannot know for certain that the group is named after a place rather than the person who discovered them or some other factor.

14. The correct answer is A. All or part of the Isle of Wight was once covered by shallow water
This is strongly implied in the final sentence. There is no mention of dinosaurs in the text (option B). There is no strong connection between the borehole depth of 1400m and the Jurassic era (option C). All that is stated is that the entire Jurassic succession is shown in boreholes of that depth. There is nothing in the text to indicate there is 'a lot' of clay on the Isle of Wight (option D). 'A lot' is a subjective term which cannot be shown with the text.

15. The correct answer is C. There are visible strata of sedimentary rock
Option A cannot be known for certain based on the text as the only indication that the Isle is an island is based on an assumption because of the area's name. While this may seem logical there are many areas known as 'islands' or similar which are not, geographically speaking, actually islands. The text speaks of six boreholes being on the island (option B) but we cannot know there is a total of six boreholes. There may be more. Option D may be chosen due to the 'Chalk Group' mentioned in the first paragraph but it should be noted that this has a capital letter and the word 'Chalk' may denote a proper name rather than a description. There is no further mention of 'chalk' in the text. The presence of visible strata can be demonstrated by the final sentence of the first paragraph where the fact that strata can be seen at various locations is noted.

16. The correct answer is A. Mercia Mudstone, Sherwood Sandstone
The Sherwood Sandstone is described as being overlain (underneath of) by Mercia Mudstone. All of the other groups, formations, or eras are mentioned, but not in the context of their relative positions to one another.

17. The correct answer is B. Reliable, amiable, careful
ESFJs tend to be amiable as they like to achieve harmony with others and place a high value on people as stated in the first paragraph 'ESFJ preferences radiate sympathy and fellowship'. They are known to be reliable as stated in the first paragraph '[they] are loyal to respected persons, institutions, or causes'. They also tend to be 'persevering, conscientious, orderly even in small matters'. Option A is wrong as ESFJs tend to more practical than theoretical. Option C is wrong as ESFJs are concerned with other people's wellbeing so being thoughtless is not a personality trait and option D is wrong because ESFJs tend to prefer harmony and are not opinionated as this could cause friction.

18. The correct answer is D. ESFJs prefer routine
Although ESFJs can adapt to routine, the last paragraph states that they enjoy variety.

19. The correct answer is D. Includes people who are not oriented to helping others
ESFJs prefer a harmonious environment where people get along and are sensitive to others. Therefore people who are not aware of other's feelings and do not help each other would not fit well into an ESFJ work environment.

20. The correct answer is B. Respond quickly to resolve without considering the consequences
ESFJs would examine the logical consequences of a situation as they are practical and use their senses. For the same reasons they would gather the evidence and they appreciate other people's opinions so would gather these as well. They would consider the impact on others as they are sensitive to these issues but would not respond quickly without considering the consequences.

21. The correct answer is B. False. Synonymy refers to works with identical or very similar meanings, not spellings.

22. The correct answer is A. True. For example, pupil is not always a synonym of student.

23. The correct answer is A. True. Synonyms can be any part of speech. Verb examples include shout and yell, bite and chew.

24. The correct answer is C. Can't tell Although the passage talks about the evolution of synonyms in the early medieval period using the words archer and bowman as examples there is no connection made with archers and the French army.

25. The correct answer is B. 'Deep blue' was chosen in preference to 'Prussian blue'
Although the text only states that 'Deep blue' was chosen, it must have been chosen over some other blue. Given that all of the other options are false, this is the best answer, and the most likely to be true. Option A is incorrect as the text states that the Penny Blue was never a real stamp. Option C is incorrect because the text states that the plate previously used for the Penny Black was used, not that it was later used for this purpose (and indeed this seems unlikely given that the stamp was being phased out). Option D is contradicted in the text.

26. The correct answer is B. The 'Penny Black' was replaced in 1841 by the 'Penny Red'

The replacement of the penny black in 1841, to become the penny red, is stated in the text. Option A is incorrect - the cancellation ink was changed from red to black. Option C is incorrect as the text states that the ink was changed. The 1841 version of the two pence blue stamp had new ink. The differences between the old and new two pence stamp are described in the 2nd paragraph (option D).

27. The correct answer is C. Proofs are used to test the colour, check the reaction of the paper, evaluate the image quality and examine the possibility of forgery
There is no mention in the text of forgery. Three proof (sample) texts are mentioned in the text (option A). The fact that paper proofs are not real postage stamps is in the text (option B). There is no specific information about changes between the Penny Black and Penny Red apart from the colour so the statement cannot be deemed true or false (option D) meaning that option C is a better answer.

28. The correct answer is A. Penny Red proof impressions were edited before stamp production
The text states that the examples printed would be indistinguishable from the later stamps indicating no edits were made. Option B is true and therefore incorrect. The use of printing plates made with different materials is mentioned in the final paragraph (option C). The reaction between various inks and the plates is also detailed in the final paragraph (option D).

29. The correct answer is A. True. 'Corporate and personal bankruptcies' are listed among the notices posted.

30. The correct answer is C. Can't tell. The passage describes the *Gazette* as not having a large circulation but this does not confirm a small readership.

31. The correct answer is C. Can't tell. The passage only states that one of the *Gazette's* officers established the first advertising agency.

32. The correct answer is A. True. His diary mentions the first publication of the *Gazette*.

33. The correct answer is C. Michael Bublé
Britney Spears and Kesha (options A and D) are both mentioned in the article but not in the context of admitting that they have used Auto-Tune technology. Nelly Furtado is not quoted but she is mentioned as being one of the few artists who do not use it. Michael Bublé admits that he uses the technology.

34. The correct answer is D. 'A particularly sinister invention'
This quote comes from Neil McCormick, a writer from *The Telegraph*. The first quote (option A) is not a criticism so does not answer the question. (Neither is option C, but that does emanate from Time magazine). Option B is stated as being a list within *Time* magazine in which Auto-Tune featured.

35. The correct answer is A. Singers will be able to spend less time recording thus freeing up studio time
Although not expressly stated it is a logical conclusion that if a machine will iron out vocals, the singer won't have to re-record as many times. Option B is incorrect as the text states that almost all singers use Auto-Tune

and that none advertise the fact. The text does not suggest that there will be 'more pop stars' as a result of this technology - just possibly that different people will achieve this aim. The text states that Michael Bublé describes everyone sounding 'like robots' as a result of Auto-Tune and there is no further information about tone.

36. The correct answer is D. Singers don't necessarily have much control over whether Auto-Tune is used in the production of their work
This can be shown in the text by the inference of the unnamed Grammy winning recording engineer who is confident that 'every singer presumes (not requests) you'll run their voice through the box' and also that Tom Lord-Alge believes that it is used on nearly every record. Similarly, Neko Case says that only he and one other artist didn't use it. Option A cannot be shown in the text as viewing figures are not mentioned. There is no strong indication that the demand for perfection comes from the public (option B) and option C cannot be shown as 'sound better' is very subjective. Although Auto-Tune may make things more 'accurate' it may adversely affect other aspects of the music.

37. The correct answer is C. The rash usually appears on the hands and feet first before spreading
The rash usually starts on the trunk and usually does not affect the hands and feet. See paragraph 2.

38. The correct answer is A. The incubation period is usually 11-21 days
The final paragraph states 'The incubation period for chickenpox is 11-21 days, usually 15-18 days' meaning that although sometimes the incubation period is 21 days, it is usually shorter, in the range of 15-18 days.

39. The correct answer is C. Skin pustules, renal complications, headaches
There are not renal complications associated with chickenpox; all the other symptoms are mentioned in paragraphs 3 and 4.

40. The correct answer is B. People who are immunocompromised tend to have more severe and persisting disease
People who are immunocompromised have 'a more fulminant illness' (paragraph 3), and the last paragraph states they may be infectious longer. A is false as patients are infectious for up to 5 days after the rash appears. C is false as people who have shingles have had a reactivation of latent zoster virus which means they have had chickenpox at some point beforehand (paragraph 1). D is false because although herpes zoster is less infectious than chickenpox, if lesions are exposed then the patient can still infect others.

41. The correct answer is C. Can't tell. The passage mentions 9 Stuart monarchs, some of whom may have been Queens.

42. The correct answer is A. True. James IV married Margaret Tudor and the birth of their son first brought the House of Stuart (Kings of Scotland) into the line of descent of the House of Tudor and therefore the English throne. This statement can be verified within the passage.

43. The correct answer is C. Can't tell. This is not explicitly stated in the text. It is possible for Charles II to be a brother, uncle or cousin of Charles I.

44. The correct answer is B. False. James IV was the father of James V and James V was the grandfather of James VI - making James IV the great grandfather of James VI & I.

1.

The side of the park with the larger lake is the larger side **No**
This is not necessarily true. We don't have this information

All three play areas can be accessed without crossing the railway bridge **Yes**
All three play areas are on the same side of the park

There are ducks in both halves of the park **Yes**
There is a lake on each side of the park and both lakes have many ducks

The smaller lake is not used for boating **No**
The text doesn't tell us which lake is used for boating

The café is closer to the church than the cricket club **No**
Although the cafe and church are on one side of the park whilst the cricket club is on the other, we cannot conclude relative distances. Two places could be immediately opposite each other by one of the bridges whilst the third be in a much further flung corner.

2.

Some people had a starter, a main course and coffee **No**
We don't know this

Some people left before dessert **No**
We only know some people left after dessert

Everyone had a main course **Yes**
The text states that everyone had a main course.

The number of cold drinks sold was equal to the number of main courses **Yes**
Everyone had a main course. Everyone had a single cold drink.

Fewer people had coffee than had a starter **No**
It is impossible to know how many people had either a starter or a dessert other than it was 'some'.

3.

World War Two ended before 1965 **Yes**
The centre was built on a site that had been heavily bombed in the war (past tense) and it opened in 1965.

There is a wide redevelopment project planned for the area **Yes**
The proposed demolishment of this centre is part of a wider redevelopment project for the area.

The Latin American community is the dominant group in the area **No**
There is a vibrant Latin American community but we cannot say the Latin American community is dominant

The shopping centre is faded and depreciating in value **No**
We know that the centre may be demolished and may make assumptions about why that is but nothing in the text indicates that the centre is run down or losing value

The Elephant and Castle shopping centre will be demolished **No**
The word 'could' is used in relation to this. It is merely a possibility.

4.

Over half of all social media users as shown are aged under 35 **No**
We don't have information about how many users are on each platform so cannot draw this conclusion.

Of the social media platforms shown, Facebook has the most representative age distribution **No**
We don't have information about the general population to conclude if these figures are representative or not

On average around a quarter of people aged 25-34 use social media **No**
We don't have information about the general population to conclude this

If people continue to use the same social media platforms as they get older then these proportions will shift in the coming years **Yes**
If all of the people aged under 25 continue to use Snapchat as they reach their 30s or 40s then the shift will be inevitable - even accounting for younger people also joining the service.

Less than 10% of all social media use is from people aged over 65 **Yes**
The chart shows this must be so as even the most popular platform with the over 65s has only 10% use from them

5. The correct answer is B. The least fuel-efficient car is the cheapest
The table can be completed. It is important to remember that fuel-efficiency is measured in miles per gallon so the higher the number the more efficient the vehicle. We know from the first point that option A is untrue. Option C is untrue as the £1600 car gets 31mpg – the most efficient car – which is black. The silver car is less efficient than the black car.

1500	Blue	25mpg
1600	Black	31mgg
1700	Red	27 mpg
1800	Silver	29 mpg

6. The correct answer is C. Gold wrapped fudge is chocolate flavour
Options A or B could be true, but we cannot complete the table. Option D is incorrect.

1	Silver	
2	Pink	Cherry
3	Gold	Chocolate
4	Green	

7. The correct answer is D. Francesca wore pink

24	White	Andy
26	Red	Rachel
28	Blue	George
29	Pink	Francesca

8. The correct answer is B. Unit B is a hotel.
This is the only certain fact – we know the hotel has direct park views (as opposed to diagonal park views described elsewhere). We know that units A and E are the business centre and shopping mall, but we don't know which is which. Unit C is the housing unit (closest to the hotel) and unit D is the leisure centre (diagonal views but not closest to the hotel).

9. The correct answer is B. Norman was awarded some points in this round
Only the two closest bowls are awarded points (dark grey and white). Olive must have been dark grey (point 2) and Norman light grey (point 1).

10. The correct answer is D. A 'basic standard of living' varies so rates should reflect the economy more generally
This option queries one of the terms of the proposition making it the most valid.

Option A introduces the welfare state, option B introduces the notion of personal dignity, option C assumes that people earning minimum wage don't need anything more.

11. The current answer is C. 25 years after quitting, the difference between 10 or 35 cigarettes per day makes negligible difference
Option A is incomplete – lower risk than what?
Option B is untrue – the relative risk is lower but far from equal
Option D is untrue as there is an increase in incidence between the 30-39 and 40+ columns.

12. The correct answer is A. Yes – achieving well at a poor school is a greater achievement than achieving well at a good school and universities should take into account the character and work ethic of the student, which overcame their circumstances.
The very notion of 'poor' and 'good' schools indicates that students who achieve equally well at either have had to work at different rates with different resources.
Statement B – introduces a social responsibility to universities that is not warranted
Statement C – a student from a poor school who gets excellent exam results shows they have academic rigour.

13. The correct answer is C. Technological progress can have unintended, detrimental consequences
There is no suggestion that simpler times were more joyful, just that there was some joy. Bookstores may not be able to stock the same vast range of books an e-reader can access but this does not mean their selection is 'very limited'. The idea that people using printed books are not concerned by inconveniences is not warranted – they just prefer the qualities of a printed book over the convenience of an e-reader.

14.

Only 3 regions have a below average percentage premium for a grade 3 home over a grade 1 home The average is given as 18% and only 3 regions report an average below that	**Yes**
The average given here is the median The average must be the mean given that the average does not fall midway in the list of figures	**No**
The premium is less in areas with generally higher house prices as people there can take their children out of the state school system and use private education instead. This may seem logical but we don't have data to support it as a conclusion	**No**
The cheapest homes in England can be found in the North East We only have average figures here and no information about range.	**Yes**
Those who pay the most to live near a Grade 1 school, rather than a Grade 3 school, live in London Although the percentage difference is smaller, the amounts are much larger in London than anywhere else.	**Yes**

15. The correct answer is B. Wider adoption of organic farming would help tackle unemployment
The text makes clear that the yield of organic farming is lower and that it is more labour intensive meaning the costs are much higher per unit of produce. There is no mention that agricultural chemicals are harmful to health, nor that the use of chemicals is the only difference between organic and intensive farming. Whilst option B may see logical it is a far more removed suggestion than option D. There is nothing in the text about unemployment.

16. The correct answer is D. The long-term trend cannot be observed using short term measurements
The long-term trend is measured by the 132 (11 year) month running mean and shows a general upwards trend over the 120 years covered. The blue line – the 12 month mean – shows a lot of fluctuation and the long-term trend isn't as immediately visible. Statement A is not true as the overall picture is one of temperature rise. Statement B cannot be demonstrated by the graph and is not suggested anywhere.

17.

A higher percentage of students took some sort of Welsh GCSE in 2002 than 2001 We only have numbers so cannot speculate about percentages	**No**
The Welsh Second Language (short) was introduced in 1999 It only appears in the data from 1999 but it's possible very small numbers took it in previous years	**No**
There have been between 35,000 and 40,000 Welsh GCSE students throughout the period shown We know the numbers of those taking the Welsh GCSE and those who didn't – which must add up to the total	**Yes**
The number of Welsh first language pupils has remained quite static at between 4,000 and 5,500	**Yes**
The largest change over this period was that more students took Welsh Second Language (short) as opposed to not taking any Welsh GCSE The numbers of Welsh Second Language (full) are reasonably constant. The biggest change in the replacement of green with light blue. (No Welsh GCSE to Welsh Second Language (short)).	**Yes**

18. The correct answer is A. Yes – Nothing quite compares to seeing other places with your own eyes.
This is the only statement that doesn't introduce unrelated concepts. Statement B contains the assumption that all travellers 'fully experience' local culture which is the converse of Statement D which suggests most travellers don't experience true local culture at all. Both are based on assumptions. Option C states something quite random and unconnected and doesn't really address the proposition directly.

19. The correct answer is B. The rarest animal to see was the rhino

Twenty groups saw lions in total. Only 2 groups saw 3 of the 4 animals. 27 groups saw just 1 animal, 30 groups saw more than 1 animal.

20. The correct answer is C. Fewer than 20 students in total take three out of the four classes offered
Students taking ballet, tap and speech = 2; Students taking ballet, tap and freestyle = 10; Students taking ballet, speech and freestyle = 0; Students taking tap, speech and freestyle = 7

21. The correct answer is B. Howard (shortest) and Justin (longest)
Ian can't have travelled the shortest distance as he travels further than Howard (point 4). Kevin can't have travelled the shortest distance as he travels further than Ian (point 2). Kevin can't have travelled the furthest as Justin travels further than him (point 3).

22. The correct answer is D. Most teams in this sample have a 10,000+ capacity stadium
Option A: many teams have won a trophy and never been relegated = 4 + 5 + 13 + 9
Option B: 13 teams (1 + 2 + 7 + 3) are outside the 'won a trophy' shape
Option C: 11 + 13 + 6 = 30 = teams who have won a trophy and play in red
8 + 4 + 5 + 10 + 9 = 36 = teams who have won a trophy and don't play in red

23. The correct answer is B.
24. The correct answer is B. A third
The total number of children in the class is 30 (we know they all forgot something) and 10 pupils forgot two things.
25. The correct answer is C. 14. There were originally 16 children who forgot their pyajamas but two of them (twins) have had their forgotten items delivered.
26. The correct answer is B. Isabel and Jonathan decide against Portugal and Spain
There is a 3 in 5 chance that the couple will select one of the three other options which are not Spain or Portugal. Compare that to the other options

- choosing to stay in a hotel - 1 in 4
- choosing Italy - 1 in 5
- deciding against a villa or an apartment - 2 in 4 or 1 in 2.

27. The correct answer is B. 28
We know that the only day where 29 children attended was Wednesday.
There were 145 possible attendances (29 children x 5 days) and 5 of the absences were due to the football match on Friday. That means there were 3 further absences which must have been distributed between Monday, Tuesday and Thursday.

28. The correct answer is D. No – there are fewer dice combinations which add up to 8 or more than those which add up to 7 or less.

1 + 1	2 + 1	3 + 2	5 + 1	2 + 6	5 + 3	6 + 4
1 + 2	2 + 2	3 + 3	5 + 2	3 + 5	5 + 4	6 + 5
1 + 3	2 + 3	3 + 4	6 + 1	3 + 6	5 + 5	6 + 6
1 + 4	2 + 4	4 + 1		4 + 4	5 + 6	
1 + 5	2 + 5	4 + 2		4 + 5	6 + 2	
1 + 6	3 + 1	4 + 3		4 + 6	6 + 3	

29. The correct answer is C. No – there is a less than 50% chance of Rachel picking a blue ball of to complete the blanket.
Once Rachel has removed the blue ball there are five balls of wool left in the bag – 2 of which are blue. There is only a 40% chance she will pick one of these.

1. The correct answer is E. 1700g
150 +675 + 150 +150 +75 + 2×200 +100 = 1700g
2. The correct answer is E. 29%
150 +675 + 150 +150 +75 + 2×200 +100 = 1700g; (500/1700) × 100 = 29.41 = 29%

3. The correct answer is B. 857g
675 × 1.27 = 857.25 = 857 g
4. The correct answer is D. 3330 seconds
30 mins × 1.85 = 55.5; 55.5 × 60 = 3330 seconds
5. The correct answer is B. Bincom
Bincom = 34/82 = 0.415
Rixypolydon = 1/7 = 0.143
Granular Silycom = 3/13 = 0.231
Yernyphosotride = 2/19 = 0.105
Polytomi = 1/50 = 0.02

6. The correct answer is D. 0.086
Bincom = 34/82 = 0.415, Rixypolydon = 1/7 = 0.143, Granular Silycom = 3/13 = 0.231, Yernyphosotride = 2/19 = 0.105, Polytomi = 1/50 = 0.02
Total = 0.914
Missing chemical = 1 - 0.914 which is 0.086

7. The correct answer is B. 194g
Chemical weight = 1200 × 0.7
Chemical weight = 840
Granular Silycom = 3/13 of 840
Granular Silycom = 840 × (3/13) or 840 × 0.231
Granular Silycom = 194.04 or = 194 g

8. The correct answer is A. £1.43
£2.30 = 2.30 ×1.07 euros
£2.30 = 2.461 euros
3.99 euros = 3.99/1.07 Pounds
3.99 euros = £3.72897
Price difference = £3.73 - £2.30 = £1.43

9. The correct answer is D. 14.16
Climbing speed = 800 feet per minute. Intended altitude = 13,000 feet. 13,000/800 = 16.25 minutes. Time = 14:16
10. The correct answer is C. 53.6 m/s
120 miles per hour = 120 × 1609 metres per hour = 193,080 metres per hour = 193,080/60/60 metres per second = 53.633 = 53.6 m/s

11. The correct answer is E. 8.4%
There are 12 people jumping (6 participants in tandem with the 6 professional parachutists).
Total weight = 12 × 70 kg = 840 kg;
% weight = (840/10,000)×100 = 8.4%

12. The correct answer is D. 2,418
The jumper will exit the aircraft at 13,000 feet = 13 (thousand) × 0.189 = 2.457 miles.
They will fall at 120 miles per hour for one minute (120 mph / 60 = 2 miles per minute.
Their height after one minute = 2.457 miles - 2 miles = 0.457 miles
To convert to feet 0.457/0.189 = 2.418 thousand feet = 2,418 feet

13. The correct answer is B. 8.262 bar
9.18 × 0.90 = 8.262 bar
14. The correct answer is E. 0.918 bar
9.18 × 0.10 = 0.918
15. The correct answer is A. OFF – ON
OFF - ON
16. The correct answer is C. 20 bar
At T10, Pc = 10% Pc = 2 bar; Max Pc = 100 % Pc = (2/10) × 100 = 20 bar
17. The correct answer is E. £938
Choosing to sit together implies that the family are also booking seats:
Flights = £219.50 x 4 people = £878, choose seats = £10 x 4 people = £40 , seats together = £20 x 4 people =£ 80, early booking = £15 x 4 people = £60
Therefore total flight cost: £878 + £40 + £80 - £60 = £938

18. The correct answer is B. £1567.30

Accommodation cost is £899, of which 70% is lost for cancellation within the 49 - 29 day bracket. 70% x £899 = £629.30
Flight costs are now non-refundable. From Q1 total flight cost is £938.
Total loss = accommodation cancellation costs + flight cancellation costs: £938 + £629.30 = £1,567.30

19. The correct answer is D. 1,206.75 km
500 mph x 1.5 hrs = 750 miles
750 m x 1.609 km = 1,206.75 km

20. The correct answer is C. £118.44
Convert sterling into euros at the Buy rate: £850 x 1.137 = 966.45 euros
Euros left on return: 966.45 - 831.71 = 134.74 euros, convert euros into sterling at the sell rate: 134.74 euros x 0.879 = £118.44

21. The correct answer is C. 60%
(18/30) × 100 = 60 %
22. The correct answer is A. 14%
Total number of seats = 30+28+35+30 = 123; total number of pupils using bus = 18+27+32+29 = 106; empty seats = 123-106 = 17; (17/123)×100 = 13.8211 = 13.82%
23. The correct answer is E. 3.57%
27 pupils were using the bus ((27/28) × 100 = 96.42875 = 96.43 %), now there are 28 people using the bus (= 100%); 100 - 96.43 = 3.57 %
24. The correct answer is A. 6%
(3/32 - 1/30) × 100 = (0.09375 - 0.033333) × 100 = 0.06042 × 100 = 6.14 = 6 %

25. The correct answer is C. 87
482 × 0.18 = 86.76 = 87
26. The correct answer is D. 27
482 × 0.14 = 67.48; 67 × 0.4 = 26.8 = 27
27. The correct answer is B. 90
482 × 0.18 = 86.76; 86.76 + 3 = 89.76 = 90
28. The correct answer is C. 47
482 × 0.08 = 38.56; 40/5 = 8; 38.56 + 8 = 46.56 = 47
29. The correct answer is E. £150
1500 × 2/3 = 1000; 1000 - 600 - 250 = £150.
30. The correct answer is A. £525
1500 × 1/3 = 500; 500 × 1.05 = £525
31. The correct answer is E. £400
Best outcome = 60% increase; 250 ×1.6 = £400
32. The correct answer is D. £1225
The low risk amount is guaranteed: 1500 × 1/3 = 500; 500 × 1.05 = £525; High risk shares worst-case scenario = 30% loss: 1500 × 2/3 = 1000; 1000 × 0.70 = 700; low risk plus high risk values = £525 + £700 = £1225
33. The correct answer is E. £13/ 1 / -
Boarding house costs 2 adults x 10 shillings x 6 nights = 120 shillings or £6 + 4 children x 10 shillings x 6 nights = 120 shillings or £6. £6 + £6 = £12
Travel costs 2 x adults + 3 x children (6 x 2) + (3 x 3) = 21 shillings of £1 / 1 shillings
£12 + £1 / 1 = £13 / 1 / -

34. The correct answer is C. £11 / - / -
Boarding house costs 2 adults x 8 shillings x 6 nights = 96 shillings or £4 / 16 / -
Plus 4 children x 4 shillings x 6 nights = 96 shillings or £4 / 16 / -
Accommodation costs = 96 shillings + 96 shillings = 192 shillings or £9 / 12 / -
Travel costs 2 x adults + 3 x children (8 x 2) + (4 x 3) = 28 shillings of £1 / 8 shillings

£9 / 12 + £1 / 8 = £11 / - / -

35. The correct answer is E. £9 / 4 / -
Boarding house costs 2 adults x 6 shillings x 6 nights = 72 shillings or £3 / 12 / -
Plus 4 children x 3 shillings x 6 nights = 72 shillings or £3 / 12 / -
Accommodation costs = 72 shillings + 72 shillings = 144 shillings or £7 / 4 / -
Travel costs 2 x adults + 4 x children (10 x 2) + (5 x 4) = 40 shillings or £2 / - / -
£7 / 4 / - + £2 / - / - = £9 / 4 / -

36. The correct answer is C. £3 / 17 / -
The most expensive holiday would be Brighton £13 / 1 / - (261 shillings)
The cheapest would be Harwich £9 / 4 / - (184 shillings)
261 - 184 = 77 shillings = 3 / 17 / -

Question Set 1 (questions 1-5)
Set A always has exactly two circles.
Set B always has exactly two crescent shapes.
The colours of the shapes are irrelevant.

1. Set B
2. Set B
3. Set B
4. Neither
5. Set A

Question Set 2 (questions 6-10)
Set A always contains one 4-sided shape, there are at least 3 shapes in total.
Set B always contains one oval shape, there are at least 3 shapes in total.

6. Neither
7. Neither
8. Set A
9. Set B
10. Neither

Question Set 3 (questions 11 – 15)
All of Set A has exactly one pair of white shapes that are identical in both shape and orientation and one pair of the same shapes - one black one white.
All of Set B has exactly one pair of black shapes that are identical in both shape and orientation.

11. Set A
12. Neither
13. Set A
14. Set A
15. Neither

Question Set 4 (questions 16-20)
Set A always contains only one white square which is always placed in the top left corner.
Set B always contains only one black square which is always placed in the top left corner.

16. Set A
17. Neither
18. Set A
19. Set B
20. Neither

Question Set 5 (questions 21-25)
Set A always contains a black triangle placed in a corner. Set B always contains a black circle placed in a corner.

21. Neither
22. Set B
23. Neither
24. Neither
25. Neither

Question Set 6 (questions 26-30)
Set A always contains only two lines in contact with each other. This contact is always at or through the middle of one line.
Set B always contains three and no more lines in contact with each other. Points of contact can be anywhere on the line.

26. Neither
27. Set B
28. Neither
29. Set B
30. Neither

31. The correct answer is D.
Each picture has one arrow pointing in one direction, two pointing in the direction one quarter clockwise turn and three pointing a further clockwise turn. (e.g. one pointing up, two pointing right, three pointing down). This pattern rotates anticlockwise one turn with each sequence.

32. The correct answer is C.
The black and light grey squares are moving around the outside of the grid in a clockwise direction. The square with vertical stripes is moving around the grid in an anti-clockwise direction. Where it occupies the same square as a grey or black square it will show over the grey or be invisible over the black. The central square in the grid has lines which rotate in direction - vertical, diagonal, horizontal, diagonal. A circle moves anti-clockwise but isn't visible when occupying the same square as black.

33. The correct answer is B
The number of circles decreases with each picture in the sequence - 9, 8, 7, 6 so we know there are 5 circles in the correct answer. The number of circles, of which we can see the entire outline, increases with each picture in the sequence - 1, 2, 3, 4 so the correct answer will have 5 circles with entirely visible outlines.

Question Set 7 (questions 34-38)
Set A always contains three shapes, one of which will be black.
Set B always contains four shapes.

34. Neither
35. Set B
36. Set A
37. Neither
38. Set B

Question Set 8 (questions 39-43)
Set A always contains at least 5 shapes with a split circle in the centre.
Set B always contains at least 4 shapes with a split circle in the bottom middle.

39. Neither
40. Neither
41. Set B
42. Set A
43. Neither

Question Set 9 (questions 44-48)
Set A always includes one white arrow pointing down.
Set B always includes one black arrow pointing up.

44. Set A
45. Set B
46. Neither
47. Neither
48. Set B

Question Set 10 (questions 49-53)
Set A always has three triangles pointing in the same direction. There are also at least two other shapes present.
Set B always has three triangles pointing in different directions. There are also at least two other shapes present.

49. Neither
50. Set A
51. Set B
52. Neither
53. Neither

54. The correct answer is C.
The shapes rotate in a clockwise direction, also rotating 90 degrees to the right. The effects - dashed, shaded, bold - rotate in an anti-clockwise direction.

55. The correct answer is A.
The black shape has a vertical line of symmetry, the white shape has a horizontal line of symmetry and the grey shape has multiple lines of symmetry.

1. The correct answer is B. Appropriate but not ideal – 2 marks (1 mark for A. A very appropriate thing to do or C. Inappropriate but not awful)
This action does ensure that any children get help from the service qualified to deal with these situations but contacting them when the doctor only has reason to suspect the patient has children could be an overreaction.

2. The correct answer is A. A very appropriate thing to do – 2 marks (1 mark for B. Appropriate but not ideal)
The patient may or may not be truthful but if she says she does have children help can immediately be organised. If she says she doesn't have children, even if the medical staff believe her to be lying, the situation is no worse than it was before.

3. The correct answer is D. A very inappropriate thing to do – 2 marks (1 mark for C. Inappropriate but not awful)
While this action does respect the patient's privacy it does nothing about the fact that others may be in danger.

4. The correct answer is B. Appropriate but not ideal – 2 marks (1 mark for A. A very appropriate thing to do or C. Inappropriate but not awful)
While extra research may reveal whether children are present or in danger it does not actually do anything to help them.

5. The correct answer is C. Inappropriate but not awful – 2 marks (1 mark for B. Appropriate but not ideal or D. A very inappropriate thing to do)
If the problem is serious, a week may be too long to wait but at least the patient can be seen.

6. The correct answer is B. Appropriate but not ideal – 2 marks (1 mark for A. A very appropriate thing to do or C. Inappropriate but not awful)
Although this seems like the 'right' thing to do, it is important to remember that the money was offered as a thank you gift and was given without compunction. It could be seen as impolite and ungrateful to refuse point-blank a well-meant gesture.

7. The correct answer is C. Inappropriate but not awful – 2 marks (1 mark for B. Appropriate but not ideal or D. A very inappropriate thing to do)
The money was not offered as a bribe or in return for anything but as a thank you. A polite 'thank you' is always appropriate. However - accepting gifts like this can set a dangerous precedent as the exchange of monetary gifts like this is closely regulated to avoid accusations of inequity.

8. The correct answer is A. A very appropriate thing to do – 2 marks (1 mark for B. Appropriate but not ideal)
This way the gratitude of the gentleman will benefit everyone on the team and there is nothing underhand.

9. The correct answer is A. A very appropriate thing to do – 2 marks (1 mark for B. Appropriate but not ideal)
The practice manager will be very familiar with not only the legality of this kind of gift but also the social and personal aspects of it. He or she will be able to advise Tai of the best course of action.

10. The correct answer is A. A very appropriate thing to do – 2 marks (1 mark for B. Appropriate but not ideal)
Although Petra is nervous about asking for help from this teacher it is entirely appropriate for her to approach him again. He is, after all, her teacher and it is his job to help her. Though she may be naturally reticent after being upset the previous time it shows maturity and resilience to approach him again.

11. The correct answer is C. Inappropriate but not awful – 2 marks (1 mark for B. Appropriate but not ideal or D. A very inappropriate thing to do)
This is likely to be the first port of call for most students in this position. However - asking your peers is unlikely to fully resolve the misunderstanding but may lead to a false sense of security. There is a risk of exchanging incorrect information.

12. The correct answer is B. Appropriate but not ideal – 2 marks (1 mark for A. A very appropriate thing to do or C. Inappropriate but not awful)
Although another teacher may be able to explain the issue Petra is struggling with they won't necessarily know the context of her problem and therefore their help, whilst useful, won't be as specifically directed and personal as the help that could be offered by her own teacher.

13. The correct answer is D. A very inappropriate thing to do – 2 marks (1 mark for C. Inappropriate but not awful)
It is important to try your best at every essay, coursework piece and assignment in any qualification. Even if any 'don't count' towards the final grade the subject matter will, most likely, be built upon in future assignments or be tested in the final exam.

14. The correct answer is A. A very appropriate thing to do – 2 marks (1 mark for B. Appropriate but not ideal)
Any work experience is valuable and will be recognised as such by the institutions receiving Oscar's application.

15. The correct answer is C. Inappropriate but not awful – 2 marks (1 mark for B. Appropriate but not ideal or D. A very inappropriate thing to do)
It is clear from the scenario that Oscar is mainly engaged in the retail activities of the chemist and any claim to be 'in the medical field' would be at best an exaggeration, and at worst a deception. He is unlikely to be able to back this up if he were to be interviewed as well.

16. The correct answer is A. A very appropriate thing to do – 2 marks (1 mark for B. Appropriate but not ideal)

This would enable Oscar to honestly say he has been involved in the medical side of the pharmacist's business and also give him more genuine insight into what is involved. It also shows initiative and eagerness on his part which should be commended.

17. The correct answer is D. A very inappropriate thing to do – 2 marks (1 mark for C. Inappropriate but not awful)
Not only could this potentially endanger patients as he may be offering advice or handing out prescriptions without proper training or knowledge but Oscar could irritate his colleagues by taking initiative which is well beyond his remit.

18. The correct answer is C. Inappropriate but not awful – 2 marks (1 mark for B. Appropriate but not ideal or D. A very inappropriate thing to do)
Laura may have reasons for not contributing. She could feel put her on the spot and may feel uncomfortable in front of the group. She may have ideas but is not as vocal as expressing them.

19. The correct answer is B. Appropriate but not ideal – 2 marks (1 mark for A. A very appropriate thing to do or C. Inappropriate but not awful)
This could be a way for Richard to find out the reasons without asking in the group which may have made Laura feel uncomfortable. It is not ideal, as Laura may not wish to disclose her reasons to Richard. What would be appropriate is for Richard to suggest to the group that everyone takes a turn to present their ideas to the group. It would be a non-confrontational way of looking at engagement from all group members.

20. The correct answer is D. A very inappropriate thing to do – 2 marks (1 mark for C. Inappropriate but not awful)
This would be confrontational as it will make Laura feel she is being singled out and make her feel the group has no confidence in her.

21. The correct answer is A. A very appropriate thing to do – 2 marks (1 mark for B. Appropriate but not ideal)
It is possible that Laura is simply a naturally quiet person. Offering the option to contribute ideas in a forum other than a group meeting would enable her (and possibly others) to input their ideas. It would also be useful to have a written record of what has been said.

22. The correct answer is D. A very inappropriate thing to do – 2 marks (1 mark for C. Inappropriate but not awful)
Ben is upset and his wheezing has been exacerbated. The doctor needs to make an attempt to calm the boy to ensure Ben is in no further harm and his breathing returns to normal.

23. The correct answer is B. Appropriate but not ideal – 2 marks (1 mark for A. A very appropriate thing to do or C. Inappropriate but not awful)
Although Ben is crying, as his wheezing has been exacerbated, the doctor needs to perform the check up to ensure Ben is in no immediate danger. It is not ideal as the doctor should calm Ben down first before attempting to place the stethoscope again.

24. The correct answer is C. Inappropriate but not awful – 2 marks (1 mark for B. Appropriate but not ideal or D. A very inappropriate thing to do)
A detailed history is probably overkill at an emergency appointment with a locum doctor. The child really does need to be examined and delaying it really only delays Ben potentially getting upset again. The conversation may elicit useful information but ultimately this is a stalling tactic in an urgent situation.

25. The correct answer is A. A very appropriate thing to do – 2 marks (1 mark for B. Appropriate but not ideal)
This is the most compassionate response which still allows the essential examination to take place. It may take a little longer but does not endanger Ben at all and may build a better trust foundation for Ben's future interactions with doctors.

26. The correct answer is D. A very inappropriate thing to do – 2 marks (1 mark for C. Inappropriate but not awful)
If the guidelines state an ID badge must be worn at all times, this is of great importance and is for patient and public safety.
27. The correct answer is A. A very appropriate thing to do – 2 marks (1 mark for B. Appropriate but not ideal)
A student ID Badge must be worn at all times as this identifies Leanne as a student and not yet qualified. By informing the hospital she will be late, her supervisor will be aware of her whereabouts and allow the session to continue.

28. The correct answer is C. Inappropriate but not awful – 2 marks (1 mark for B. Appropriate but not ideal or D. A very inappropriate thing to do)
This may inconvenience Leanne's friend a great deal. It is better for her to try and solve the issue herself rather than imposing on her friends.

29. The correct answer is B. Appropriate but not ideal – 2 marks (1 mark for A. A very appropriate thing to do or C. Inappropriate but not awful)
This ensures that the patient can be seen quickly without any breach of protocol; however if the problem genuinely is urgent then tomorrow may not be soon enough.

30. The correct answer is D. A very inappropriate thing to do – 2 marks (1 mark for C. Inappropriate but not awful)
It is unlikely that the receptionist has any real ability to discern whether the patient's problem is serious or not and, even if they have, taking their information over the phone breaches confidentiality

31. The correct answer is D. A very inappropriate thing to do – 2 marks (1 mark for C. Inappropriate but not awful)
Rescheduling another patient's appointment at the last moment for another patient is highly inappropriate.

32. The correct answer is A. A very appropriate thing to do – 2 marks (1 mark for B. Appropriate but not ideal)
Ultimately the doctors want Laura to succeed and will assist her in gaining the clinical skills she needs. They may be able to offer advice and resources which could help her, or they may be able to boost her confidence in her own abilities having worked alongside her. When you are a student it is rarely inappropriate to ask for support.

33. The correct answer is B. Appropriate but not ideal – 2 marks (1 mark for A. A very appropriate thing to do or C. Inappropriate but not awful)
This course of action would give Laura practical advice and a visual image of how the procedure should be done. It may supplement the theoretical knowledge Laura already has and give her some confidence or insight. It is not ideal as it also may not do these things.

34. The correct answer is D. A very inappropriate thing to do – 2 marks (1 mark for C. Inappropriate but not awful)
Whilst it is common to practice non-invasive procedures (temperatures, blood pressure) on one another as medical students there are many more potential problems in an invasive procedure such as drawing blood. To do so without supervision could put her course mates at risk.

35. The correct answer is C. Inappropriate but not awful – 2 marks (1 mark for B. Appropriate but not ideal or D. A very inappropriate thing to do)
Reviewing academic and theoretical information is unlikely to help or harm (hence it isn't an awful course of action) as it is clinical skills Laura needs support with.

36. The correct answer is C. Inappropriate but not awful – 2 marks (1 mark for B. Appropriate but not ideal or D. A very inappropriate thing to do)
It is entirely possible that Laura is more skilled than she believes and the procedures will be fully supervised. It's not good to attempt procedures you feel ill equipped to do but sometimes our feelings are not a good barometer of our actual ability.
37. The correct answer is B. Appropriate but not ideal – 2 marks (1 mark for A. A very appropriate thing to do or C. Inappropriate but not awful)
Calvin is absolutely correct that the class is important and it is right that he should encourage his colleague to pull together and get on with it. However – this also displays something of a lack of compassion.

38. The correct answer is A. A very appropriate thing to do – 2 marks (1 mark for B. Appropriate but not ideal)
Reassurance and an attempt to calm may be all that is necessary to help Jake into the lesson. If not, it's still the kindest course of action

39. The correct answer is C. Inappropriate but not awful – 2 marks (1 mark for B. Appropriate but not ideal or D. A very inappropriate thing to do)
While this doesn't address the problem it also does allow Jake the autonomy to deal with the situation in his own way. Presumably he understands the implications and issues and may just need some time

40. The correct answer is B. Appropriate but not ideal – 2 marks (1 mark for A. A very appropriate thing to do or C. Inappropriate but not awful)
It would probably be sensible for Jake to seek support around this issue and it is appropriate for Calvin to suggest this. It's not ideal though as Jake may not wish to disclose his feelings at this point to the lecturer. It would be better if Calvin had suggested it rather than asked him to do it.

41. The correct answer is D. A very inappropriate thing to do – 2 marks (1 mark for C. Inappropriate but not awful)
This is ultimately very unhelpful.

42. The correct answer is C. Inappropriate but not awful – 2 marks (1 mark for B. Appropriate but not ideal or D. A very inappropriate thing to do)
This could be seen as forming an alliance against Charlotte and is unlikely to result in good group work. However - it may enable Mark and Susie to check they're on the same page (or otherwise). It's possible that Susie is perfectly happy with the situation.

43. The correct answer is D. Not important at all – 2 marks (1 mark for C. Of minor importance)
At present Oliver is unlikely to do well in this class as his lectures are being so disrupted. It is unlikely any action will make the situation worse.

44. The correct answer is A. Very important – 2 marks (1 mark for B. Important)
As Oliver is finding it difficult to concentrate it seems likely that his studies will suffer if the situation goes unchanged. This should be foremost in Oliver's mind as he decides what to do.

45. The correct answer is D. Not important at all – 2 marks (1 mark for C. Of minor importance)
Whilst Oliver may not welcome upsetting his class mates he will want to prioritise his studies and do well in this class which will necessitate some action.

46. The correct answer is C. Of minor importance – 2 marks (1 mark for B. Important or D. Not important at all)
It is technically true that the lecturer should take charge of the situation but as this doesn't seem to be happening Oliver should feel no qualms about taking action if he wishes to do well in his studies.

47. The correct answer is B. Important – 2 marks (1 mark for A. Very important or C. Of minor importance)

While offensive jokes should always be avoided, it's even more important if the target of the jokes is present as individual people may be upset.

48. The correct answer is D. Not important at all – 2 marks (1 mark for C. Of minor importance)
Heidi must react to her own conscience.

49. The correct answer is C. Of minor importance – 2 marks (1 mark for B. Important or D. Not important at all)
Heidi should be aware that she is inconveniencing other people if she pulls out but the higher principle is not causing offense by being unkind.

50. The correct answer is A. Very important – 2 marks (1 mark for B. Important)
While we all must do things we find uncomfortable from time to time this usually pertains to the effort required to do the right thing rather than that required to do something you feel is wrong.

51. The correct answer is B. Important – 2 marks (1 mark for A. Very important or C. Of minor importance)
The fact that Harry has other doctors in his family (possibly including his brother) gives credence to the story.

52. The correct answer is C. Of minor importance – 2 marks (1 mark for B. Important or D. Not important at all)
While 'previous good character' should be taken into account it is important that any allegations or rumours are investigated anyway.

53. The correct answer is D. Not important at all – 2 marks (1 mark for C. Of minor importance)
If these events were told by anyone action would be recquired. There is no reason to take the word of a student as more or less reliable than anyone else.

54. The correct answer is C. Of minor importance – 2 marks (1 mark for B. Important or D. Not important at all)
A 'problem patient' may be suspected of making something like this up. However – if the story has enough elements in it which ring true then proper investigations need to take place. It's possible the story has been embroidered so those investigations must be thorough.

55. The correct answer is D. Not important at all – 2 marks (1 mark for C. Of minor importance)
While this is true it is important to apply current knowledge and practice whilst it is still current.

56. The correct answer is A. Very important – 2 marks (1 mark for B. Important)
It is imperative that students are taught up to date material

57. The correct answer is B. Important – 2 marks (1 mark for A. Very important or C. Of minor importance)
There may be good and bad ways to do this but substandard teaching should not be allowed to continue unchecked

58. The correct answer is A. Very important – 2 marks (1 mark for B. Important)
However highly regarded or rewarded a career is, if it isn't something you really enjoy or want to do then it is likely to be a poor choice.

59. The correct answer is C. Of minor importance – 2 marks (1 mark for B. Important or D. Not important at all)
It is clear that not everyone has the ability to pursue, for example, medicine. However - it does not follow that everyone with the appropriate ability should pursue the most challenging path available to them. There are many other factors to consider besides the competitiveness to gain entry on a course. In the long run medicine will not be served by people who are clever, but indifferent, becoming doctors.

60. The correct answer is C. Of minor importance – 2 marks (1 mark for B. Important or D. Not important at all)
No-one likes to upset or disappoint people who they care for, and who care for them. However - ultimately those people would prefer to see their daughter or student happy and fulfilled in life.

61. The correct answer is A. Very important – 2 marks (1 mark for B. Important)
Ria's preferred career is hardly mundane or low-skilled. It is important to remember than many careers are important, skilled, interesting and useful.

62. The correct answer is B. Important – 2 marks (1 mark for A. Very important or C. Of minor importance)
Being aware of your own limitations is important, especially so in medicine. However - this would also be the case had Shaun just recently qualified as a doctor.

63. The correct answer is A. Very important – 2 marks (1 mark for B. Important)
If there is someone needing medical attention, and the most qualified person available is a Shaun, then the few months left of his training becomes less relevant.

64. The correct answer is D. Not important at all – 2 marks (1 mark for C. Of minor importance)
In the case of a genuine emergency it is important to put patient welfare first and liability second.

65. The correct answer is B. Important – 2 marks (1 mark for A. Very important or C. Of minor importance)
While 'final exams' and qualification are significant milestones, it is important to remember that learning happens throughout your training and doesn't magically appear after graduation. This does not give anyone 'carte blanche' to begin practicing medicine when they are not qualified to do so but should give med students some confidence if an emergency arises.

66. The correct answer is A. Very important – 2 marks (1 mark for B. Important)
We all make mistakes and while some of them have more long ranging consequences than others it is important to learn from them and move forward.

67. The correct answer is C. Of minor importance – 2 marks (1 mark for B. Important or D. Not important at all)
It is reasonable to expect proper teaching from a teacher and anyone who is paid and qualified to teach. When accepting teaching from someone who isn't qualified then there may be a risk involved.

68. The correct answer is B. Important – 2 marks (1 mark for A. Very important or C. Of minor importance)
Even when mistakes are made there is usually a great deal of 'good' as well. It is important to be able to recognise and appreciate the things you have done well in as well as learning from your errors.

69. The correct answer is A. Very important – 2 marks (1 mark for B. Important)
The fact that these exams are only mocks is very important. This gives Vivienne's friends a chance to re-learn the formula and do better in their finals.

27/44

Full Mock Test 3 Verbal Reasoning (21 minutes for this section)

Carbohydrates that a person eats are converted by the liver and muscles into glycogen for storage. Glycogen burns rapidly to provide quick energy. Runners can store about 2,000 kcal worth of glycogen in their bodies, enough for about 18-20 miles of running. Many runners report that running becomes noticeably more difficult at that point. When glycogen runs low, the body must then obtain energy by burning stored fat, which does not burn as readily. When this happens, the runner will experience dramatic fatigue and is said to "hit the wall". The aim of training for the marathon (26 miles), according to many coaches, is to maximise the limited glycogen available so that the fatigue of the "wall" is not as dramatic. This is accomplished in part by utilising a higher percentage of energy from burned fat even during the early phase of the race, thus conserving glycogen.

Carbohydrate-based 'energy gels' are used by runners to avoid or reduce the effect of "hitting the wall", as they provide easy to digest energy during the run. Energy gels usually contain varying amounts of sodium and potassium and some also contain caffeine. They need to be consumed with a certain amount of water. Recommendations for how often to take an energy gel during the race range widely.

Alternatives to gels include various forms of concentrated sugars, and foods high in simple carbohydrates that can be digested easily. Many runners experiment with consuming energy supplements during training runs to determine what works best for them. Consumption of food while running sometimes makes the runner sick.

1. All of the following statements are true except:

A. Eating while running can cause the runner problems
B. Energy gels contain a carefully balanced set of nutrients
C. Energy gels should not be consumed on their own
D. Energy gels contain glycogen

2. According to the text which of the following statements is true?

A. Runners can store enough glycogen in their body to complete a marathon
B. Runners can store enough glycogen in their body to run most of a marathon
C. Runners can burn fat as readily as carbohydrates
D. Runners burn their fat stores before their carbohydrates

3. An unsuitable snack for a runner during a marathon would be:

A. Fruit (high in simple carbohydrates, little fat)
B. A whole grain cereal bar (contains complex carbohydrates)
C. Jelly babies (high in fat and sugar)
D. Carbohydrate gel (contains nutrients and caffeine)

4. All of the following statements are true except:

A. During training, runners should try various types of supplement
B. Runners should only take supplements once they 'hit the wall'
C. Running becomes difficult once the body has burned through its store of glycogen
D. Burning fat provides energy but not as efficiently as burning glycogen

The human body contains chemical compounds such as water, carbohydrates, fatty acids and nucleic acids. These compounds in turn consist of elements such as carbon, hydrogen, oxygen, nitrogen, calcium etc. All these compounds and elements occur in various forms and combinations (e.g. hormones, vitamins, phospholipids, and hydroxyapatite), both in the human body and in the plant and animal organisms that humans eat.

The human body consists of elements ingested, digested, absorbed, and circulated through the bloodstream to feed the cells of the body. Digestive juices break chemical bonds in ingested molecules and modulate their

confirmations and energy states. Though some molecules are absorbed into the bloodstream unchanged, digestion releases them from the matrix of foods. Unabsorbed matter, along with some waste products of metabolism, is eliminated from the body in the faeces.
Nutritional studies must consider the state of the body before and after experiments, as well as the chemical composition of the whole diet and of all material excreted from the body. Comparing the food to the waste can help determine the specific compounds and elements absorbed and metabolised in the body. The effects of nutrients may only be discernible over an extended period.
In general, eating a wide variety of fresh, unprocessed foods has proven favourable for health compared to diets based on processed foods. In particular, the consumption of whole-plant foods slows digestion and allows better absorption, and a more favourable balance of essential nutrients per calorie, resulting in better management of cell growth and maintenance as well as better regulation of appetite and blood sugar. Regularly scheduled meals are more wholesome than haphazard ones.

5. An apple a day is good for you.

A. True
B. False
C. Can't tell

6. Nutritional studies should last at least a fortnight.

A. True
B. False
C. Can't tell

7. Processed foods are bad for you.

A. True
B. False
C. Can't tell

8. Hydroxyapatite contains both hydrogen and oxygen molecules.

A. True
B. False
C. Can't tell

Petty, G. (2009) *Teaching today: a practical guide*, 4th edn, Oxford, Oxford University Press, pp. 231–2.
Group work is interactive. It gives students a chance to use the methods, principles and vocabulary that they are being taught. Shy students who will not contribute to the full class can usually be coaxed into contributing to a group. What is more, there's a built-in self-checking and peer-tutoring aspect to most group work, where errors in understanding are ironed out, usually in a very supportive atmosphere. Students can often do together what they could not achieve alone, with each member of the group providing part of the 'jigsaw' of understanding.
Group work involved learners in task-centred talking. As well as being an enjoyable activity, this provides huge opportunities for learning. It requires that learners process the new material and make personal sense of it. Good group work hands the responsibility over to the students.
Students get a chance to practice high-order mental skills such as creativity, evaluation, synthesis and analysis. They also practice 'common skills' such as the ability to work with and communicate with others. In addition, group work gives students a universally welcomed opportunity to get to know each other. It can also arouse group loyalty, especially if there is an element of competition between groups.
Groups can, however, by hijacked by a determined individual with some group members becoming passengers. Difficulties with groups can be overcome by using well devised tasks, good teaching methods and ensuring groups take responsibility for their work.

9. Which of the following statements is true?

A. Group work ensures that all individuals are engaged
B. Group work allows students to improve only their high order mental skills
C. Group work allows quieter students the opportunity to participate
D. Group work allows group members to compete against each other

10. Which is not a confirmed advantage of group work?

A. Groups allow students to work with different students and get to know them better
B. Peer tutoring and self-checking
C. Students become responsible for their own learning
D. Groups are easier to manage for the teacher

11. Which of the following interactions is not an intra-group interaction?

A. Feedback to other students
B. Analysing information
C. Competition
D. Contributing to others learning

12. Which of the following would not be beneficial to the facilitation of working in groups?

A. The tasks should be well devised
B. High order mental skills
C. Teacher allocation of tasks to individuals
D. Time should be given to allow students to analyse information

Flowering plants (angiosperms) are the most diverse group of land plants. They can be distinguished from gymnosperms, the only other seed-producing plants, by characteristics including flowers, endosperm, and the production of seed-bearing fruits.
Flowers are the reproductive organs of flowering plants and the feature most distinguishing them from other seed plants. Flowers aid angiosperms by enabling a wider range of adaptability and broadening the ecological niches open to them.
Flower parts such as stamen are much lighter than the corresponding organs of gymnosperms and have contributed to the diversification of angiosperms with adaptations such as particular pollinators.
The male gametophyte in angiosperms is significantly smaller than those of gymnosperm seed plants. This decreases the time from pollination to fertilisation, which begins very soon after pollination. The shorter time leads to angiosperms setting seeds faster than gymnosperms.
The closed carpel of angiosperms also allows adaptations to specialised pollination syndromes and controls. Once the ovary is fertilised, the carpel and some surrounding tissues develop into a fruit that often serves to attract seed-dispersing animals. The resulting cooperative relationship presents another advantage.
The small female gametophyte may be an adaptation allowing for more rapid seed set, eventually leading to such flowering plant adaptations as annual life cycles, allowing the flowering plants to fill more niches.
Endosperm formation generally begins after fertilisation and before the first division of the zygote. Endosperm is a highly nutritive tissue that can provide food for the developing embryo and sometimes for the seedling when it first appears.
These distinguishing characteristics have made angiosperms the most diverse and numerous land plants and commercially important to humans.

13. Flowers are angiosperms.

A. True
B. False
C. Can't tell

14. Gymnosperms and angiosperms both have stamens.

A. True
B. False
C. Can't tell

15. Angiosperms produce seed.

A. True
B. False
C. Can't tell

16. Gymnosperms have large female gametophytes.

A. True
B. False
C. Can't tell

The most common size of sail ship of the line was the "74" (named for its 74 guns), originally developed by France in the 1730s. Until this time the British had 6 sizes of ship of the line, and they found that their smaller 50- and 60-gun ships were becoming too small for the battle line, while their 80s and over were 3-deckers and therefore unwieldy and unstable in heavy seas. Their best were 70-gun 2-deckers of about 46 metres (150 ft) long on the gun deck, while the new French 74s were around 52 metres (170 ft). In 1747 the British captured a few of these French ships during the War of Austrian Succession.

In the next decade Thomas Slade (surveyor of the navy from 1755) broke away from the past and designed several new classes of 51- to 52-metre 74s to compete with these French designs, starting with the Dublin and Bellona classes. Their successors gradually improved handling and size through the 1780s. Other European navies also ended up building 74s as they had the right balance between offensive power, cost, and manoeuvrability. Larger vessels were still built, as command ships, but they were more useful only if they could get close to an enemy, rather than in a battle involving chasing or manoeuvring. The 74 remained the favoured ship until 1811, when Seppings's method of construction enabled bigger ships to be built with more stability.

In the Royal Navy, smaller two-deck 74- or 64-gun ships of the line that could not be used safely in fleet actions had their upper decks removed (or razeed), resulting in a very stout, single-gun-deck warship called a razee. The resulting razeed ship could be classed as a frigate and was still much stronger. The most successful razeed ship in the Royal Navy was HMS Indefatigable, commanded by Sir Edward Pellew.

17. Which of these statements is most likely to be true?

A. Thomas Slade designed the first '74s' for the Royal Navy in the 1730s
B. Larger ships were too unstable to be used in the battle line
C. The '74' was superseded after 1811 by newer designs
D. The HMS Indefatigable is an example of a successful '74'

18. Which of these statements is true?

A. The least common size of sail ship of the line was the "74"
B. The best British ships before 1750 were the '70s'
C. Sir Edward Pellew was the most successful commander of a '74'
D. The Dublin class of ships were almost 50 metres long

19. Which of these statements is false?

A. Up to 1730 the British navy had 6 different sizes of ships of the line
B. Larger ships were used as command vessels
C. Some smaller ships were converted into strong frigates
D. Some French ships were captured during the revolutionary wars from which the British '74s' were developed

20. Which of these statements is most likely to be false?

A. Later construction methods enabled larger ships to be built without sacrificing stability
B. '74s' had the right balance of power, cost, and manoeuvrability
C. The '74s' were the popular design up to the end of the Napoleonic wars in 1815
D. Ships of the line were developed mostly by European powers

In mathematics, a prime number is a natural number that has exactly two distinct natural number divisors: 1 and itself. An infinitude of prime numbers exists, although the density of prime numbers within natural numbers is 0. The property of being prime is called primality.
Verifying the primality of a given number n can be done by trial division, dividing n by all integer numbers m smaller than or equal to the square root of n, thereby checking whether n is a multiple of m, and therefore not prime but a composite. For big primes, increasingly sophisticated algorithms which are faster than this technique have been devised.
There is no known formula that yields all the prime numbers and no composites. However, the distribution of primes and the statistical behaviour of primes in the large can be modelled. The first result in that direction is the prime number theorem which says that the probability that a given, randomly chosen number n is prime is inversely proportional to its number of digits, or the logarithm of n. This statement has been proven since the end of the 19th century. The unproven Riemann hypothesis dating from 1859 implies a refined statement concerning the distribution of primes.
Many fundamental questions around prime numbers remain open. For example, Goldbach's conjecture which asserts that any even natural number bigger than two is the sum of two primes, or the twin prime conjecture which says that there are infinitely many twin primes (pairs of primes whose difference is two), have been unresolved for more than a century, notwithstanding the simplicity of their statements.

21. 125 is a prime number.

A. True
B. False
C. Can't tell

22. Riemann lived in the mid-19th century.

A. True
B. False
C. Can't tell

23. Goldbach's conjecture is supported by the number 20.

A. True
B. False
C. Can't tell

24. The prime number theorem suggests that random numbers over 10,000,000 are less likely to have primality than a number under 100,000.

A. True
B. False
C. Can't tell

Stigma is a Greek word that in its origins referred to a type of marking or tattoo that was cut or burned into the skin of criminals, slaves, or traitors in order to visibly identify them as blemished or morally polluted people. These individuals were to be avoided or shunned, particularly in public places.
Social stigmas can occur in many different forms. The most common stigma concerns culture, obesity, gender, race and diseases. Many people who have been stigmatised feel as though they are transforming from a whole

person to a tainted one. They feel different and devalued by others. This can happen in the workplace, educational settings, health care, the criminal justice system, and even in their own family. For example, the parents of overweight women are less likely to pay for their daughters' college education than are the parents of average-weight women.

Stigma may also be described as a label that associates a person to a set of unwanted characteristics that form a stereotype. It is also affixed. Once people identify and label a person's 'differences' others will assume that is just how things are and the person will remain stigmatised until the stigmatising attribute is undetected. A considerable amount of generalisation is required to create stigmatised groups, meaning that someone is attributed to a general group, regardless of how well they actually fit into that group. However, the attributes that society selects differ according to time and place. What is considered out of place in one society could be the norm in another. When society categorizes individuals into certain groups the labelled person is subjected to status loss and discrimination. Society will start to form expectations about those groups once the cultural stereotype is secured.

Stigma may affect the behaviour of those who are stigmatised. Those who are stereotyped often start to act in ways that their stigmatisers expect of them. It not only changes their behaviour, but it also shapes their emotions and beliefs. Members of stigmatized social groups often face prejudice that causes depression (i.e. deprejudice). These stigmas put a person's social identity in threatening situations, like low self-esteem. Because of this, identity theories have become highly researched. Identity threat theories can go hand-in-hand with labelling theory.

Members of stigmatized groups start to become aware that they aren't being treated the same way and know they are probably being discriminated against. Studies have shown that by 10 years of age, most children are aware of cultural stereotypes of different groups in society, and children who are members of stigmatised groups are aware of cultural types at an even younger age.

25. Based on the text which adage do you think most likely is a summary of 'labelling theory'?

A. A chip on your shoulder
B. A leopard cannot change its spots
C. Give a dog a bad name and hang him
D. Actions speak louder than words

26. When a person finds themselves subject to some form of stigma, which description is not a response suggested by the passage?

A. Beginning to act in the way that fits the stereotype they're subject to
B. Feeling angry and defensive
C. Development of depression
D. Loss of sense of 'belonging'

27. What doesn't the recognition of cultural stereotypes by young children suggest to us?

A. Children are unaware of the subtleties of behaviour
B. Children witness evidence of prejudice and discrimination
C. Stereotypes are strongly reinforced in many areas of society
D. Parents may inadvertently, or deliberately, pass on their prejudices

28. Which statement accurately likens stigma in modern usage compared to the original meaning of the word from ancient Greece?

A. Stigma requires a visible characteristic
B. Stigmatised people are shunned in public places
C. Stigma is a permanent state
D. A stigmatised person is polluted or blemished

In 1785, the "Protestant Presbyterian Church of Wilmington" was incorporated by the State Legislature. The church seems to have continued its semi-independent existence until April 4, 1817, when it was received into the Fayetteville Presbytery of the Presbyterian Church.
Fire destroyed the first three buildings erected by this congregation. The first two buildings, constructed in 1818 and 1821, were located on Front Street, between Dock and Orange. The cornerstone of the 1821 building is now at the foot of the stairs of the Kenan tower. The third building, which was constructed on this present site, was dedicated on 28 April 1861 (just weeks after the start of the Civil War), and burned on New Year's Eve, 1925. It was succeeded by the present building, which was completed in 1928.
The Lectern Bible, which is displayed on the front of the lectern, is one of the few physical links left to this congregation from its past. It was the pulpit Bible of the 1861 church and escaped the 1925 fire only because it had been stolen from the pulpit when the Union Army occupied Wilmington during the Civil War. Descendants of the Union officer into whose hands it eventually passed returned it to the church in 1928.
The present church building was designed by the noted architect Hobart Upjohn. His plans included architectural styles from three different periods: the Norman, as represented in the chapel; the English Decorated, in the sanctuary and the Elizabethan, in the church school building. The large clerestory windows have as their unifying theme the "I Am's" of Christ.
The organ was built by Ernest M. Skinner, one of America's master organ builders. It was built to suit the structure of the church building, and since a recent renovation, should sound just as it did when Skinner finished work on it. The organ is a memorial to James Sprunt, who was a ruling elder in this church. The windows in the Kenan Memorial Chapel were created by Owen Bonawits of New York and are of antique stained glass treated so that they are truly antique in colour. These windows represent the twelve apostles.

29. Which of these statements is most likely to be true?

A. The Norman, English Decorated and Elizabethan architectural styles can be seen in the chapel, school and sanctuary respectively
B. The clerestory window illustrates the 'I Am' statement of Jesus
C. Fire destroyed the third building during the civil war
D. The present building was completed three years after the previous one was destroyed

30. Which of these statements is true?

A. Part of the 1821 building is included in the foundations of the present building
B. The lectern Bible was stolen from the 1821 building but returned in 1928
C. The organ commemorates a former elder of the church
D. The windows of the Kenan Memorial Chapel are dedicated to Owen Bonawits

31. Which of these statements is false?

A. For about 22 years the church was independent of outside authority
B. The present building is the second on this site
C. Designing this church established Hobart Upjohn as an architect
D. The organ renovation has re-established its original sound quality

32. Which of these statements is likely to be untrue?

A. For more than 40 years, the congregation worshipped on Front Street
B. The lectern Bible is one of many links to the history of the church displayed in the current building
C. The church survived the depredations of the Civil War and continued in use for more than 60 years
D. The windows depicting the apostles are treated to show an authentic antique colour

Shoe polish (or boot polish), usually a waxy paste or a cream, is a consumer product used to polish, shine, waterproof, and restore the appearance of leather shoes or boots, thereby extending the footwear's life. In some regions-including New Zealand-"nugget" is used as a common term for solid waxy shoe polish, as opposed to liquid shoe polishes.

Various substances have been used as shoe polish for hundreds of years, starting with natural substances such as wax and tallow. Modern polish formulae were introduced early in the 20th century and some products from that era are still in use today. Today, shoe polish is usually made from a mix of natural and synthetic materials, including naphtha, turpentine, dyes, and gum arabic, using straightforward chemical engineering processes. Shoe polish can be toxic, and, if misused, can stain skin.

The popularity of shoe polish paralleled a general rise in leather and synthetic shoe production, beginning in the 19th century and continuing into the 20th. The World Wars saw a surge in demand for the product, in order to polish army boots.

33. Shoe polish was first used in the 19th century.

A. True
B. False
C. Can't tell

34. Polishing leather shoes makes them last longer.

A. True
B. False
C. Can't tell

35. Manufacturing modern shoe polish requires complex chemical engineering processes.

A. True
B. False
C. Can't tell

36. Shoe polish manufacture produces toxic waste products.

A. True
B. False
C. Can't tell

Some people choose to be vegetarian or vegan for environmental reasons.

The use of large industrial monoculture that is common in industrialised agriculture, typically for feed crops such as corn and soy is more damaging to ecosystems than more sustainable farming practices such as organic farming, permaculture, arable, pastoral, and rain-fed agriculture. Other concerns include the waste of natural resources, such as food, water, etc.

Animals that feed on grain or rely on grazing require more water than grain crops. According to the United States Department of Agriculture, growing crops for farm animals requires nearly half of the US water supply and 80% of its agricultural land. Animals raised for food in the U.S. consume 90% of the soy crop, 80% of the corn crop, and 70% of its grain. In tracking food animal production from the feed through to the dinner table, the inefficiencies of meat, milk and egg production range from a 4:1 energy input to protein output ratio up to 54:1. The result is that producing animal-based food is typically much less efficient than the harvesting of grains, vegetables, legumes, seeds and fruits, though this might not be true to the same extent for animal husbandry in the developing world where factory farming is almost non-existent, making animal-based food much more sustainable.

Some have described unequal treatment of humans and animals as a form of species bias such as anthropocentrism or human-centeredness. Val Plumwood (1993, 1996) has argued that anthropocentrism plays a role in green theory that is analogous to androcentrism in feminist theory and ethnocentrism in anti-racist theory. Plumwood calls human-centredness "anthropocentrism" to emphasise this parallel. By analogy with racism and sexism, Melanie Joy has dubbed meat-eating "carnism."

37. All of the following statements are true except:

A. If more people avoided animal products in their diet then there would be less pressure on the environment
B. About 20% of agricultural land in the US is used for growing crops
C. Non-industrial animal farming is more energy efficient than factory farming
D. Industrial farming may be unsustainable in the long term

38. Which of the following could be a real life example based on information in the text?

A. 54,000 kilo-calories inputted to produce 1000 kilo-calories of food
B. Each 10 calories of end-product required 600 calories of energy for production
C. 5,000 calories worth of fruit requires less than 5,000 calories of energy for production
D. 25,000 kilo-calories inputted to produce 1,000 kilo-calories of food protein

39. What is not a logical conclusion to draw about the work of Plumwood?

A. Meat eating could be called 'carnism'
B. Animals and humans are of equal worth
C. As racism and sexism have come to be unacceptable so should human-centeredness
D. Environmental theory can be understood better with the concept of anthropocentrism

40. Which of the following statements is true?

A. Animals in the US consume 70% of the grain crop
B. Organic farming does not damage ecosystems
C. Industrialised farming relies on sufficient rainfall
D. Western culture places higher value on humans than animals

The principal applications of political correctness concern the practices of awareness and toleration of the sociologic differences among people of different races and genders; of physical and mental disabilities; of ethnic group and sexual orientation; of religious background, and of ideological worldview. Specifically, the praxis of political correctness is in the descriptive vocabulary that the speaker and the writer use in effort to eliminate the prejudices inherent to cultural, sexual and racist stereotypes with culturally neutral terms, such as the locutions, circumlocutions, and euphemisms presented in the Official Politically Correct Dictionary and Handbook (1993) such as:

- "intellectually disabled" instead of mentally retarded
- "African-American" instead of black and Negro, in the US
- "Native American" instead of Indian, in the US
- "First Nations" instead of Indian, in Canada
- gender-neutral terms such as "firefighter" instead of fireman and firewoman; 'police officer' instead of policeman and policewoman
- value-free terms describing physical disabilities, such as "visually impaired" instead of blind and "hearing impaired" instead of deaf
- value-free cultural terms, such as "holiday season" and "winter holiday", instead of Christmas

Opponents of such compound-descriptor words and prolix usages, apply the terms politically correct, political correctness, and PC as pejorative and obscurantist criticism, denoting, and connoting apparently excessive deference to particular social sensibilities, at the expense of common-sense considerations of language, thought, and action. Conversely, opponents of political correctness then employed the term politically incorrect to communicate that they were unafraid to ignore the social constraints inherent to politically-correct speech. From such opposition emerged the culturally liberal television talk-show *Politically Incorrect* (1993-2002) and the culturally conservative book series of *The Politically Incorrect Guide to...* a given subject, such as the US constitution, capitalism, and the Bible. In these cultural and sociological matters, the term denotes and connotes that the speaker and the writer use language and proffer ideas, and practice behaviours that are unconstrained by a perceived "liberal" orthodoxy, and by over-sensitive concerns about expressing political biases that might offend people who do not share such cultural perspectives.

41. What human quality or difference seems least likely to be part of the 'politically correct' agenda?

A. Differences in height
B. Differences in levels of intelligence
C. Differences in religion
D. Differences in political opinion

42. Which statement is likely to be the best description of the underlying aim of the political correctness movement?

A. To ensure that everyone held inoffensive opinions
B. To protect vulnerable groups from prejudice and discrimination
C. To ensure that offence was not caused through careless language
D. To stop the use of stereotypes

43. Which of the following descriptions would be most likely to be defined as not being politically correct?

A. A homosexual Native American
B. A greetings card wishing someone 'Happy Holidays'
C. A hearing impaired African-American
D. A physically disabled former policeman

44. How did the movement for 'political correctness' backfire as described in the article?

A. The left-wing media countered it
B. Some left- and right-wing media countered it
C. The right-wing media countered it
D. It made being 'politically incorrect' appear inoffensive

Full Mock Test 3 Decision Making (31 minutes for this section)

1. Working people who earn more than £11,000 per year must pay income tax at a fixed percentage. Those who earn over £50,000 per year pay an additional percentage of income tax. Some people, who have inconsistent (or numerous sources of) income, must fill in a tax return annually. Most employed people don't need to fill in a tax return.

Select the words 'Yes' or 'No' if the conclusion does or doesn't follow

A man earning £50,000 will pay more tax as a proportion of their total earnings than someone earning £40,000	Yes / No
Employed people usually have consistent income from a single source	Yes / No
Unemployed people never have to fill in a tax return	Yes / No
All income tax payers earn more than £11,000 per annum	Yes / No
John earns £45,000 from his employment. He also owns some rental properties which earn him £10,000 profit per year. John has to pay higher rate income tax.	Yes / No

2. Being fully compliant with health and safety rules costs most businesses 10% of their profits. The risk of a health and safety infraction which will cost them more than 10% of their profits is calculated at 2% per annum. A drop in profits of more than 10% will reduce the total share value of the business by 7%.

Select the words 'Yes' or 'No' if the conclusion does or doesn't follow

There will be, on average, a significant health and safety infraction every fifty years	Yes / No
A company that is fully compliant with health and safety rules will lose 7% of its value.	Yes / No
If a company is 50% compliant with health and safety rules it will cost them 5% of their profits	Yes / No
Company X was sued by an employee who was injured at work due to health and safety rules being ignored. The resulting fine was 10.5% of the profits for the year. Company X lost more than 5% in total share value that year.	Yes / No
A company that decides to risk not being compliant with health and safety rules is likely to make higher profits and retain share value than one that is fully compliant	Yes / No

3. If you hold a passport to country A you can travel freely to countries B, C and D without a visa. If you hold a passport to country B you can travel freely to country A, you must get a visa to travel to county C and you are not allowed to visit country D. Passport holders in country C cannot visit any other country without having a visa. Passport holders of country D can travel freely without a visa to countries A and C, but cannot travel to country B without a special visa which is usually only given to high ranking officials.

Select the words 'Yes' or 'No' if the conclusion does or doesn't follow

Amerdeep lives in country D and has just returned from a trip to country B. It is likely that Amerdeep is an influential person of high rank. Yes / No

Bilal has two visa stamps in his passport based on his travel between these four countries. He must be from country C. Yes / No

A group of friends who live in the four different countries wish to meet for a reunion holiday. The single best country for them to meet in to avoid complicated visa applications is country A. Yes / No

There is a strained political relationship between countries B and D Yes / No

Having no visa requirements for entry increases tourism to any country. Country A has the biggest tourism sector. Country C has the second largest. Yes / No

4. Of all the artists performing at the festival, none were older than 50 playing in a band
Select the words 'Yes' or 'No' if the conclusion does or doesn't follow

Only people younger than 50 played at the festival Yes / No

Most of the performers were young Yes / No

Every member of every performing band was under the age of 50 Yes / No

All the people under 50 performing at the festival were in a band Yes / No

Any over 50s who performed at the festival were not part of a band Yes / No

5. Four couples go on holiday for their silver wedding anniversary. The four men – Alan, James, Lloyd, Mick and the four women Isobel, Jean, Karen and Sue each find one thing to complain about though: foreign food, rude staff, small beds or the heat.

- Alan does not like foreign food but Karen (not his wife) loves it!
- Isobel and Lloyd have found the staff to be very polite
- Jean is content with the temperature and the size of the bed and isn't married to James who is upset about one of these two things.
- The couple complaining about the heat are not Mick and Sue

Which of the following is definitely true?

A. Jean isn't enjoying the foreign food
B. Lloyd is complaining that it's too hot
C. Sue thinks the bed is too small
D. James has found the staff to be rude

6. A maths teacher is marking a set of exam papers. The papers have been anonymised. Each student has taken two papers.
His 'students' have been classified as EE184, H800, H817 and H880b
The paper 1 scores are 52, 56, 60 and 68
The paper 2 scores are 66, 68, 70 and 72

- The lowest paper 1 score was not the same student as the lowest paper 2 score
- The highest paper 1 score was the same student as the highest paper 2 score
- EE184 scored in the 60s for both papers
- H800 scored 56 for paper 1 but didn't score 66 for paper 2
- H880b scored 16 more points in paper 2 than in paper 1

Which of the following statements must be true

A. H880b scored 72 in paper 2
B. H817 got the highest overall score
C. EE194 made the smallest improvement between papers 1 and 2
D. H800 made the biggest improvement between papers 1 and 2

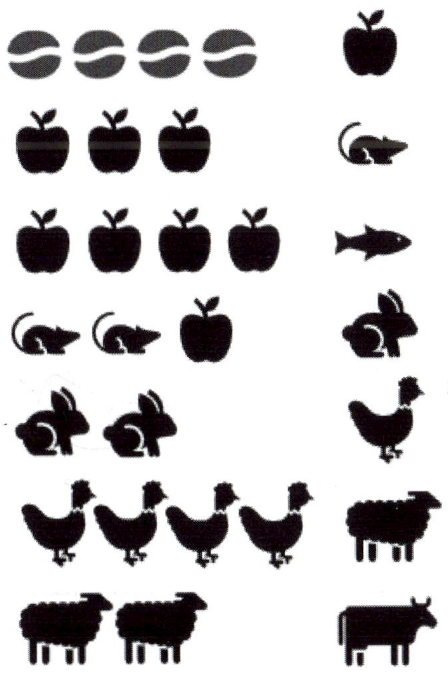

7. An archaeologist is interpreting some ancient artefacts and believes she has found a rudimentary currency system using cocoa beans as the basic unit.

Imagine that a person had raised two chickens with which they want to buy some fish for a celebration dinner. How many fish could they buy?

A. 1
B. 2
C. 3
D. 4
E. 5

8. The plan shows an allotment plot in which a gardener grows root vegetables (potatoes, carrots and parsnips), leafy vegetables (broccoli, cabbage and herbs) and fruit (redcurrants, raspberries and strawberries).

- Square 5 contains a root vegetable.
- All three fruit crops are in a single row
- Broccoli and carrots are both located in a corner plot
- Squares 2 and 4 have leafy vegetable crops

1	2	3
4	5	6
7	8	9

What could be growing in Plot 8?

A. Redcurrants
B. Potatoes
C. Cabbage
D. Parsnips

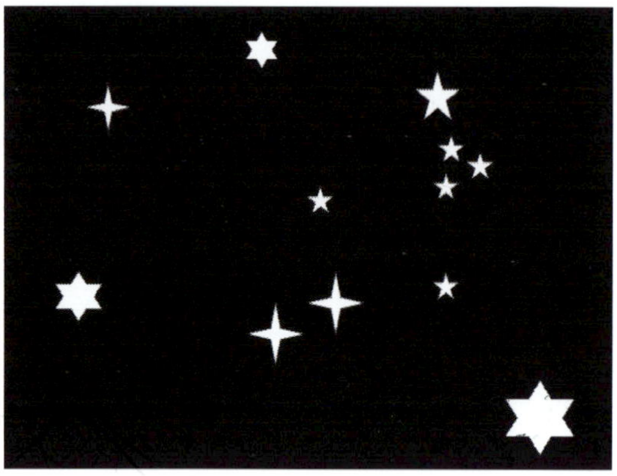

9. An astronomer is representing a small segment of night sky.
The larger the star is in the picture the larger it is.
The more points it has the closer it is to earth.

Which of the following must be true?

A. The largest star is also the closest
B. The three furthest stars are mid-sized
C. The smallest stars are furthest away
D. A six-pointed star is bigger than a four-pointed star

10. Tattoos and body art have become much more commonplace in the last decade. It is expected that up to 30% of people aged between 18 and 30 will have a tattoo by the time they reach 30. There is concern that choices made in youth may be regretted later as, traditionally, tattoos have been assumed to be the preserve of rebels, prisoners and gang members.
Young people should be cautioned against permanent body art such as a tattoo

A. Yes – having a tattoo will make other people assume they're of poor character
B. Yes – any permanent choice should be approached with caution
C. No – lots of young people are now having tattoos so the old assumptions no longer apply
D. No – the people may be young, but they are adults and allowed to make their own choices

11. The use of smartphones has gone from zero to almost everyone in the space of one generation. There is no definitive knowledge about the long term impact of smartphone use given the short time they have been here. Some speculation about damage to eyes, concentration, social relationships and potentially body tissue due to the radiation has taken place.
Until we know smartphones pose no danger there should be steps taken to reduce our dependence on them

A. Yes – no amount of convenience is worth a serious illness such as a brain tumour
B. Yes – all consumer products must be rigorously tested before being declared completely safe
C. No – the world has changed in numerous ways since the advent of the smart phone, there is no way to attribute any ill effect to the smart phone
D. No – there is no way that any consumer product can be declared to be completely safe so the suggestion is impractical

12. It is possible to study for GCSE and A-level qualifications on your own if given access to good enough resources.

A. Yes – a motivated student will be able to learn everything necessary to get good grades
B. Yes – the exams rely on fact recall and comprehension
C. No – group work and discussion are an imperative part of study
D. No – students of typical GCSE / A-level age are not sufficiently self-disciplined

13. An extra UK bank holiday should be introduced to move towards equalising the number of public holidays enjoyed by other similar countries.

A. Yes – it is important that the UK does not fall behind in this regard
B. Yes – UK workers would probably enjoy an extra day for leisure and relaxation
C. No – working more than other countries gives the UK a competitive advantage
D. No – bank holidays are to remember or celebrate specific events and should not just be invented

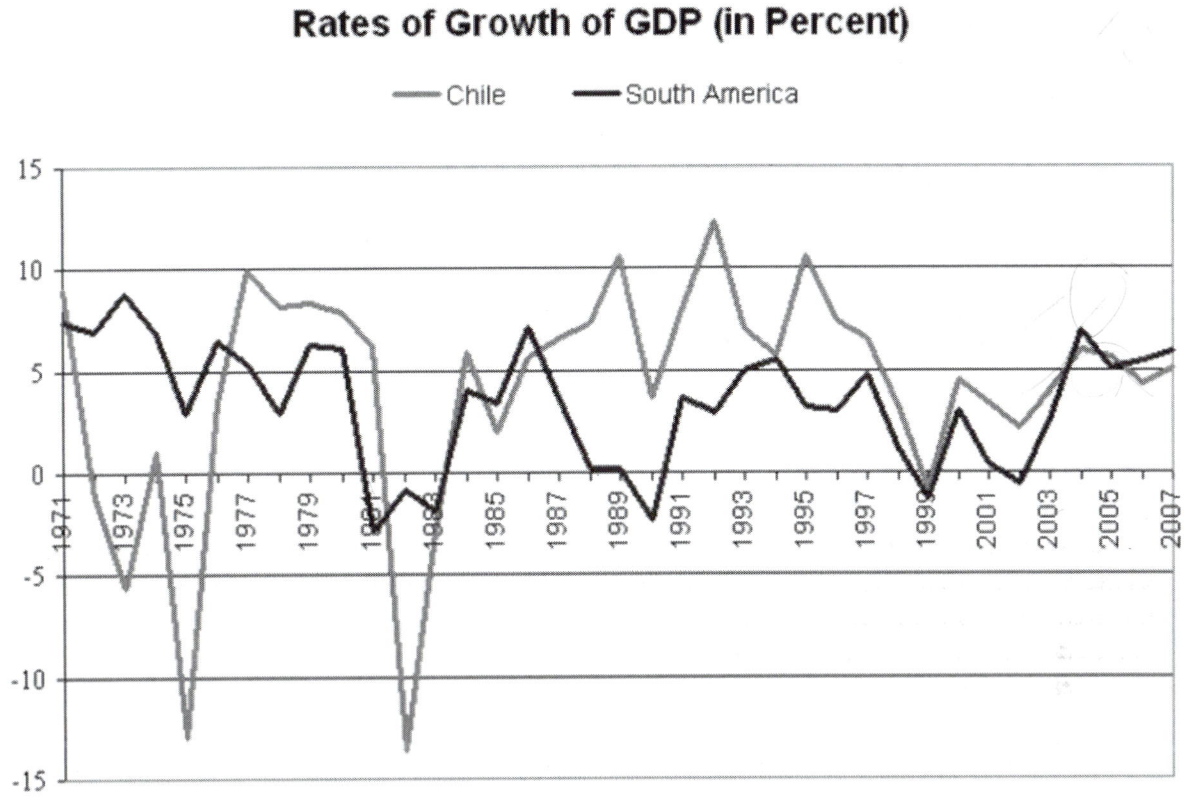

14. Select the words 'Yes' or 'No' if the conclusion does or doesn't follow

Chile spent fewer years in negative growth than South America as a whole	Yes / No
The biggest year of change for South America was 1980	Yes / No
Chile is one of the more volatile economies in South America	Yes / No
Another South American country must have had negative growth in 1988	Yes / No
The overall trend for Chile, and the continent as a whole, is upward	Yes / No

15. A reliance on caffeine-based drinks such as coffee or cola should be considered an addiction like smoking, drug abuse or alcoholism.

Select the strongest argument

A. Yes – substance dependence is a problem regardless of the substance
B. Yes – people should be able to access support to withdraw from the use of addictive substances
C. No - caffeine is naturally occurring in many food stuffs and isn't a harmful 'drug'
D. No - caffeine is not harmful in the way that other addictive substances are

16. Some health professionals believe that people would benefit from 10 portions of fruit and vegetables every day. The current official recommendation is for intake of only 5 which is only half of that amount. Should the recommended amount be increased?
Select the strongest argument

A. Yes – it is irresponsible to let people believe that 5 portions a day will lead to peak health if they really require 10
B. Yes – if more people eat more fruit and vegetables it will benefit farmers and retailers as well as their own personal health
C. No - people struggle to reach the current recommended intake and will be demoralised if this is doubled
D. No – changing official recommendations based on the beliefs of some people is irresponsible and further research is needed first

17. Several studies have shown that diesel cars, unlike petrol cars, spew out high levels of what are known as nitrogen oxides and dioxides, together called NOx. Nitrogen dioxide (NO_2) is particularly nasty: recent studies have shown it can cause or exacerbate many health conditions, such as inflammation of the lungs, which can trigger asthma and bronchitis, and increased risk of heart attacks and strokes. Particulate matter, which is belched out from diesel exhausts, has been shown to cause cancer. This has long been recognised, and modern diesel cars are fitted with extremely effective filters that stop almost all this carcinogenic soot from escaping into the atmosphere.

Select the words 'Yes' or 'No' if the conclusion does or doesn't follow.

Petrol cars are better for the environment and health	Yes / No
Modern diesel cars have less impact on the health of people than older ones	Yes / No
Inhaling NO_2 is a primary cause of heart attacks and strokes	Yes / No
Diesel cars release a few different compounds and pollutants into the atmosphere	Yes / No
The pollutants mentioned are the sole cause of multiple respiratory, cardiovascular and neurological complaints	Yes / No

18. There should be many more available spaces at medical school so that more aspiring doctors can be trained.
Select the strongest argument:

A. Yes – an ageing population will need an increasing number of doctors
B. Yes – plenty of very capable people don't get a place who could be excellent doctors
C. No - it's important that only the very best people become doctors
D. No – more money should be put into health promotion instead so fewer doctors are needed

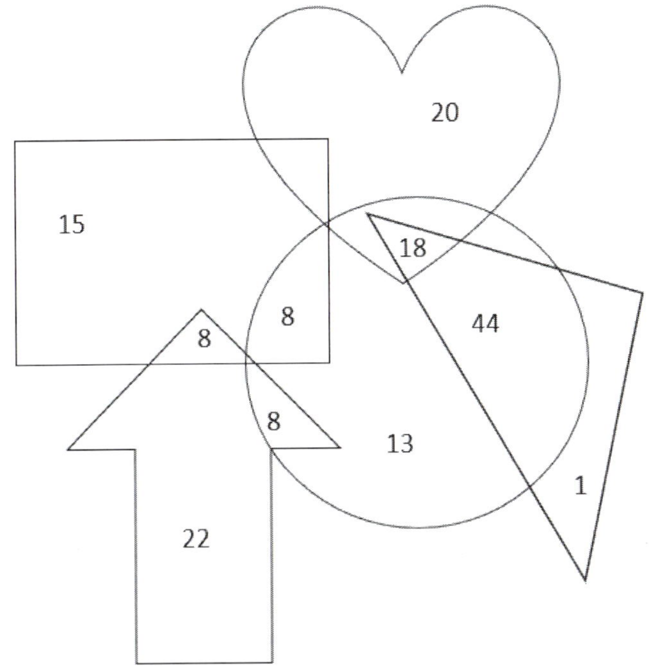

Commuters' methods of travel

- **Rectangle = cycle**
- **Arrow = drive**
- **Triangle = walk**
- **Circle = train**
- **Heart = bus**

19. Which of the following statements is true?

A. Twice the number of commuters who only drive only walk

B. Fewer commuters exclusively cycle than use three modes of transport

C. The number of commuters who use two modes of transport is three times the number who use two

D. The same number of commuters walk as catch the bus

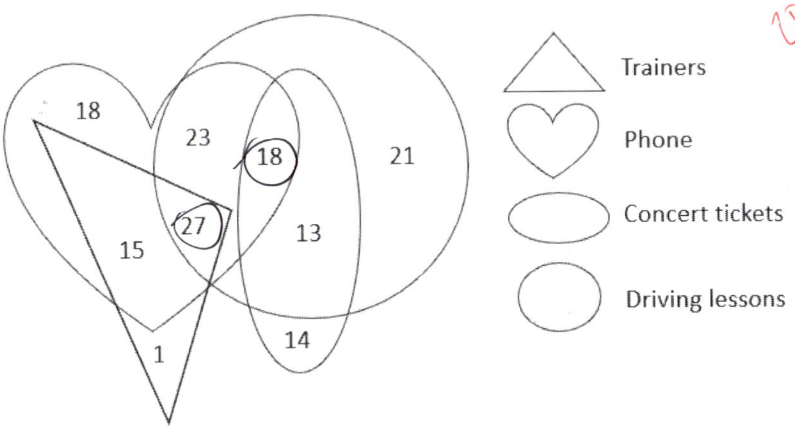

A group of teenagers were asked what they are saving up to buy.

20. Based on the diagram, which combination represents a total of 45 students?

A. Those saving for one thing only

B. Those saving for three things

C. Those saving for two things

D. Those saving for more than one thing

21. There is one old person's home with five centenarians – two ladies and three gentlemen! They each attribute a different reason for their longevity! Can you deduce how old the ladies Daisy and Jasmine, and gentlemen Daniel, Laurence and Max are; and which of them says that family, laughter, tea, bubble bath or olive oil is their secret?

- The oldest member of the group attributes his longevity to drinking lots of tea
- Daisy is six years older than Jasmine. Neither of them think olive oil is useful for anything – the person who does credit olive oil is the youngest man in the group.
- Bubble bath is (apparently) two years more effective than laughter
- The 105-year-old is older than Laurence but younger than Max

Which of the following statements must be true:

A. Jasmine enjoys bubble baths

B. Daisy is 109

C. The 103-year-old uses olive oil

D. Max laughs a lot

22. A group of children are swapping football stickers.

- Joe swaps three team photo stickers for one club badge
- Tim swaps two team photo stickers for a stadium sticker
- Harry swaps three club badges for a trophy sticker
- Gareth swaps two stadium stickers and a club badge for sticker which makes up part of a 3 x 3 grid of stickers which form a page sized photo on the front cover

Pete only has club badges and wants to get the whole front cover. How many stickers will he need?

A. 7
B. 13
C. 21
D. 63

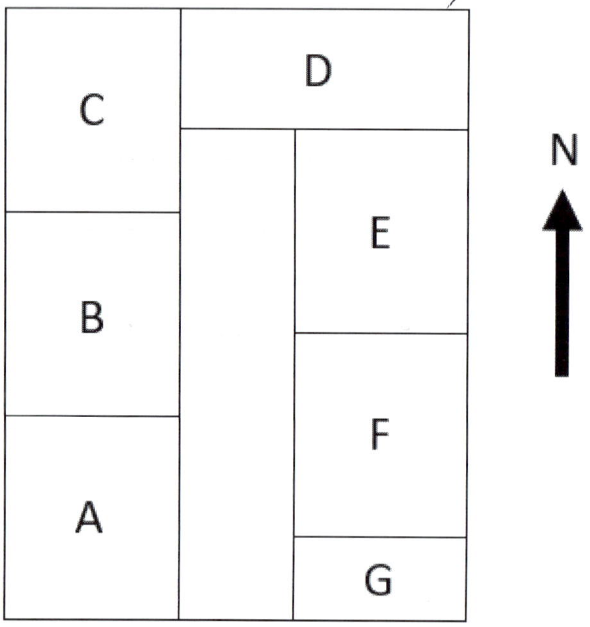

23. Five friends (Becky, Naomi, Priyanka, Sanduni and Shabnam) share this flat. There is four bedrooms (two friends share a room), a bathroom, and a kitchen.
The living room doesn't get much sunshine in the evening as it is on the eastern edge of the flat. The kitchen has both a northern and a western wall. Becky, Priyanka and Sanduni pay slightly less rent than the others as two of them share the long thin room, and the other has the smallest room. Naomi is next to the bathroom, which is next to the kitchen.

Which of the following statements must be true?

A. Sanduni and Priyanka share room D
B. The living room is room F
C. Naomi's door is directly opposite room G
D. Shabnam's room is next to the living room.

A conference in Hong Kong is made up of the following attendees:

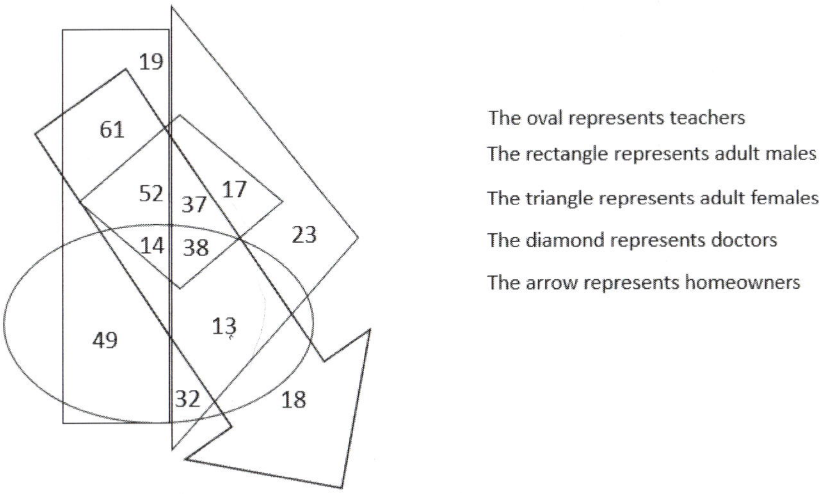

24. Which of the following statements is false?

A. The conference has more doctors in total than teachers.
B. Adult male homeowners outnumber adult female doctors.
C. There are 24 more female doctors who are also teachers and homeowners than there are male doctors who are also teachers and homeowners.
D. The number of male doctors who are also homeowners is equal to the number of female doctors who are also homeowners.

A cleaning product brand conducted a survey on the household chores members of the public do every day.

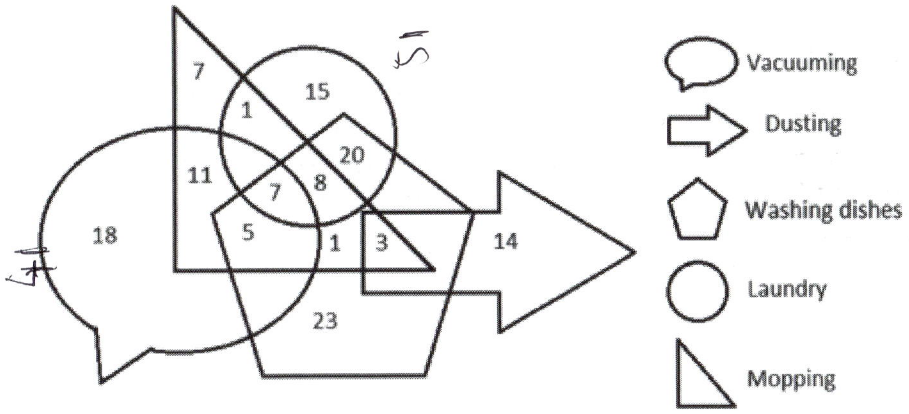

25. Based on the diagram, which of the following statements is false?

A. The amount of people who only wash dishes and do laundry every day is 7% of the total amount of people who vacuum every day.
B. 16 more people do laundry every day than vacuum.
C. The number of people who vacuum and mop and wash dishes every day is a third of the number of people who do laundry only.
D. 6% more people dust, wash dishes and do laundry every day than those who mop, dust and vacuum.

26. Maddie has two cars. She wishes to keep the best one and sell the other. Her first car, which is grey, has been reliable for 40 out of the last 50 weeks. Her second car, which is black, has been reliable for 18 of the last 20 weeks. According to insurance company statistics – a grey car is 15% less likely to be involved in an accident than average. A black car is involved in 5% more accidents than average. The average chance of a car being in an accident in any given year is 2%.
Considering all of this information – which car should Maddie sell?

A. The grey car – as it is less reliable and the difference in the chance of an accident amounts to only 4 in 1000
B. The grey car - as it is less reliable and the difference in the chance of an accident amounts to 4% of 2%.
C. The black car – as it is statistically more likely to be in an accident
D. The black car – as the difference in likelihood of an accident counters the difference in reliability.

27. 10% of customers who enter the supermarket buy a bottle of wine
25% of customers who enter the supermarket spend more than £50
25% of the customers who spend more than £50 will have bought a bottle of wine.
40% of the customers who spend less than £10 buy a bottle of wine
A bottle of wine costs an average of £7.
Which of the following statements is true?

A. Many customers entering the supermarket buy just a bottle of wine
B. Most supermarket customers spend between £10 and £50.
C. Customers spending more than £50 will spend more than 10% of their spend on wine
D. Customers spending under £10 spend more than 50% of their spend on wine

28. Anna drinks coffee every day.
Research study 1 shows that 300 out of 3000 people who drink coffee every day also overuse headache medication. Research study 2 shows that 80% of people who overuse headache medication are female. Considering only the information from study 1 and 2, is Anna more likely to overuse headache medication than a man who drinks coffee every day.

A. Yes, she has an 80% likelihood of overusing headache medication
B. Yes, she has a 90% likelihood of overusing headache medication, 80% due to her gender and 10% due to being a daily coffee drinker
C. No, because people who drink coffee every day have a 3% chance of overusing headache medication
D. No, because men and women who drink coffee every day have an equal likelihood of overusing headache medication

29. Drivers of red cars have a 10% annual chance of being stopped for speeding. Around 200 of every 20000 drivers of blue cars are stopped for speeding in the same time period. Drivers of red cars are 80% male. Drivers of blue cars are 20% female.
Is a woman who is stopped for speeding more likely to be driving a red car than a blue one?

A. Yes, women are more likely to drive a red car
B. Yes, drivers of red cars are stopped 10 times more often than blue cars
C. No, most drivers of red cars are male
D. No, the number of women who drive blue cars is greater than the number that drive red ones

Full Mock Test 3 Quantitative Reasoning (24 minutes for this section)

The table shows the items bought by Fiona during a shopping spree

Item	Number Bought
T-shirts	7
Jeans	2
Skirts	4
Dresses	1
Tops	6
Shoes (pairs)	5
Hats	2

Amount spent = £1,482.63

1. What percentage of the items bought where skirts? Give the answer to the nearest whole number

A. 7%
B. 6%
C. 15%
D. 4%
E. 14%

2. The tops cost an average of £23 each. What percentage of the amount spent was on tops? Round the answer to 3 significant figures.

A. 1.55%
B. 1.56%
C. 9.30%
D. 9.31%
E. 16.20%

3. If the total amount spent on shoes was 30% of the total amount spent, how much did each pair of shoes cost on average? Give the answer to the nearest whole penny.

A. £444.79
B. £88.96
C. £44.48
D. £444.78
E. £89

4. Later in the day Fiona bought 3 pairs of earrings for a total of £238.97. On average, what percentage of the total amount spent that day was spent per pair of earrings? Give the answer to 1 decimal place.

A. 16.1%
B. 13.9%
C. 13.8%
D. 5.4%
E. 4.6%

£1721.6

Recipe for short-crust pastry – makes 300g

Ingredients:

- 200g plain flour
- pinch of salt
- 110g butter
- 2-3 tbsp very cold water

5. How much butter would you need to make 1kg of pastry

A. 300g
B. 330g
C. 367g
D. 370g
E. 400g

6. You have 500g of plain flour. How much pastry could you make?

A. 500g
B. 600g
C. 700g
D. 750g
E. 1kg

7. You would like to make 3 pies with the pastry, each requiring 250g of pastry. How much butter will you need to buy?

A. 220g
B. 275g
C. 330g
D. 380g
E. 425g

8. You are having a party and decide to make 4 pies a day for a week to make sure you have enough. How many 1kg bags of flour must you buy to have enough for all the pastry?

A. 3
B. 4
C. 5
D. 6
E. 7

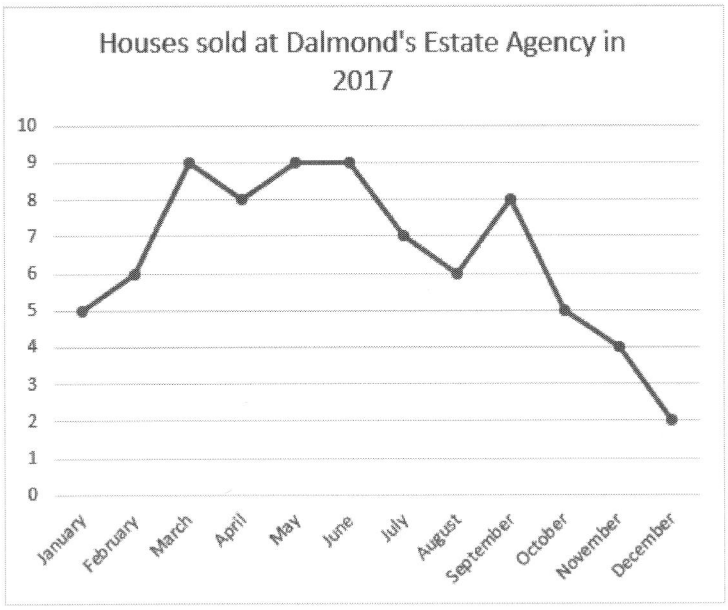

9. How many houses were sold in the first quarter?

A. 11
B. 28
C. 9
D. 20
E. 4

10. When was the biggest monthly change in sales?

A. February to March and September to October
B. September to October
C. June to July
D. February to March
E. January to February and November to December

11. What percentage of sales was made in the summer months (June to August inclusive)?

A. 32%
B. 28%
C. 48%
D. 22%
E. 4%

12. What were the mean monthly sales in 2007?

A. 6
B. 6.5
C. 7
D. 7.5
E. 9

Degree results for degree course H800

Result	Number of students achieving result
1st	3
2:1	24
2:2	38
3rd	17
Pass	4
Fail	6

13. What percentage of students achieved a 2:1 grade?

A. 24%
B. 26%
C. 23%
D. 25%
E. 27%

14. What percentage of students didn't fail?

A. 92%
B. 86%
C. 93%
D. 7%
E. 6%

15. 60% of those with a 2.2 grade are female. How many males achieved a 2.2? Give the answer to the nearest whole number.

A. 38
B. 15
C. 23
D. 9
E. 17

16. After appeals to the exam board, 16% of those with a 3rd had their grade changed to a 2.2. How many students now have a 2.2 grade? Give the answer to the nearest whole number.

A. 42
B. 43
C. 45
D. 3
E. 41

	Initial gross profit earned each week	Revised gross profit earned each week
Fresh fruit and vegetables	550	350
Pre-packed goods	602	645
Household consumables	255	263
Tools and gadgets	198	211
Cards, gifts and trinkets	395	385
TOTAL	**2000**	**1854**

Joe runs a small general store. Last year he installed an electronic till which is linked to his computer so he can determine every week what gross profit he has made on every category of goods.

He has noticed that the amount of shelf space devoted to each category is not proportionate to the profits earned by those goods. He decides to adjust his display to reflect the profitability.

Joe has 150m of shelf space available.

17. How much shelf space should Joe set aside for pre-packed food? Give your answer to the nearest metre

A. 45
B. 41
C. 36
D. 46
E. 40

18. After a few weeks Joe notices that profitability has fallen when he expected it to rise. He notes that part of the reason for reduced profit on fruit and vegetables is the shelves being empty part way through the day. He decides to allocate 80m to fruit and vegetables and adjust other categories in line with the revised profitability figures.

How much space will now be allocated to pre-packed Food?

A. 9
B. 12
C. 35
D. 30
E. 18

19. Joe re-visits the calculations a few weeks later and discovered that profitability on fruit and vegetables has almost doubled to £1,066 while the other categories have fallen by about 5% from the initial figures.

How much profit is Joe now recording?

A. 1904
B. 2442
C. 2815
D. 1815
E. 2014

20. Which product category is likely to bring in closest to £20,000 per year?

A. Fresh fruit and vegetables
B. Pre-packed goods
C. Household consumables
D. Tools and gadgets
E. Cards, gifts and trinkets

A nutritionist decides to investigate the salt contents in various foods. He discovers that 82% of microwave meals have more than seven times the recommended daily allowance (RDA) of salt, and 17% of the Lighter Options range of pasta dishes contained 5% more salt than the RDA. Upon further investigation he also discovered that all 7 of the ice cream tubs he examined contained 0.2% salt. Following his food investigations, he interviewed 182 people and determined that the diets of 83% of them had more than 3 times the RDA of 6g of salt.

21. How many interviewees were consuming more than three times the RDA of salt?

A. 2
B. 151
C. 83
D. 182
E. 147

22. What salt content was in 17% of the Lighter Options pasta dishes?

A. 6.3g
B. 6g
C. 1.2g
D. 3g
E. 30g

23. All the ice creams under investigation come to a total weight of 3100 grams. What was the average weight of salt per ice cream tub? Give the answer to 2 decimal places.

A. 6.20g
B. 0.89g
C. 88.57g
D. 0.12g
E. 8.86g

24. The studies also showed that 6% of microwaves meals contained 8 times or more of the RDA of salt, while 10% contained less than 0.5 times the RDA of salt. If 150 microwave meals were in the study, how many meals contained more than 42g of salt, but less than 48g of salt?

A. 76
B. 114
C. 2
D. 90
E. 123

Breed	Age at Sale (months)
Dalmatian	8
Labrador	6
Beagle	3
Collie	4
Yorkshire Terrier	4
Spaniel	6
Alsatian	6
Whippet	8
Bulldog	2
Boxer	3
Siberian Husky	1

The table shows the ages of puppies sold at a pet store.

25. What is the range of ages at sale in months?

A. 8
B. 7
C. 5
D. 4
E. 6

26. What is the mean value of age at sale, to the nearest whole month?

A. 4
B. 6
C. 8
D. 5
E. 7

27. What is the mode value of age at sale?

A. 8
B. 5
C. 7
D. 4
E. 6

28. What is the median value of age at sale?

A. 6
B. 7
C. 8
D. 4
E. 5

The following standard ratios apply:

width to height ratio = 5:3

weight (kg) to volume (m^3) ratio = 6:13

Oxidiser to fuel mixture ratio = 4.6:1.5

29. If the height of a television screen is 23.47 cm, what is its width? Give your answer to 2 decimal places.

A. 14.08 cm
B. 14.67 cm
C. 117.35 cm
D. 39.12 cm
E. 46.94 cm

30. If the volume of a vessel is 6 cubic metres, what is its weight? Give your answer to 2 decimal places.

A. 2.77 kg
B. 13.00 kg
C. 1.89 kg
D. 4.11 kg
E. 0.46 kg

31. There are two oxidiser tanks filled with 310 g of oxidiser per tank. How much fuel will be required to make the propellant mixture? Give your answer to 2 decimal places.

A. 101.09 g
B. 202.17 g
C. 950.67 g
D. 475.33 g
E. 67.39 g

32. If the density of liquid in a tank is 495 kilograms per cubic metre and the depth of the liquid is 6 metres, what is the density to depth ratio?

A. 615:8
B. 55:1
C. 99:5
D. 165:2
E. 83:1

GIC No.:	8247708B				March
Gross Salary: 184 hours (1st - 31st March)					
					£949.44
Deductions:					
Student Loan Payment (@ £22 per £600 gross salary)					£22.00
Government Insurance Contribution (GIC) (12% gross salary)					£xxxx
Income Tax (19.3% gross salary)					£183.23
Payroll No.:	84281			Net Salary	**£xxxx**
Ban No.: 53784	Sort Code	12-23-56			

The table shows some details of an employee's payslip for March. Unfortunately, a computer error missed off some of the payment details (shown as xxxx)

33. What is the net salary? In other words, how much will the employee receive after deductions?

A. £949.44
B. £744.20
C. £630.27
D. £747.71
E. £654.90

34. The gross salary comprises basic salary plus allowances. A London-weighting allowance has been included in the gross salary, as 4% of the basic salary. Assuming no other allowances, what was the Basic Salary this month?

A. £911.46
B. £36.52
C. £949.44
D. £237.36
E. £912.92

35. What tax is paid on the hourly gross salary? Give the answer to the nearest penny.

A. 99p
B. 27p
C. £1.52
D. £1.00
E. 19p

36. In the next month the employee receives a gross pay rise of 3 %, but the tax also rises by 0.5%. What net salary will the employee now receive?

A. £648.36
B. £649.83
C. £630.27
D. £14.67
E. £644.94

Full Mock Test 3 Abstract Reasoning (13 minutes for this section)

Set A

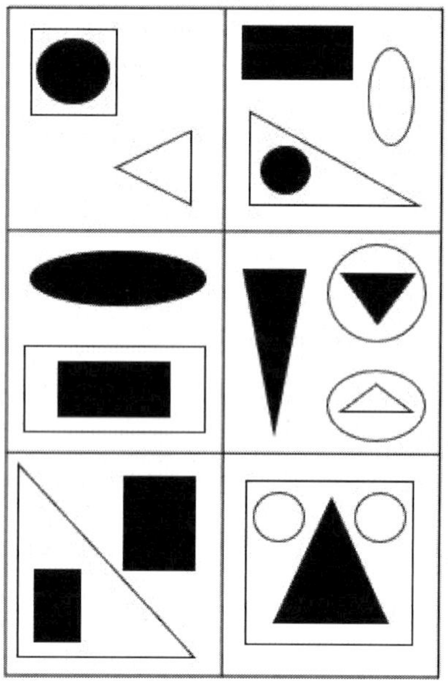

Set B

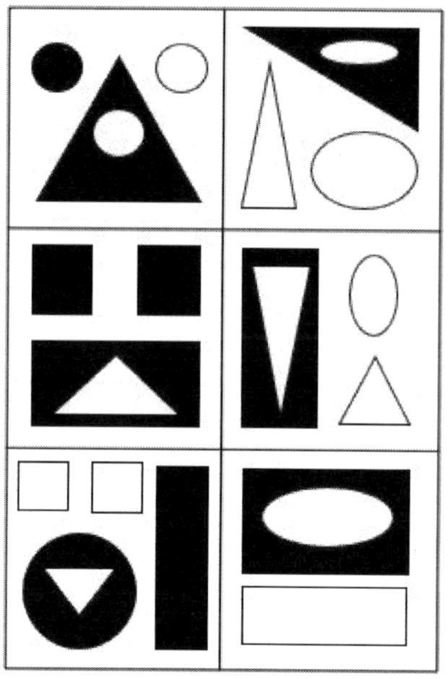

1 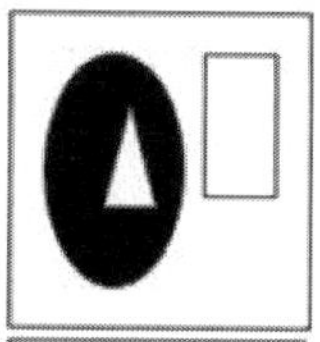
Set A
Set B
Neither

2 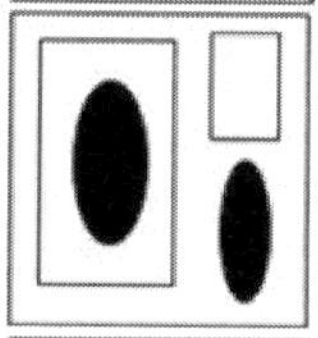
Set A
Set B
Neither

3 
Set A
Set B
Neither

4 
Set A
Set B
Neither

5 
Set A
Set B
Neither

To which of the two sets do the following shapes belong?

Set A

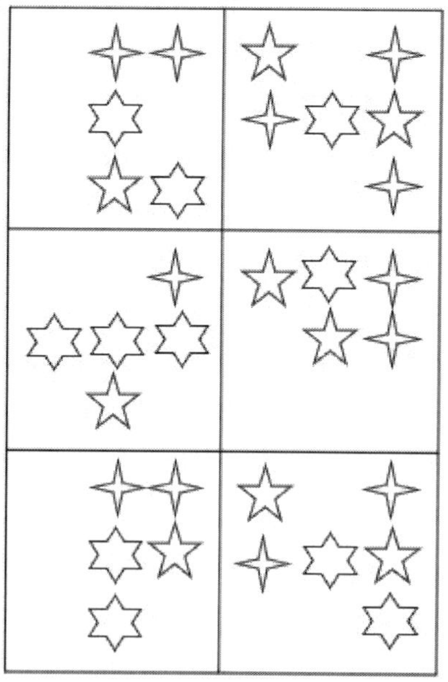

Set B

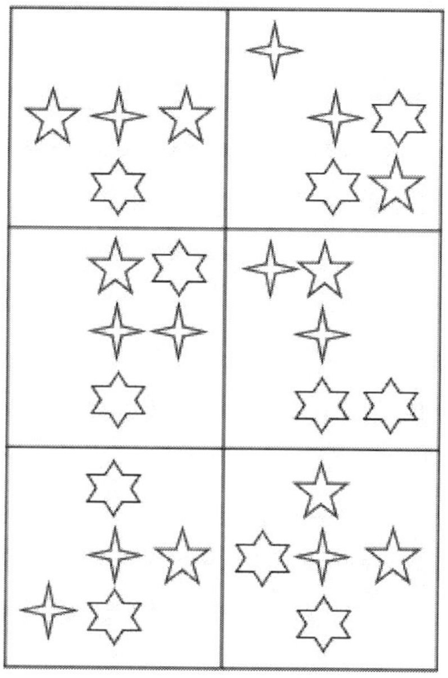

6 
Set A
Set B
Neither

7 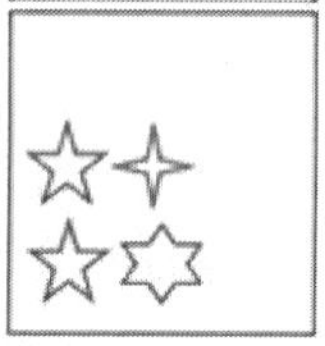
Set A
Set B
Neither

8 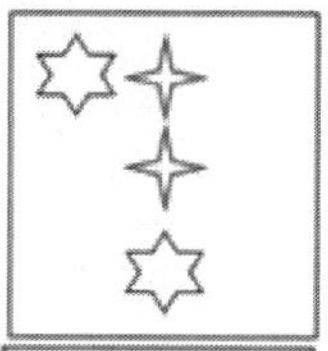
Set A
Set B
Neither

9 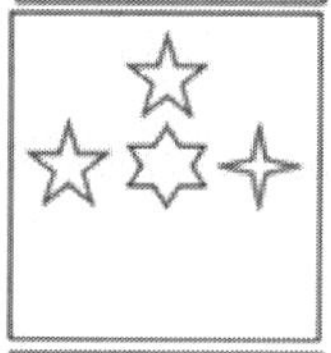
Set A
Set B
Neither

10 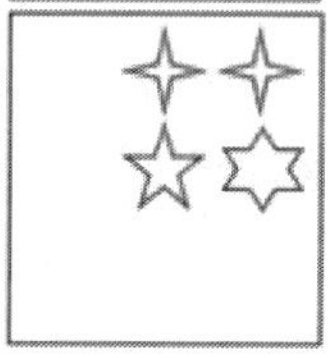
Set A
Set B
Neither

Set A

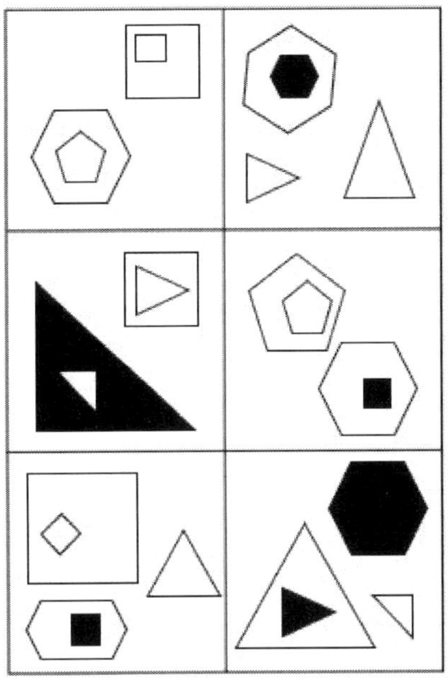

Set B

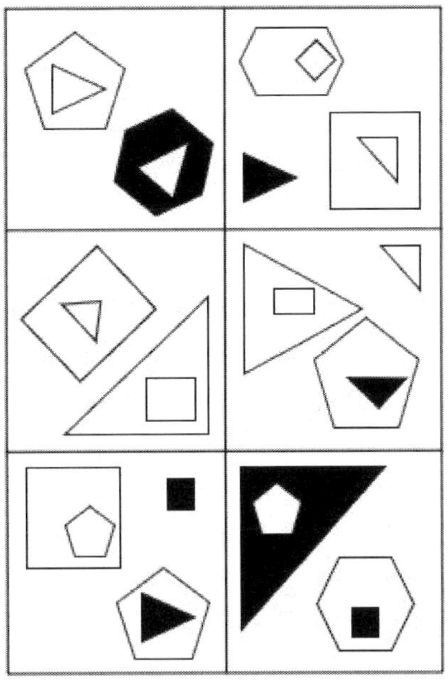

11 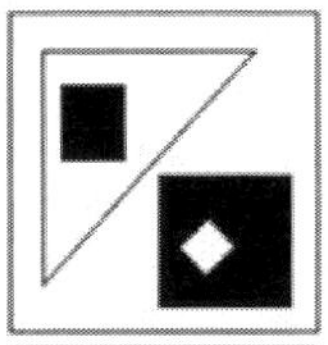
Set A
Set B
Neither

12 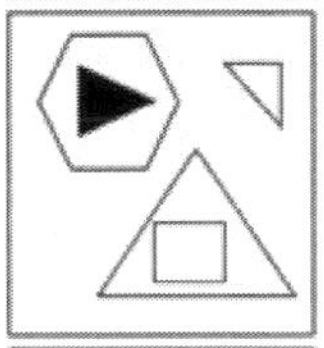
Set A
Set B
Neither

13 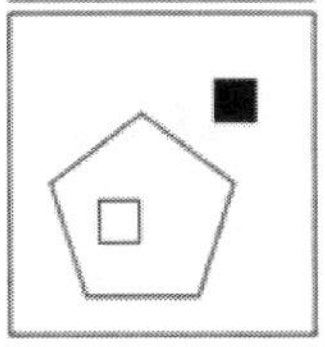
Set A
Set B
Neither

14 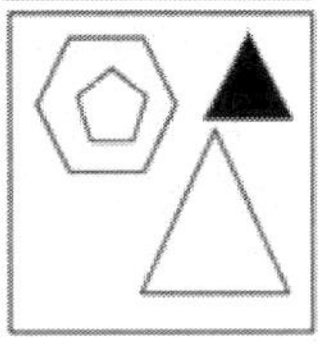
Set A
Set B
Neither

15 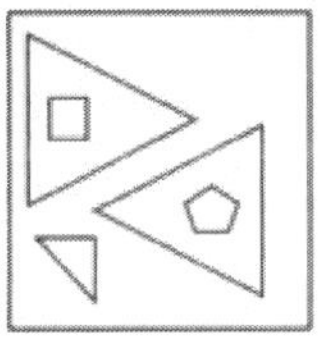
Set A
Set B
Neither

To which of the two sets do the following shapes belong?

Set A

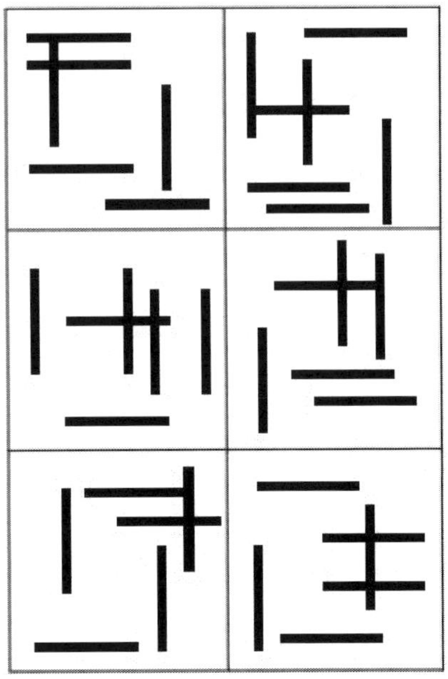

Set B

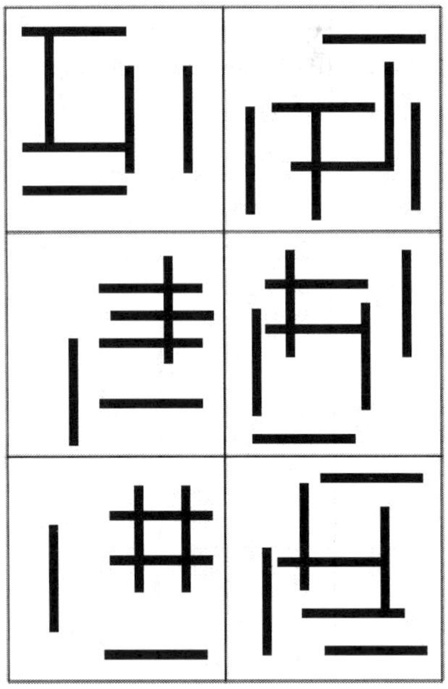

16 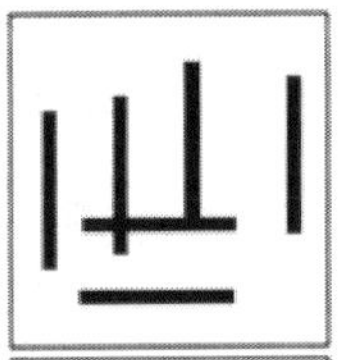
Set A
Set B
Neither

17 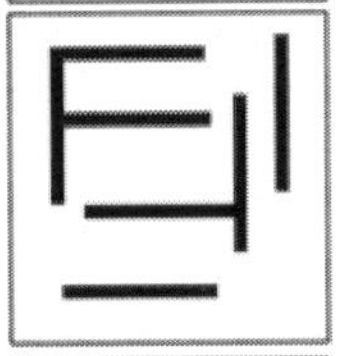
Set A
Set B
Neither

18 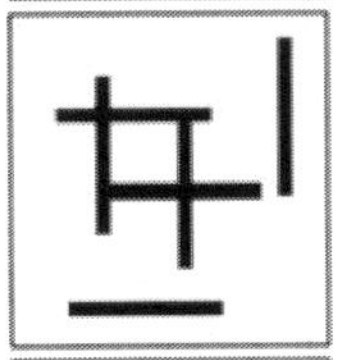
Set A
Set B
Neither

19 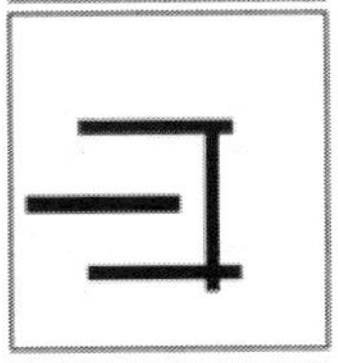
Set A
Set B
Neither

20 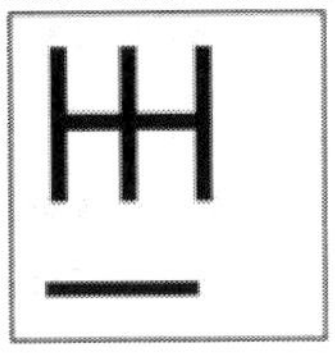
Set A
Set B
Neither

Set A Set B

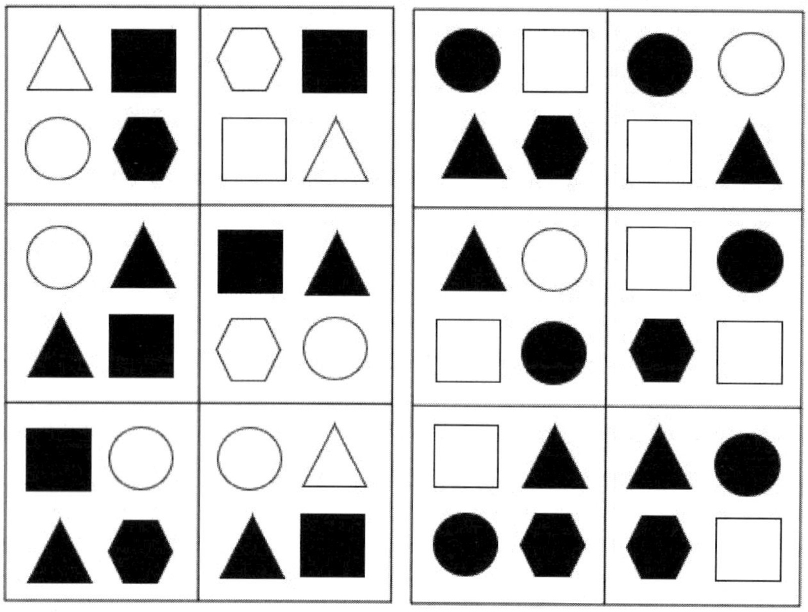

21 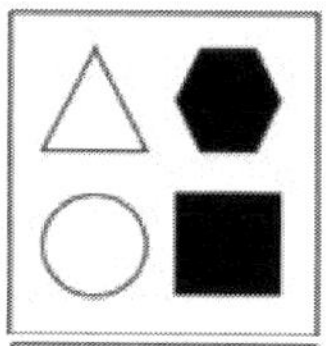
Set A
Set B
Neither

22 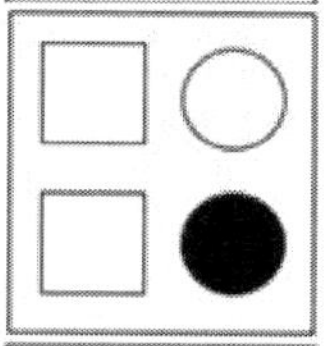
Set A
Set B
Neither

23 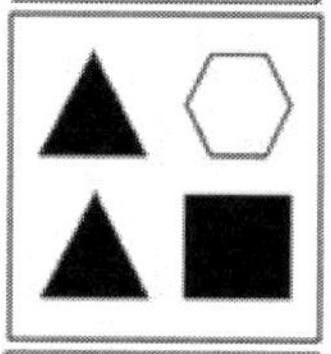
Set A
Set B
Neither

24 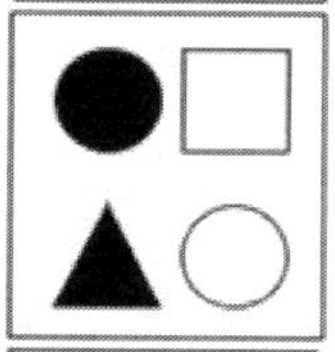
Set A
Set B
Neither

25 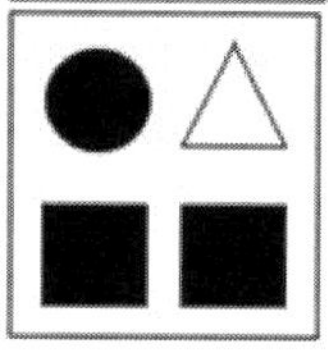
Set A
Set B
Neither

To which of the two sets do the following shapes belong?

26 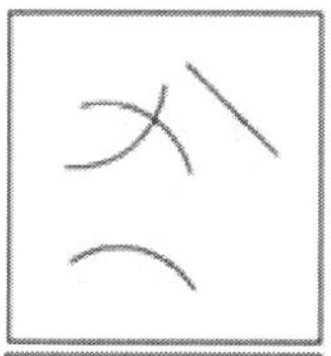
Set A
Set B
Neither

27 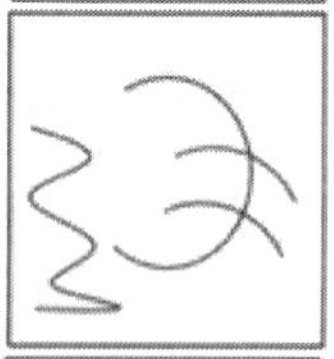
Set A
Set B
Neither

28 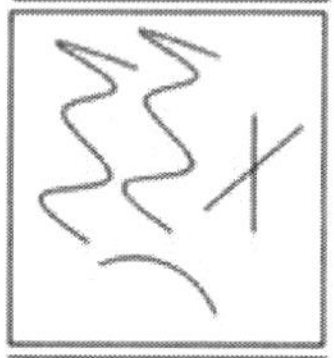
Set A
Set B
Neither

29 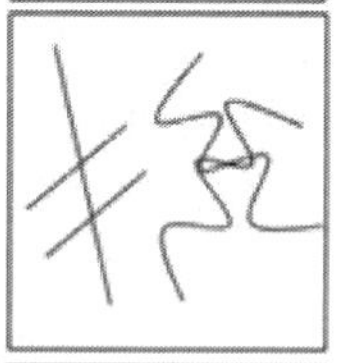
Set A
Set B
Neither

30 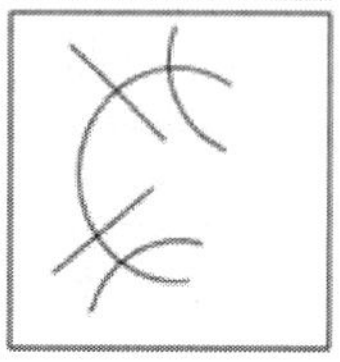
Set A
Set B
Neither

Set A Set B

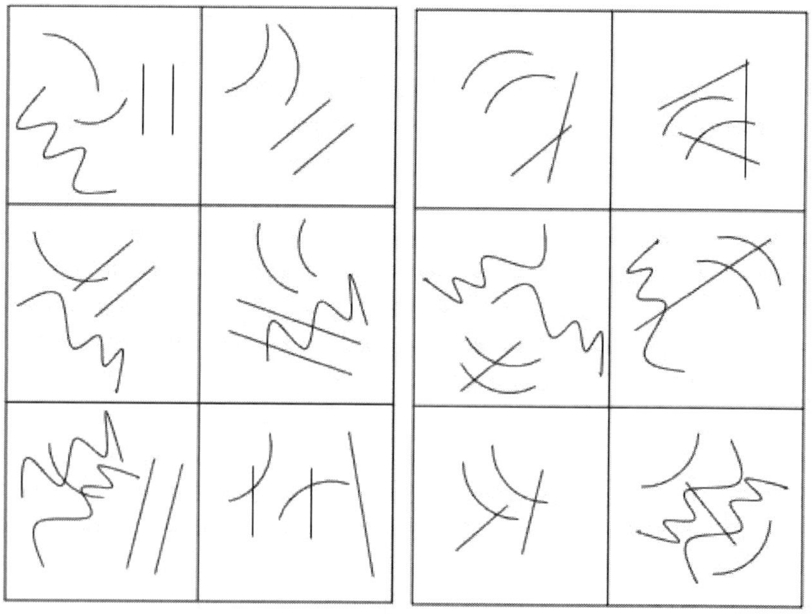

31

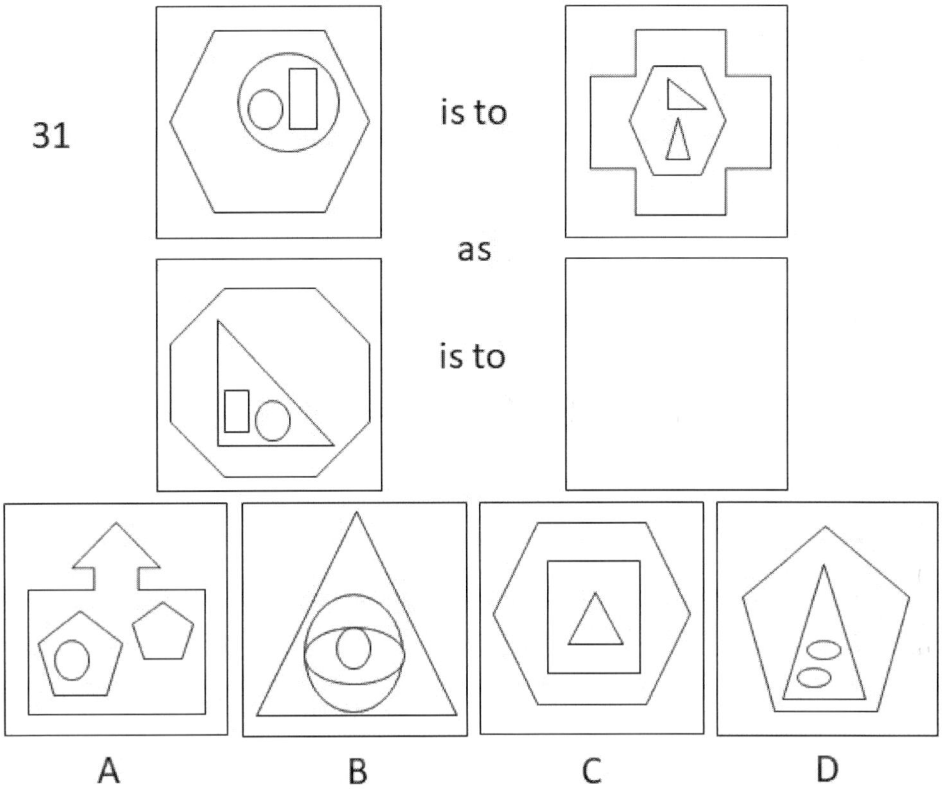

32

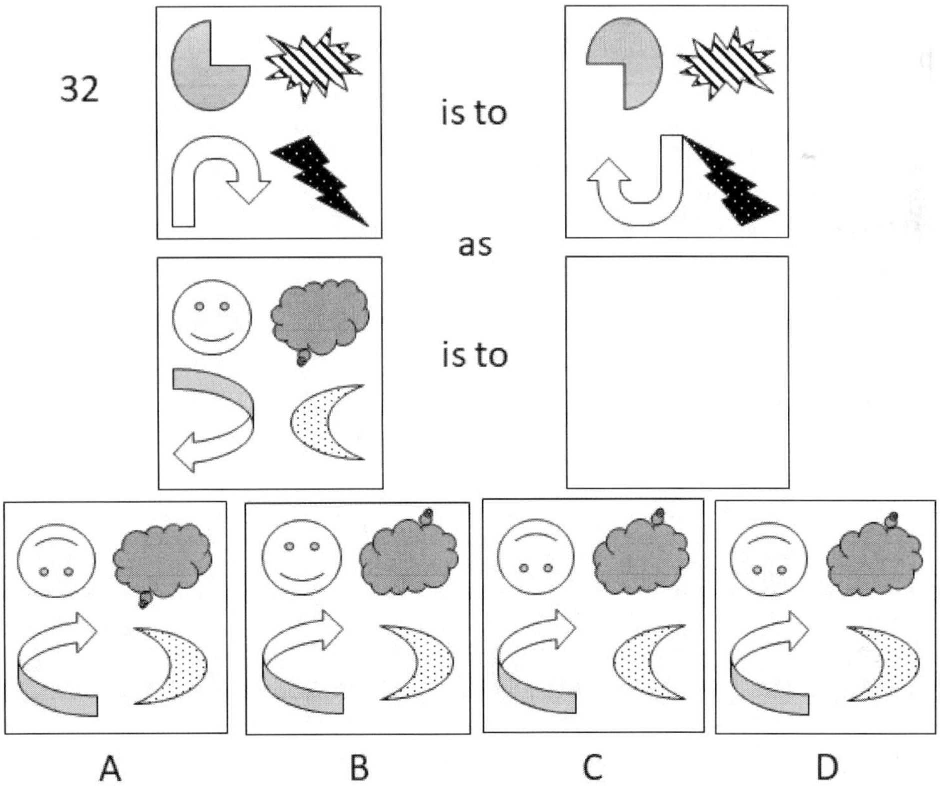

33

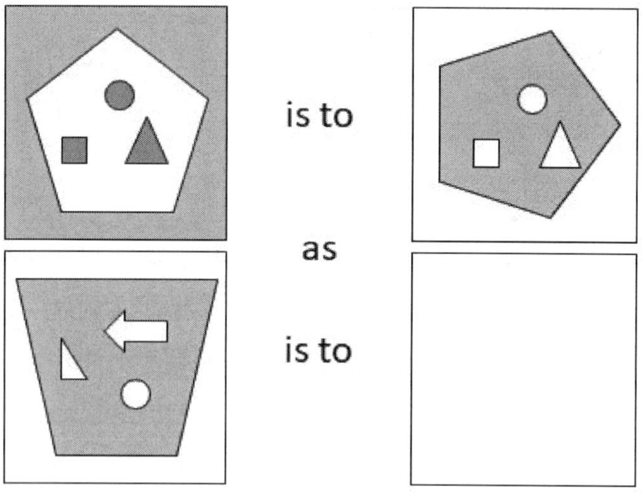

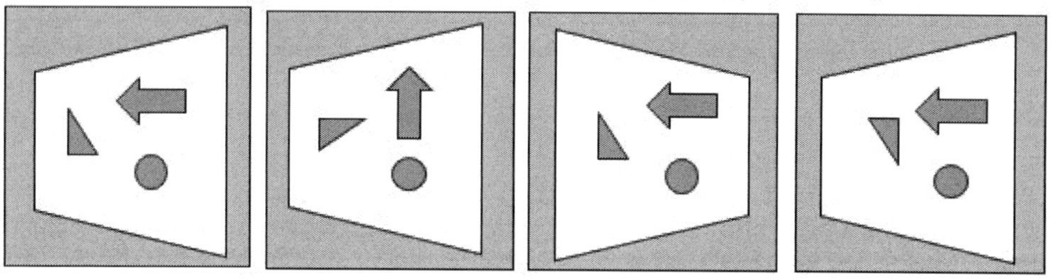

A B C D

34

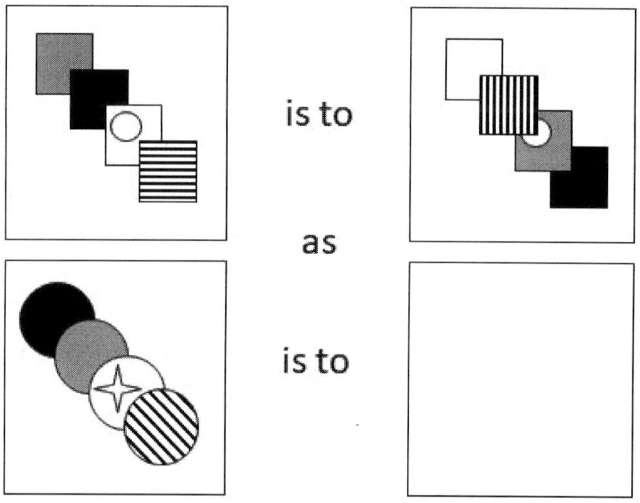

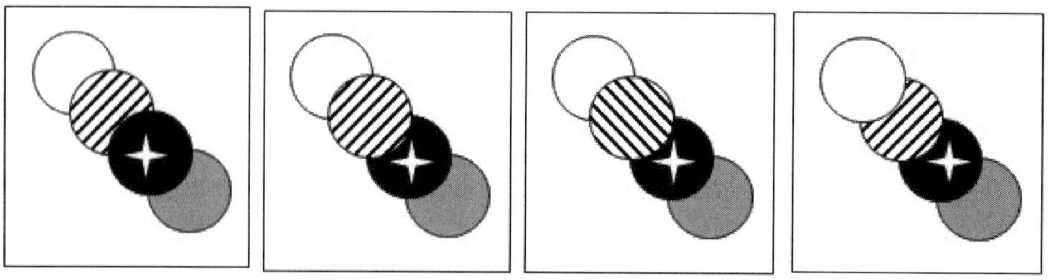

A B C D

35

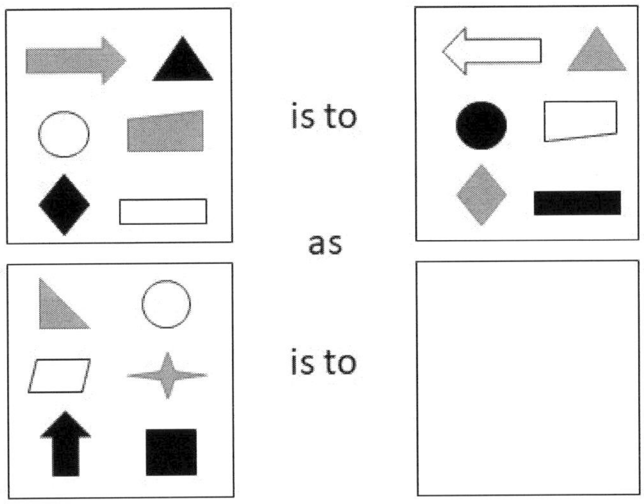

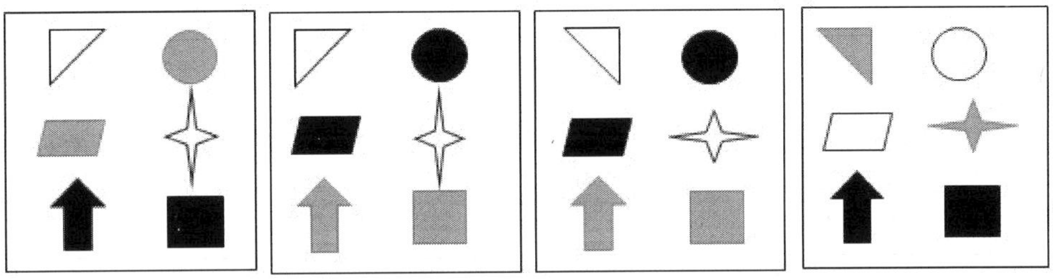

A B C D

Set A Set B

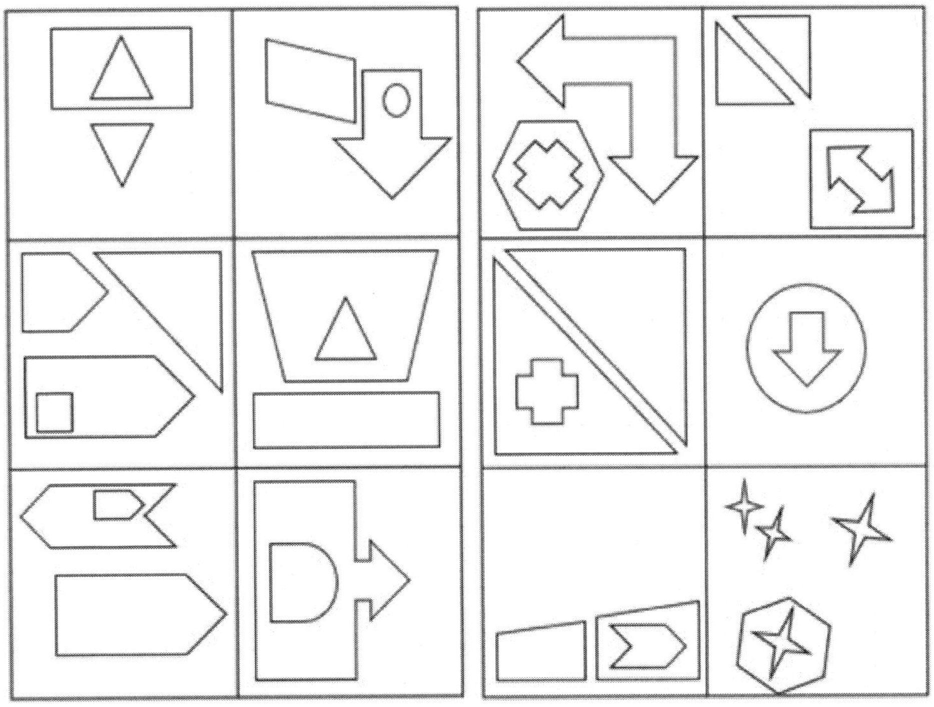

Which of the following belongs in Set A

36

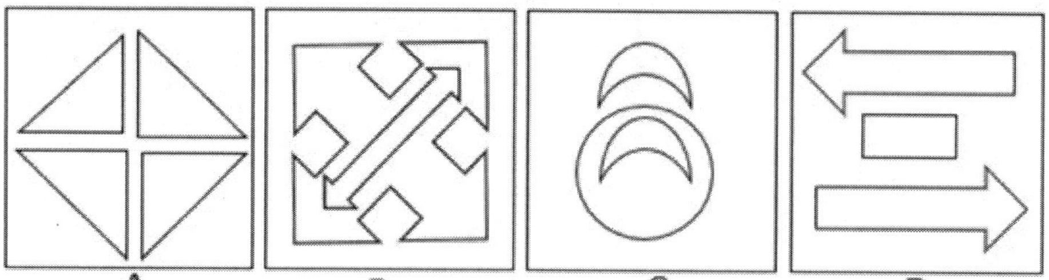

A B C D

Which of the following belongs in Set A

37

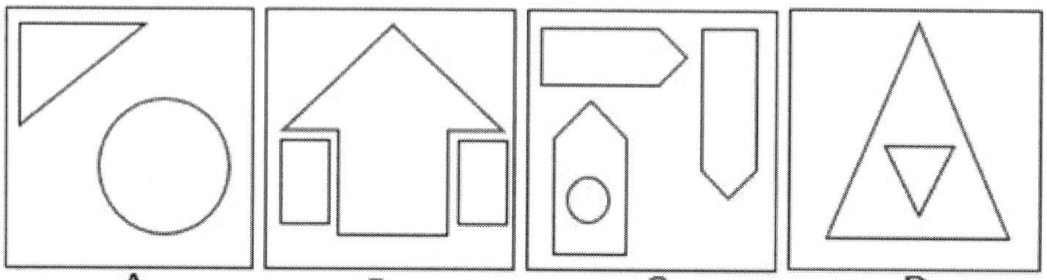

A B C D

Which of the following belongs in Set A

38

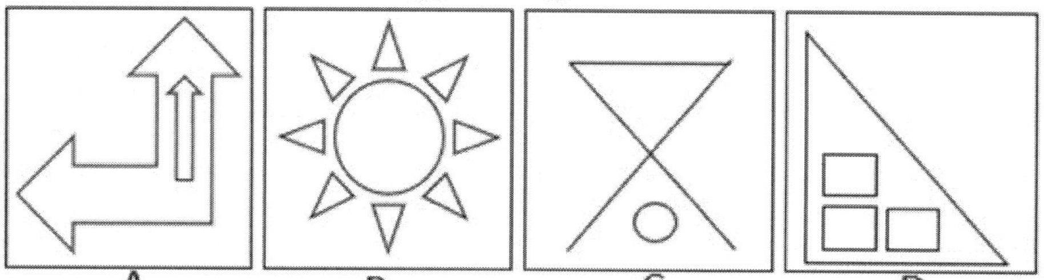

A B C D

Which of the following belongs in Set B

39

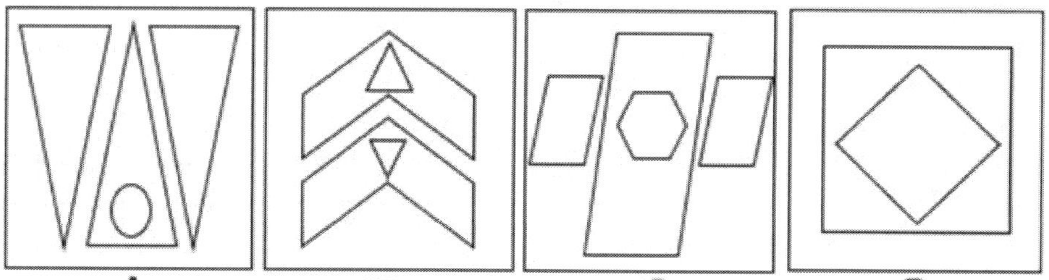

A B C D

Which of the following belongs in Set B

40

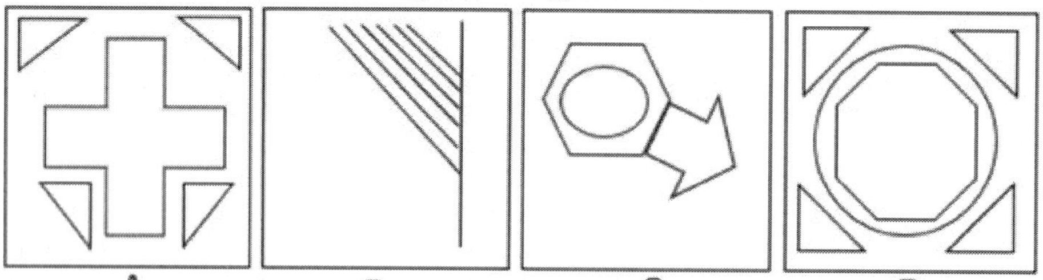

A B C D

Set A Set B

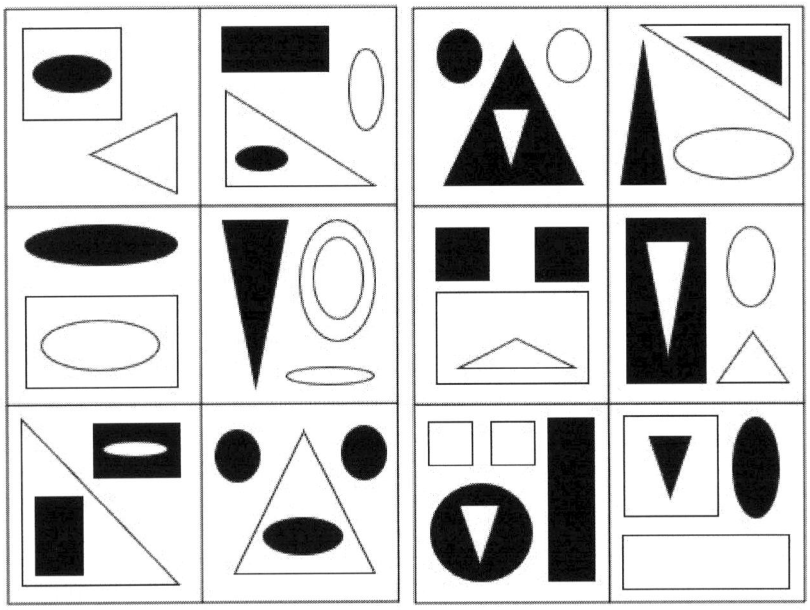

41 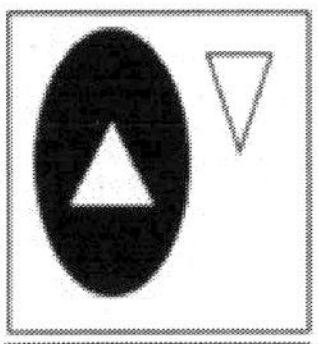
Set A
Set B
Neither

42 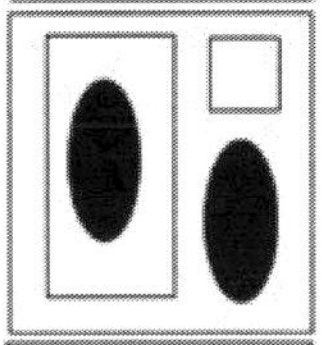
Set A
Set B
Neither

43 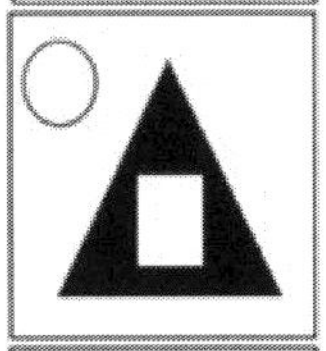
Set A
Set B
Neither

44 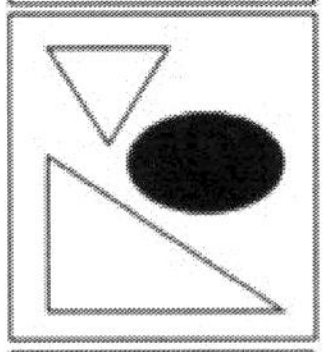
Set A
Set B
Neither

45 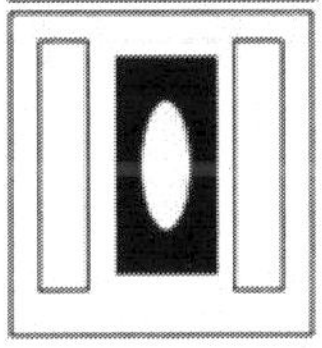
Set A
Set B
Neither

To which of the two sets do the following shapes belong?

46 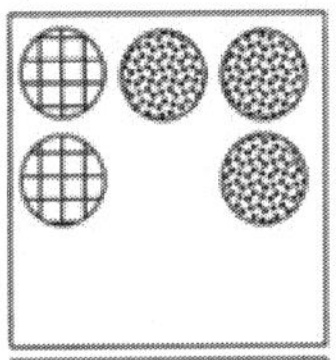
Set A
Set B
Neither

47 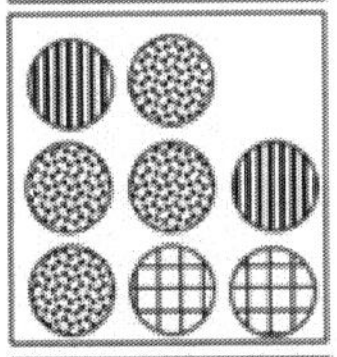
Set A
Set B
Neither

48 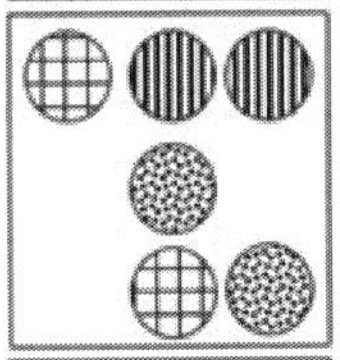
Set A
Set B
Neither

49 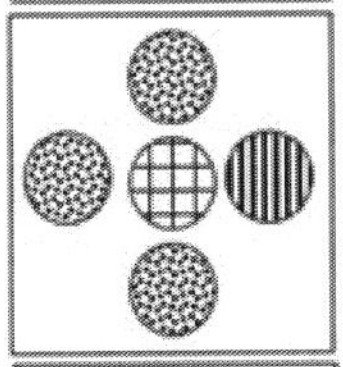
Set A
Set B
Neither

50 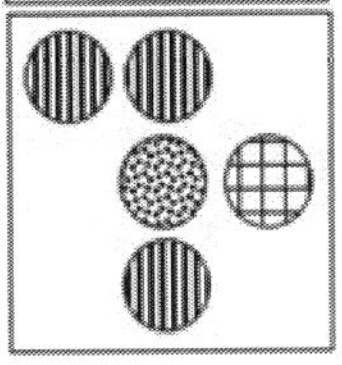
Set A
Set B
Neither

Set A Set B

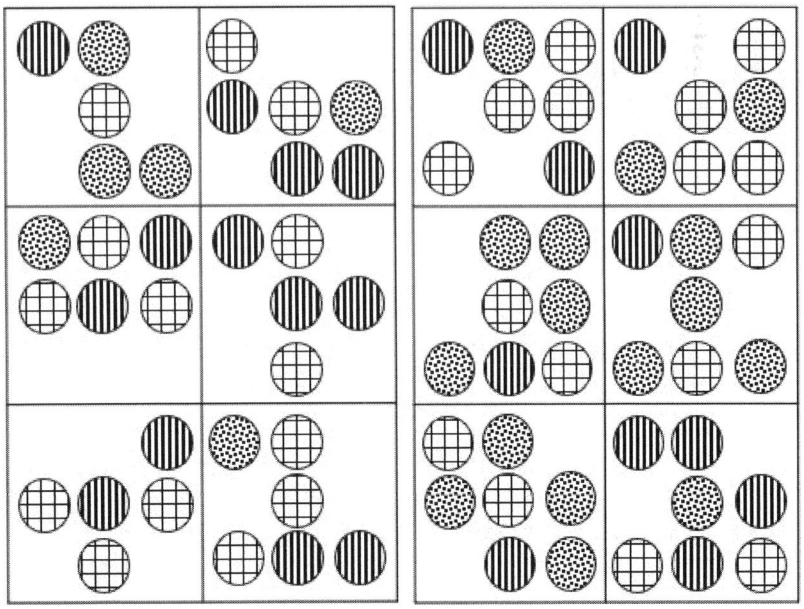

Set A Set B

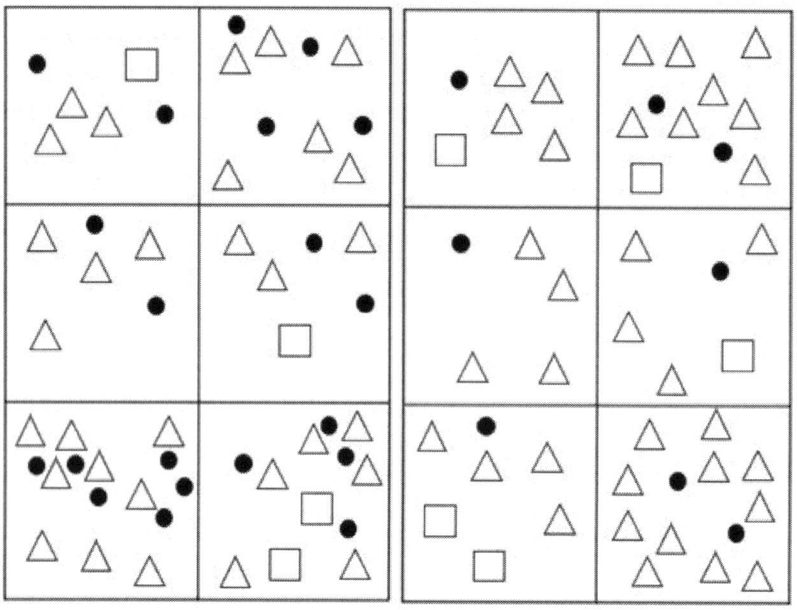

To which of the two sets do the shapes belong?

51
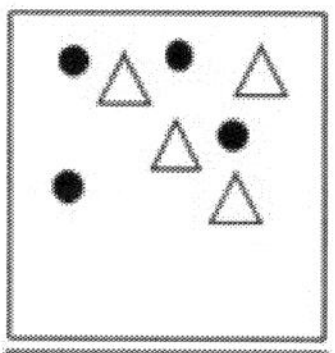
Set A
Set B
Neither

52
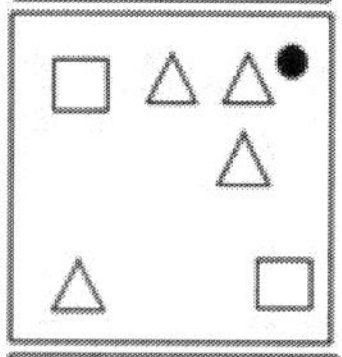
Set A
Set B
Neither

53
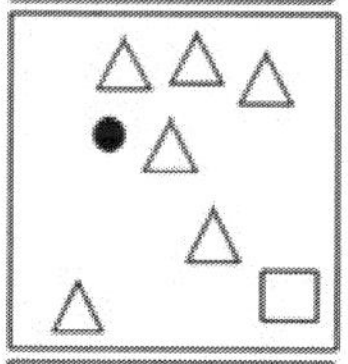
Set A
Set B
Neither

54
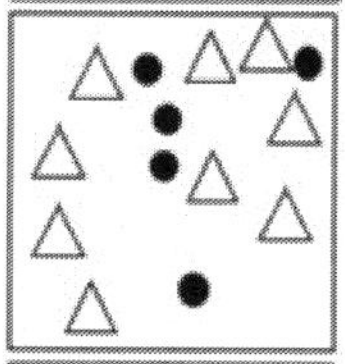
Set A
Set B
Neither

55
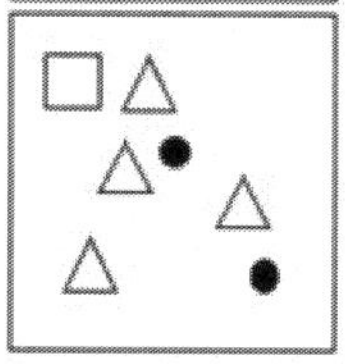
Set A
Set B
Neither

Full Mock Test 3 Situational Judgement (26 minutes for this section)

Sasha is a medical student who is completing a placement in a local hospital. She is observing a consultant, Dr Reeves, while he completes a ward round. Dr Reeves is talking to a patient, while writing him a prescription for a strong painkiller, which a nurse will administer. Dr Reeves is then urgently called to attend to another patient and leaves the ward. Sasha has a look at the notes and realises that the patient has contraindications to the medication prescribed by Dr Reeves.

How appropriate are each of the following responses by Sasha in this situation?

1. Cross out the prescription from the patient's notes

A. A very appropriate thing to do
B. Appropriate, but not ideal
C. Inappropriate, but not awful
D. A very inappropriate thing to do

2. Retake some medical history from the patient regarding the contraindications

A. A very appropriate thing to do
B. Appropriate, but not ideal
C. Inappropriate, but not awful
D. A very inappropriate thing to do

3. Talk to the nurse who is supposed to administer the medication

A. A very appropriate thing to do
B. Appropriate, but not ideal
C. Inappropriate, but not awful
D. A very inappropriate thing to do

4. Encourage the patient to refuse the medication as a mistake may have been made

A. A very appropriate thing to do
B. Appropriate, but not ideal
C. Inappropriate, but not awful
D. A very inappropriate thing to do

A patient is demanding to see a consultant. The nurse taking care of him asks Dr Williams to attend to the patient. When Dr Williams arrives at the patient's bed with the nurse, the patient tells the doctor he wants the nurse to leave the room. When Dr Williams asks why, he mentions that the nurse was rude to him earlier and was ignoring his requests to see a consultant. The nurse does not say anything in response.

How appropriate are each of the following responses by Dr Williams in this situation?

5. Ask the patient to elaborate about the nurse's behaviour

A. A very appropriate thing to do
B. Appropriate, but not ideal
C. Inappropriate, but not awful
D. A very inappropriate thing to do

6. Ask the nurse to leave the room

A. A very appropriate thing to do
B. Appropriate, but not ideal
C. Inappropriate, but not awful
D. A very inappropriate thing to do

7. Brush off the comment but speak with the nurse afterwards in private

A. A very appropriate thing to do
B. Appropriate, but not ideal
C. Inappropriate, but not awful
D. A very inappropriate thing to do

8. Immediately ask the nurse what has happened

A. A very appropriate thing to do
B. Appropriate, but not ideal
C. Inappropriate, but not awful
D. A very inappropriate thing to do

A student, Emily, is talking to her friend, Mia, about some feedback she has been given by one of the doctors at the hospital. Emily says that the doctor told her that her communication skills are very poor and that she is not interacting well with the patients. Emily feels that the feedback is not fair and the teacher has something against her.

How appropriate are each of the following responses by Mia in this situation?

9. Advise Emily to talk to other students also working with the same doctor

A. A very appropriate thing to do
B. Appropriate, but not ideal
C. Inappropriate, but not awful
D. A very inappropriate thing to do

10. Advise Emily that she should use the feedback to improve her communication skills

A. A very appropriate thing to do
B. Appropriate, but not ideal
C. Inappropriate, but not awful
D. A very inappropriate thing to do

11. Advise Emily to talk to the doctor and ask for more detailed feedback

A. A very appropriate thing to do
B. Appropriate, but not ideal
C. Inappropriate, but not awful
D. A very inappropriate thing to do

Kayla, a junior doctor, is checking a patient's notes. The patient, Adrian, is due to undergo urgent surgery at 11am the next morning. Upon checking the notes, Kayla realises that she has forgotten to order a specific blood test and the results are required before the surgery can take place. Kayla goes to the laboratory but finds it closed an hour ago and won't open again until 9am in the morning. She is worried that there will not be enough time to do the test before Adrian is due in theatre.

How appropriate are each of the following responses by Kayla in this situation?

12. Ask the surgeon to postpone the operation to later in the day

A. A very appropriate thing to do
B. Appropriate, but not ideal
C. Inappropriate, but not awful
D. A very inappropriate thing to do

13. Contact the surgical team and explain what has happened

A. A very appropriate thing to do
B. Appropriate, but not ideal
C. Inappropriate, but not awful
D. A very inappropriate thing to do

14. Talk to Adrian and ask him if he would mind the operation being rescheduled for a different day

A. A very appropriate thing to do
B. Appropriate, but not ideal
C. Inappropriate, but not awful
D. A very inappropriate thing to do

15. Talk to one of the laboratory staff as soon as they open in the morning to see if the test can be done before the operation

A. A very appropriate thing to do
B. Appropriate, but not ideal
C. Inappropriate, but not awful
D. A very inappropriate thing to do

Two medical students, Ivy and Leo, are shadowing GP's for the week. They both walk into the waiting room to call their next patients when Leo makes a comment saying that the receptionist is lazy and doesn't seem to do much other than sit around all day. Ivy realises that the receptionist and many of the patients have heard what Leo said. The receptionist looks very hurt by Leo's comment.

How appropriate are each of the following responses by Ivy in this situation?

16. Ask Leo to apologise to the receptionist

A. A very appropriate thing to do
B. Appropriate, but not ideal
C. Inappropriate, but not awful
D. A very inappropriate thing to do

17. Apologise to the receptionist on Leo's behalf

A. A very appropriate thing to do
B. Appropriate, but not ideal
C. Inappropriate, but not awful
D. A very inappropriate thing to do

18. Speak to Leo in private and explain that his comment was hurtful and rude

A. A very appropriate thing to do
B. Appropriate, but not ideal
C. Inappropriate, but not awful
D. A very inappropriate thing to do

19. Tell Leo that if he has a complaint, he should discuss it with his supervisor

A. A very appropriate thing to do
B. Appropriate, but not ideal
C. Inappropriate, but not awful
D. A very inappropriate thing to do

Fae is struggling with her A level work and has asked her friend Gabriella, who is doing the same courses but a year ahead, if she can borrow her notes and essays from the previous year so she can do additional revision work. Fae knows Gabriella gets good marks and wants to see if her work helps her understand the subject matter any better.

How appropriate are the following actions by Fae?

20. Give Gabriella a memory stick and ask if she can have a copy of all of last year's work?

A. A very appropriate thing to do
B. Appropriate, but not ideal
C. Inappropriate, but not awful
D. A very inappropriate thing to do

21. Explain to Gabriella that she's struggling and see if she offers help?

A. A very appropriate thing to do
B. Appropriate, but not ideal
C. Inappropriate, but not awful
D. A very inappropriate thing to do

22. Reassure Gabriella that she only wants to read the work to help her understanding and not to cheat?

A. A very appropriate thing to do
B. Appropriate, but not ideal
C. Inappropriate, but not awful
D. A very inappropriate thing to do

Pierre is a junior doctor. His younger sister has an ear infection and his mother asks if he can write her a prescription for antibiotics.

How appropriate are the following actions by Pierre?

23. Write the prescription after examining his sister?

A. A very appropriate thing to do
B. Appropriate, but not ideal
C. Inappropriate, but not awful
D. A very inappropriate thing to do

24. Ask his mother to make an appointment with their own GP?

A. A very appropriate thing to do
B. Appropriate, but not ideal
C. Inappropriate, but not awful
D. A very inappropriate thing to do

25. Refuse to help explaining about the rules regarding treating your own family?

A. A very appropriate thing to do
B. Appropriate, but not ideal
C. Inappropriate, but not awful
D. A very inappropriate thing to do

26. Ask a colleague to examine his sister and write the prescription?

A. A very appropriate thing to do
B. Appropriate, but not ideal
C. Inappropriate, but not awful
D. A very inappropriate thing to do

Bethany is a medical student who is observing the morning clinic of a GP on her placement. Bethany notices that the GP does not always expressly ask if the patient is happy for her to sit in on the consultation.

How appropriate are the following actions by Bethany?

27. Quickly introduce herself to the patient before the GP has a chance to begin the consultation.

A. A very appropriate thing to do
B. Appropriate, but not ideal
C. Inappropriate, but not awful
D. A very inappropriate thing to do

28. Mention her concern to the GP between consultations

A. A very appropriate thing to do
B. Appropriate, but not ideal
C. Inappropriate, but not awful
D. A very inappropriate thing to do

29. Do nothing, consent is the responsibility of the practice.

A. A very appropriate thing to do
B. Appropriate, but not ideal
C. Inappropriate, but not awful
D. A very inappropriate thing to do

30. Ask the practice receptionists to alert patients to her presence and explain that they can ask not to be observed before they come into the doctor's room

A. A very appropriate thing to do
B. Appropriate, but not ideal
C. Inappropriate, but not awful
D. A very inappropriate thing to do

Jamie is a medical student on placement with a GP surgery. He calls 'Mr Smith' into the room and begins to explain about the diabetes blood test results he has to discuss with him. Mr Smith looks puzzled and explains that he is not diabetic and that he's come to discuss a knee injury. Jamie realises he has the wrong Mr Smith.

How appropriate are the following actions by Jamie?

31. Apologise to the Mr Smith who is in the room and ask him about his knee.

A. A very appropriate thing to do
B. Appropriate, but not ideal
C. Inappropriate, but not awful
D. A very inappropriate thing to do

32. Apologise to the Mr Smith who is in the room, ask him to return to the waiting room and see if the correct Mr Smith is there.

A. A very appropriate thing to do
B. Appropriate, but not ideal
C. Inappropriate, but not awful
D. A very inappropriate thing to do

33. Ask for patients by first and surnames routinely

A. A very appropriate thing to do
B. Appropriate, but not ideal
C. Inappropriate, but not awful
D. A very inappropriate thing to do

34. Apologise to the diabetic Mr Smith about the breach of his confidentiality

A. A very appropriate thing to do
B. Appropriate, but not ideal
C. Inappropriate, but not awful
D. A very inappropriate thing to do

Kristina is a junior doctor on a very busy shift in A&E. Several seriously ill patients have been admitted by ambulance and consequently the wait for non-urgent cases has been unusually long. Mrs Stokes, an elderly lady who has presented with an earache, has been waiting for 6 hours to be seen and is very angry with Kristina.

How appropriate are the following actions by Kristina?

35. Apologise to Mrs Stokes but explain that earache is not urgent and that she should have gone to see her GP.

A. A very appropriate thing to do
B. Appropriate, but not ideal
C. Inappropriate, but not awful
D. A very inappropriate thing to do

36. Explain that the unit has a zero-tolerance policy on aggression towards staff and warn Mrs Stokes that she will call security if she doesn't calm down.

A. A very appropriate thing to do
B. Appropriate, but not ideal
C. Inappropriate, but not awful
D. A very inappropriate thing to do

37. Explain that many urgent cases have come into the unit and that the doctors had to concentrate on the really sick people.

A. A very appropriate thing to do
B. Appropriate, but not ideal
C. Inappropriate, but not awful
D. A very inappropriate thing to do

38. Apologise for Mrs Stokes' wait and proceed with the consultation

A. A very appropriate thing to do
B. Appropriate, but not ideal
C. Inappropriate, but not awful
D. A very inappropriate thing to do

Melvin has been writing a blog about his time at university. He records his ideas and reflections about the course and university life. Unexpectedly - one post he wrote about a lecture has gone viral and has been viewed almost 50,000 times. Melvin is afraid the university will object to some of the 'frank' descriptions he has given of the university and course.

How appropriate is the following action by Melvin

39. Go and ask for advice from the Student Union

A. A very appropriate thing to do
B. Appropriate, but not ideal
C. Inappropriate, but not awful
D. A very inappropriate thing to do

40. Take down the blog altogether

A. A very appropriate thing to do
B. Appropriate, but not ideal
C. Inappropriate, but not awful
D. A very inappropriate thing to do

41. Look into ways to monetise his new popularity by selling banner ads, etc.

A. A very appropriate thing to do
B. Appropriate, but not ideal
C. Inappropriate, but not awful
D. A very inappropriate thing to do

George is completing his UCAS application and reads the personal statement of one of his friends - Dean. Dean's personal statement contains a lot of details that George knows are not true. Dean tells George that everyone exaggerates in their personal statement and that George would be at a disadvantage if his was completely honest.

How appropriate are the following actions by George?

42. Ask for advice on how to make his achievements and experience sound more impressive

A. A very appropriate thing to do
B. Appropriate, but not ideal
C. Inappropriate, but not awful
D. A very inappropriate thing to do

43. Make small embellishments; for example, say he regularly reads a journal when he's only read two editions.

A. A very appropriate thing to do
B. Appropriate, but not ideal
C. Inappropriate, but not awful
D. A very inappropriate thing to do

44. Contact UCAS and report that Dean's statement contains many lies.

A. A very appropriate thing to do
B. Appropriate, but not ideal
C. Inappropriate, but not awful
D. A very inappropriate thing to do

45. Ask for advice from his teachers on how to write a good personal statement and do online research

A. A very appropriate thing to do
B. Appropriate, but not ideal
C. Inappropriate, but not awful
D. A very inappropriate thing to do

Adam is a 4th year medical student currently on a urology placement. He is shadowing a consultant who is called in to oversee the treatment of a 20-year old patient. Upon seeing the patient, Adam realises that the patient is his close friend's boyfriend.

How appropriate are each of the following responses by Adam in this situation?

46. Decide that this is just another patient and that relationships from his personal life should not affect his learning and carry on with the consultation as normal.

A. A very appropriate thing to do
B. Appropriate, but not ideal
C. Inappropriate, but not awful
D. A very inappropriate thing to do

47. Inform the consultant immediately about the relationship and ask for his/her advice on the issue.

A. A very appropriate thing to do
B. Appropriate, but not ideal
C. Inappropriate, but not awful
D. A very inappropriate thing to do

48. Introduce himself to the patient and inform him of Adam's friendship with the patient's partner.

A. A very appropriate thing to do
B. Appropriate, but not ideal
C. Inappropriate, but not awful
D. A very inappropriate thing to do

Jack and Sarah are working on a coursework together. They need to put together a report on the treatment of macular degeneration in the eye. They split up the work evenly and meet after 2 weeks to compile their work together. After reading Sarah's work, Jack realises that Sarah has not put in any effort and has plagiarised most of the work she has done.

When deciding the subsequent course of action, how important is it for Jack to consider the following?

49. Sarah is the top student in the year.

A. Very important
B. Important
C. Of minor importance
D. Not important at all

50. The coursework must be submitted by both of them so the consequences would affect Jack as well.

A. Very important
B. Important
C. Of minor importance
D. Not important at all

51. The work that Sarah has plagiarised is from a little-known journal.

A. Very important
B. Important
C. Of minor importance
D. Not important at all

52. Jack is dating Sarah's friend.

A. Very important
B. Important
C. Of minor importance
D. Not important at all

53. Reporting Sarah could result in her studies being severely affected.

A. Very important
B. Important
C. Of minor importance
D. Not important at all

Jessica is a fourth-year medical student currently on placement in the psychiatric ward. In a closed group on Facebook, Jessica reads a post in which two of her fellow course-mates are discussing a patient on her ward. Although they do not reveal the patient's name, the post does state some details about the patient suggesting his identity.

When deciding the subsequent course of action, how important is it for Jessica to consider the following?

54. The patient's confidentiality.

A. Very important
B. Important
C. Of minor importance
D. Not important at all

55. The post is on a closed Facebook group.

A. Very important
B. Important
C. Of minor importance
D. Not important at all

56. The manner in which the patient is discussed.

A. Very important
B. Important
C. Of minor importance
D. Not important at all

57. Jessica is flat mates with one of the people involved.

A. Very important
B. Important
C. Of minor importance
D. Not important at all

58. The patient has an illness that severely affects their self-awareness and so would not know that someone is discussing them elsewhere.

A. Very important
B. Important
C. Of minor importance
D. Not important at all

Tamil is helping at the local youth club for 10-12 year-olds. He wants to take the group of children to a local rock-climbing centre for an activity evening. He sends letters out to each of the children's parents or carers. Two children fail to bring back their signed letters.

When deciding the subsequent course of action, how important is it for Tamil to consider the following?

59. Children aged 10-12 need parental consent to take part in this kind of activity

A. Very important
B. Important
C. Of minor importance
D. Not important at all

60. The climbing centre is very well run and have never had an accident

A. Very important
B. Important
C. Of minor importance
D. Not important at all

61. Rock climbing is a dangerous activity

A. Very important
B. Important
C. Of minor importance
D. Not important at all

62. It is a shame for those two children to miss out on the activity

A. Very important
B. Important
C. Of minor importance
D. Not important at all

Vivien receives an email from one of her teachers which is clearly not meant for her. The email is quite personal and reveals details of holiday plans, a complaint about another of Vivien's teachers and information about another student's private life.

When deciding the subsequent course of action, how important is it for Vivien to consider the following?

63. The email was not meant for Vivien

A. Very important
B. Important
C. Of minor importance
D. Not important at all

64. The teacher may not know what has happened

A. Very important
B. Important
C. Of minor importance
D. Not important at all

65. Maintaining confidentiality is the right thing to do even when it's not legally required

A. Very important
B. Important
C. Of minor importance
D. Not important at all

66. The other student referred to may benefit from help from Vivien

A. Very important
B. Important
C. Of minor importance
D. Not important at all

Louisa, a medical student is at a charity gala held by an animal welfare charity that she supports. During the presentation at the gala, a speaker comes onto the stage and makes an announcement asking if there are any medically qualified people as there has been a medical emergency backstage. No one steps forwards and Louisa suspects there are no medically qualified people. People are starting to become anxious and the speaker is anxiously awaiting a response. Louisa must decide if she is to step forward and respond to the call.

When deciding the subsequent course of action, how important is it for Louisa to consider the following?

67. Someone else who is qualified may go forward?

A. Very important
B. Important
C. Of minor importance
D. Not important at all

68. She may not be able to help even if she did respond?

A. Very important
B. Important
C. Of minor importance
D. Not important at all

69. No one in the room knows she's a medical student

A. Very important
B. Important
C. Of minor importance
D. Not important at all

Full Mock Test 3 Answers

1. The correct answer is D. Energy gels contain glycogen
The energy gels are carbohydrate based (first line of paragraph 2.) These carbohydrates are then stored as glycogen but glycogen is not consumed from the gel.

2. The correct answer is B. Runners can store enough glycogen in their body to run most of a marathon
Paragraph 1 states 'Runners can store about 2,000 kcal worth of glycogen in their bodies, enough for about 18-20 miles of running' but this is not enough glycogen to complete a marathon.

3. The correct answer is B. A whole grain cereal bar (contains complex carbohydrates)
The last paragraph states 'Alternatives to gels include various forms of concentrated sugars, and foods high in simple carbohydrates that can be digested easily'. Complex carbohydrates take longer to digest and do not provide the instant energy that simple carbohydrates can.

4. The correct answer is B. Runners should only take supplements once they 'hit the wall'
The second paragraph states that 'Carbohydrate-based 'energy gels' are used by runners to avoid or reduce the effect of "hitting the wall", as they provide easy to digest energy during the run' implying that these gels should be taken throughout the race, not just at the point that the runner's glycogen stores have been used up.

5. The correct answer is C. Can't tell. The text states only that in general, unprocessed foods have proven more favourable to health than processed foods. A wide variety is recommended which may preclude a daily apple.

6. The correct answer is C. Can't tell. The text says that the effects of nutrients may only be discernible over an extended period, logically they may also be discernible in the short term.

7. The correct answer is C. Can't tell. The text states only that in general, unprocessed foods have proven more favourable to health than processed foods.
5kg of unprocessed red meat a day might be better for health than 5kg of processed red meat a day while both are still bad for you.

8. The correct answer is C. Can't tell. While this is implied by the structure of the name, the composition of hydroxyapatite is not defined in the text.

9. The correct answer is C. Group work allows quieter students the opportunity to participate
As stated in the first paragraph, 'shy students who will not contribute to the full class can usually be coaxed into contributing to a group'.

10. The correct answer is D. Groups are easier to manage for the teacher
Although groups are smaller than teaching an entire class, care must be taken to ensure that individuals do not take over the group and others do not participate. As stated in the last paragraph 'difficulties with groups can be overcome by using well-defined tasks, good teaching methods and ensuring groups take responsibility for their work' implying that the teacher must put as much effort into group work as they would into a didactic session.
The other statements are defined in the passage as benefits of group work

11. The correct answer is C. Competition
Paragraph 3 mentions competition as something that is beneficial between groups. Feedback to other students, analysis of information and contributing to others' learning are described as benefits of group work and would all occur within the group.
12. The correct answer is C. Teacher allocation of tasks to individuals

Students should be allowed the opportunity to form the dynamics of their group themselves. The first paragraph states that 'Students can often do together what they could not achieve alone, with each member of the group providing part of the 'jigsaw' of understanding'. Paragraph 2 states "Good groupwork hands the responsibility over to the students."

13. The correct answer is B. False. Flowering plants are angiosperms. Flowers are their reproductive organs.

14. The correct answer is B. False. Gymnosperm do not have flowers - stamen are a flower part and are compared to the corresponding organs of gymnosperms.

15. The correct answer is A. True. Gymnosperms are "the only other seed-producing plant".

16. The correct answer is C. Can't tell. The text clearly compares male gametophytes in angiosperms and gymnosperms but does not define the size or relative size of female gymnosperm gametophytes.

17. The correct answer is C. The '74' was superseded after 1811 by newer designs
This is stated in the text towards the end of the second paragraph.
Option A is incorrect as the French were developing the 74 in the 1730s, the British surveyor Slade worked on a British competitor from 1747 onwards.
Option B is incorrect as the text describes how larger ships were used in the line, but were less useful for chasing or manoeuvring.
Option D is incorrect as HMS Indefatigable was a razeed ship and not a 74.

18. The correct answer is B. The best British ships before 1750 were the '70s'
This is stated early in the first paragraph.
Option A states exactly the opposite to the text in the first line.
Option C assumes that Sir Edward Pellew commanded a '74'. He may have done so but the text does not tell us so. HMS Indefatigable was a frigate.
Option D says that the Dublin class fell short of 50 metres but the text tells us, in the middle of the first paragraph, that it was 51 or 52 metres long

19. The correct answer is D. Some French ships were captured during the revolutionary wars from which the British '74s' were developed
Option D is a false statement. The ships were captured during the War of Austrian Succession not the Revolutionary wars. Options A and B are stated in the first paragraph. Option C is described in the final paragraph.

20. The correct answer is C. The '74s' were the popular design up to the end of the Napoleonic wars in 1815
Option C is a false statement. The last two lines of the first paragraph say that the Seppings method became more popular in 1811. No mention is made in the text of the Napoleonic wars or 1815.

21. The correct answer is B. False. 125 is divisible by 5 and 25 as well as 1 and itself.

22. The correct answer is C. Can't tell. The text does not give any biographical detail about Riemann, or even whether this is a personal name, rather than a place name.

23. The correct answer is A. True. 20 is an even natural number bigger than two that is the sum of two primes - 7 and 13.

24. The correct answer is A. True. The theorem says that the probability that a given, randomly chosen number n is prime is inversely proportional to its number of digits.

25. The correct answer is C. Give a dog a bad name and hang him

This idiom, like labelling theory is implied, is about how when someone is classified about something, however unjustified, it is hard for them to shake off that label. The other idioms are not appropriate - option A is about people with unjustified annoyance, option B is about the inability of someone to change their actual nature and option D is about the difference between someone's speech and their actions.

26. The correct answer is B. Feeling angry and defensive
All of the other options are mentioned within the text. The way in which people shift their behaviour and attitudes to fit the stereotype they are subject to is detailed. The frequency of depression is also referred to. The fact that people who have been placed in a stigmatised group lose their sense of wholeness and feel different and devalued is also mentioned.

27. The correct answer is A. Children are unaware of the subtleties of behaviour
The fact that children are aware of different groups and their relative status in society from a young age suggests many things. It certainly indicates that children are a lot more aware of subtle cues than we may assume.

28. The correct answer is B. Stigmatised people are shunned in public places
The text describes the places in which stigmatised people may be made to feel excluded or devalued - these places include many that are 'public' such as the workplace and educational settings. Option A is not accurate as the text includes 'invisible' factors such as culture and disease as potential triggers for stigma in modern usage. Option C likewise is not accurate as the text clearly describes some factors that need not be permanent (e.g. obesity) compared to the scarring suffered by the stigmatised in ancient Greece. Similarly, option D is inaccurate because it is so value laden. When describing modern stigma, the text is careful to stress that people may feel polluted or blemished but does not state that they actually are.

29. The correct answer is D. The present building was completed three years after the previous one was destroyed
This is shown in the text. Option A is incorrect as the English Decorated style is in the sanctuary and the Elizabethan in the school rather than the other way around as in the statement. Option B is incorrect because the text mentions a series of windows rather than just one. The construction of the building began in 1861 (weeks after the start of the civil war) but didn't burn down until 1925 (option C) and while the text does not preclude the possibility of the war lasting 65 years it seems unlikely.

30. The correct answer is C. The organ commemorates a former elder of the church
The organ is a memorial to James Sprunt who was a ruling elder in the church. Option A is incorrect as the stone is only placed 'at the bottom of the stairs', not necessarily in the foundations. Option B is incorrect because the building the Lectern Bible was stolen from was dated 1861. Option D is incorrect - the windows were created by Bonawits and don't commemorate him.

31. The correct answer is C. Designing this church established Hobart Upjohn as an architect
The text described Upjohn as a noted architect meaning he was already established. Option A is incorrect – the church was 'semi independent' from 1785 to 1817 which is than 32 years. Option B is true and thus incorrect. Similarly option D is stated in the text and therefore is incorrect.

32. The correct answer is B. The lectern Bible is one of many links to the history of the church displayed in the current building
The text states that there are few links. Option A is true - the site on Front Street had a church there from 1818 and the new, present, site was dedicated in 1861. Option C is likely to be true - we have the dates of the dedicated of the site in 1861 and the date the church burned down in 1925. The description of the windows and their features is in the text (option D).

33. The correct answer is C. Can't tell. Shoe polish may have become popular in the 19th century but its first use is not mentioned in the passage, although the passage states that polishes have been in use for "hundreds

of years" this could be 200 years making it first used in the 19th century or longer making it before the 19th century.

34. The correct answer is A. True. It is used to "polish, shine, waterproof, and restore the appearance of leather shoes or boots, thereby extending the footwear's life."

35. The correct answer is B. False. It is manufactured using "straightforward chemical engineering processes".

36. The correct answer is C. Can't tell. Waste products of manufacture are not detailed in the passage.

37. The correct answer is A. If more people avoided animal products in their diet then there would be less pressure on the environment
80% of US agricultural land is used for growing feed crops, not all crops. Option A is correct as the opening sentence states that people become vegetarian for environmental reasons and then the text describes how animal-based food is damaging the environment. Option C is incorrect because the contrast with animal-husbandry is made in the text saying that animal-based food in the developing world is much more sustainable - we can assume this is true from an energy input/output point of view because of the position of the sentence. Option D is true, and thus incorrect, because the whole text is about how unsustainable industrial agriculture is given the energy inefficiencies.

38. The correct answer is D. 25,000 kilo-calories inputted to produce 1,000 kilo-calories of food protein
The ratios mentioned regarding the production of food states that there is a range of ratios for 4:1 to 54:1 of inefficiencies based on energy input to protein output. Option A doesn't specify protein output over the more general energy. Option B is outside of the range described in terms of ratio. Option C is about fruit for which there is no efficiency information stated in the text.

39. The correct answer is Meat eating could be called 'carnism'
While this is in the text it is attributed to Melanie Joy, not Plumwood

40. The correct answer is D. Western culture places higher value on humans than animals
Although not stated explicitly this is clearly what is referred to in the final paragraph where descriptions of 'human-centeredness' are given. Option A is incorrect because 70% of the grain crop is consumed by animals raised for meat. The environmental impact of organic farming is described as 'less' than that of industrialised agriculture, not nothing at all. Rain based agriculture is described as an alternative method to industrialised agriculture so it is reasonable to assumed that it is not as reliant on the vagaries of weather.

41. The correct answer is D. Differences in political opinion
None of these qualities is specifically mentioned. However - height and intelligence could fall under the category of physical or intellectual (dis)ability. Religious background is mentioned to it is reasonable to assume that personal religious practice or conviction would be part of the political correctness remit. However - there is no specific mention of political opinion, the closest thing being 'ideological worldview' which is not synonymous.

42. The correct answer is C. To ensure that offence was not caused through careless language
'Political correctness' as described in the text as being an exercise in language and word change, not a drive to change opinions (option A). Similarly, it is unreasonable to conclude that changing the words used, in any sphere, would end prejudice and discrimination entirely and clearly this is a wider remit than that described in the text (option B). Option D also describes a wider scope and remit than that described in the text.

43. The correct answer is D. A physically disabled former policeman
Option D is not gender neutral. The term 'homosexual' is not defined as being politically incorrect or politically correct in the text but sexual orientation is so we can reasonable infer than there are politically acceptable

terms for people of homosexual orientation. However - the text is explicit in making general terms gender neutral.

44. The correct answer is B. Some left- and right-wing media countered it
The text describes how a 'culturally liberal television talk-show' and a 'culturally conservative book series' both were produced with 'Political Incorrectness' as their core theme. Options A and C are incorrect as both imply that the entirety of media outlets which lean left (or right) countered the movement when no such suggestion is made. There is no information about whether 'political incorrectness' as a backlash against 'political correctness' was found offensive.

1

A man earning £50,000 will pay more tax as a proportion of their total earnings than someone earning £40,000 A person earning £50,000 will pay tax on 39,000, whereas a person earning £40,000 will pay tax on £29,000. The tax rate will be the same but the proportion of non-taxable income is less for the lower earner.	**Yes**
Employed people usually have consistent income from a single source Most employed people don't have to fill in a tax return, tax returns are completed by people with inconsistent income or numerous sources of income	**Yes**
Unemployed people never have to fill in a tax return Unemployed does not mean 'without income'. There is no mention of the unemployed and their tax status in the text	**No**
All income tax payers earn more than £11,000 per annum The text only says that income tax must be paid by workers earning over this threshold. It does not say that everyone who pays income tax earns at this level from employment.	**No**
John earns £45,000 from his employment. He also owns some rental properties which earn him £10,000 profit per year. John has to pay higher rate income tax. John's income is over £50,000 (albeit from multiple sources). He is likely to have to fill in a tax return as well.	**Yes**

2.

There will be, on average, a significant health and safety infraction every fifty years 2% per annum equates to 1 in 50	**Yes**
A company who is fully compliant with health and safety rules will lose 7% of its value. The reduction in value described is for when profits drop by more than 10%	**No**
If a company is 50% compliant with the health and safety rules it will cost them 5% of their profits There is nothing to suggest the figures are linear	**No**
Company X was sued by an employee who was injured at work due to health and safety rules being ignored. The resulting fine was 10.5% of the profits for the year. Company X lost more than 5% in total share value that year. The loss of 7% value is something that is stated as 'will happen' if an infraction costing more than 10% of health and safety compliance rules are ignored.	**Yes**
A company that decides to risk not being compliant with health and safety rules is likely to make higher profits and retain share value than one which is fully compliant	**Yes**

The risk is only 2% per annum meaning that it is likely that any company ignoring the rules will get away with it and not risk profits or share value as a result.

3.

Amerdeep lives in Country D and has just returned from a trip to country B. It is likely that Amerdeep is an influential person of high rank. People from country D require a special visa to visit country B. This special visa is usually only given to high ranking officials.	**Yes**
Bilal has two visa stamps in his passport based on his travel between these four countries. He must be from country C. Residents of country A need no visas. Residents of country B only need a Visa to visit country C. Residents of country D only need a special visa to visit country B. Country C residents need a visa for every other country.	**Yes**
A group of friends who live in the four different countries wish to meet for a reunion holiday. The single best country for them to meet in to avoid complicated visa applications is country A. Country A requires one friend to get a visa (the one from country C). Country C requires one friend to get a visa (the one from country B). A is not the best option – it is the joint best.	**No**
There is a strained political relationship between countries B and D This seems to be implied but it is not a logical conclusion	**No**
Having no visa requirements for entry increases tourism to any country. Country A has the biggest tourism sector. Country C has the second largest. Passport holders of countries A and D can travel into country C without a visa.	**Yes**

4.

Only people younger than 50 played at the festival There could have been people over 50 performing in other capacities than in a band	**No**
Most of the performers were young We have no information about how many bands played (which were younger than 50) compared to other performers.	**No**
Every member of every performing band was under the age of 50	**Yes**
All the people under 50 performing at the festival were in a band	**No**
Any over 50s who performed at the festival were not part of a band	**Yes**

5. The correct answer is A. Jean isn't enjoying the foreign food
We know from the third point that Jean must be complaining about either the food or the staff rudeness. We know that she is married to Alan as we know she isn't married to James and the other two couples are given in the second and fourth points. We know from the first point that Alan does not like the food. The full table cannot be completed and whilst we know who is married to whom we cannot know for certain who is complaining about the bed and who is complaining about the heat.

6. The correct answer is B. H817 got the highest overall score

H817 scored best in both exams so must have got the highest score overall. The largest improvement between papers was H880b who improved their score by 16 points (compared to 14 for H800). The smallest improvement was for H817 who improved their score by 4 points (compared to 6 for EE194).

7. The correct answer is D. 4 fish.
Two chickens are worth 4 rabbits which are worth 32 beans each – 64 beans.
1 fish is worth 16 cocoa beans = 4 fish.

8. The correct answer is A. Redcurrants
We know all the fruit is in a row, but it can't be the central row as square 5 has a root vegetable. As square 2 in the top row contains a leafy vegetable, we know the three fruit crops must be grown is squares 7, 8 and 9.

9. The correct answer is B. The three furthest stars are mid-sized
The text shows that distance is denoted by points and size is denoted by size. The three four pointed stars (furthest away) are neither the largest or smallest on the picture.

10. The correct answer is C. No – lots of young people are now having tattoos so the old assumptions no longer apply
The increasing popularity of tattoos is stated in the text. Option A is the direct opposite and assumes that the reputation of tattoos will continue even when they are commonplace. Option B is true but vague. Option D does not address the proposition as no-one is suggesting an outright ban. Adults are cautioned away from things all the time.

11. The correct answer is D. No – there is no way that any consumer product can be declared completely safe so the suggestion is impractical.
Option A minimises the impact of the Smart Phone whilst maximising the potential impact. There is no mention of cancer or tumours in the statement. Option B makes an assumption which cannot be supported and creates the impossible aim of 'completely safe'. Option C correctly identifies issues of correlation and causation but doesn't address the proposition. Option D acknowledges that 'no danger' is impossible.

12. The correct answer is A. Yes – a motivated student will be able to learn everything necessary to get good grades
Option B assumes that fact recall and comprehension are the foundation of the exams. Option C makes an assumption about the importance of group work and discussion. Option D makes an assumption about the character of young people.

13. The correct answer is B. Yes – UK workers would probably enjoy an extra day for leisure and relaxation
Option A assumes some holiday competition which the UK should aim to win! Option C does the opposite and assumes that working more gives an advantage. Option D introduces the notion of meaning which is absent in the text. Option B mirrors the word 'enjoy' suggesting that it most accurate answers what was originally proposed.

14.

Chile spent fewer years in negative growth than South America as a whole There are four points where Chile goes below the zero-growth line and 6 where the continent as a whole is below it	**Yes**
The biggest year of change for South America was 1980 In 1980 the continent went from about 7% growth to -3% growth	**Yes**
Chile is one of the more volatile economies in South America We can't know this from this chart. There may be other more volatile countries	**No**

Another South American country must have had negative growth in 1988 **Yes**
As Chile was seeing growth and South America was on the zero line there must have been other countries experiencing negative growth to bring down the average

The overall trend for Chile, and the continent as a whole, is upward **No**
The chart is very chaotic with no clear trend

15. The strongest argument is option B. Yes – people should be able to access support to withdraw from the use of addictive substances
If someone seeks support they should be taken seriously and offered help. Option A makes everything a problem – all people are dependent on oxygen for example. Option B makes a false claim that all naturally occurring things must be good yet tobacco is also naturally occurring. Option D also offers a false claim but in the other direction.

16. The strongest argument is option D. No - Changing official recommendations based on the beliefs of some people is irresponsible and further research is needed first
This responds to the vague words such as 'some' and 'believe' in the original proposition. Option A takes the benefits of fruit and vegetables – and their ability to bring people to 'peak health' much further than the proposition suggests. Option B introduces and economic benefit which is not warranted. Option C assumes that people currently struggle to consume 5 portions a day.

17.

Petrol cars are better for the environment and health **No**
This text speaks of one environmental impact and one impact on health which is caused predominantly by diesel engines. There is no suggestion that petrol cars don't have any similar unique issues.

Modern diesel cars have less impact on the health of people than older ones **Yes**
Modern diesel cars are fitted with effective filters which stop almost all carcinogenic soot from escaping into the atmosphere

Inhaling NO2 is a primary cause of heart attacks and strokes **No**
The risk is increased but there is no information about how many heart attacks and strokes are caused as a direct result of NO2, nor of the proportion of heart attacks and strokes.

Diesel cars release a few different compounds and pollutants into the atmosphere **Yes**
The compounds mentioned – nitrogen oxides and dioxides – are both plural. Additional – the particulate matter can also be released by diesel engines.

The pollutants mentioned are the sole cause of multiple respiratory, cardiovascular and neurological complaints **No**
The study cited said it can cause – or exacerbate – a number of complaints. There is enough uncertainty and conditions in the text for a confident 'yes' to be illogical.

18. The best answer is B. Yes – plenty of very capable people don't get a place who could be excellent doctors
Option A introduces the idea of an ageing population and assumes that such a population will need more doctors. Option C makes a statement with no qualification or explanation. Option D suggests that health promotion would lead to a need for fewer doctors without explanation and also assumes that it's an either / or situation.

19. The correct answer is B. Fewer commuters exclusively cycle than use three modes of transport
A. Twice the number of commuters who only drive only walk 22 car only, 1 only walks. 44 walk and train
B. Correct – 15 cycle only, 18 use three modes of transport (walk, train and bus)
C. 2 modes is 68, 3 is 18. More than 3 times the number
D. Total who walk is 63, total who catch the bus is 38

20. The correct answer is B. Those saving for three things
A. Those saving for one thing only are 21 for driving lessons, 14 for concert tickets, 1 for trainers and 18 for a phone, a total of 54
B. There are two categories saving for three things with 27 and 18 in each, a total of 45
C. This category includes 13 for concert + driving, 23 for driving + phone and 15 for trainers and phone, a total of 51
D. This is category B and C together which is 96

21. The correct answer is C. The 103-year-old uses Olive oil
Age 101, Jasmine, Family
Age 103, Laurence, Olive oil
Age 105, Daniel, Laughter
Age 107, Daisy, Bubble bath
Age 109, Max, Tea

22. The correct answer is C.21
An individual sticker in the grid is worth two stadium stickers (worth two team photo stickers each) and a club badge (worth 3 steam photo stickers each). The grid is 3x3 so nine stickers are needed in total. This requires the equivalent of 63 team photo stickers. Pete only has club badges so will need 21 of these as each of them is worth three team photo stickers.

23. The correct answer is D. Shabnam's room is next to the living room.
Rooms G and D are occupied by Becky, Priyanka and Sanduni although we don't know which two share or who is in which room. We know the living room is either room E or F but don't know which one. We can deduce that Naomi sleeps in room A and the kitchen must be room C and therefore the bathroom is room B and Naomi sleeps next to the bathroom. We don't know, from this plan, where her door is so it may not be directly opposite room G. The only other flat mate must sleep in whichever of room E and F is NOT the living room. Either way Shabnam is next door to the living room.

24. The correct answer is D. The number of male doctors who are also homeowners (52) is equal to the number of female doctors who are also homeowners (37). False
The conference has more doctors (158) in total than teachers (146). True
Adult male homeowners (61) outnumber adult female doctors (17). True
There are 24 more female doctors who are also teachers and homeowners (38) than there are male doctors who are also teachers and homeowners (14). True

25. The correct answer is D. 6% more dust, wash dishes and do laundry every day than those who mop, dust and vacuum. False
The amount of people who only wash dishes and do laundry every day is 7% of the total amount of people who vacuum every day. True
16 more people do laundry (51) every day than vacuum (35). True
The number of people who vacuum and mop and wash dishes every day (5) is a third of the number of people who do laundry only (15). True

26. The correct answer is A. The Grey Car – as it is less reliable and the difference in the chance of an accident amounts to only 4 in 1000

Grey – 80% reliability. 2% x .85 = 1.7% accident
Black – 90% reliability. 2 x 2.05 = 2.1% accident

27. The correct answer is B. Most supermarket customers spend between £10 and £50.
As only 10% of customers, overall, buy a bottle of wine but 25% and 40% of over £50 and under £10 shoppers do respectively we can conclude that most shoppers – who bring the average down – must spend between these two amounts.
We only know that 40% of those spending less than £10 buy a bottle of wine. This may not equate to a large number

28. The correct answer is D. No, because males and females who drink coffee every day have an equal likelihood of overusing headache medication
A is incorrect as the study shows that 80% of those that overuse headache medication are female not that 80% of females overuse headache medication.
B is incorrect as the study shows that 80% of those that overuse headache medication are female not that 80% of females overuse headache medication.
C is incorrect as 300 out of 3000 is 10% not 3%.
D is correct as 10% of daily coffee drinkers (no gender specified) take more headache medications than recommended.

29. The correct answer is B. Yes, drivers of red cars are stopped 10 times more often than blue cars
A is incorrect as women are equally likely to drive a red car as a blue one
B is correct as 200 out of 20000 drivers of blue cars is 1%
C is incorrect as there are the same proportion of female drivers of both red and blue cars
D is incorrect as women are equally likely to drive a red car as a blue one - absolute numbers are not given

1. The correct answer is C. 15% - (7+2+4+1+6+5+2) = 27; (4/27) × 100 = 14.8 = 15%

2. The correct answer is D. 9.31% - 23 × 6 = £138; (138/ 1482.63) × 100 = 9.30778 = 9.31%

3. The correct answer is B. £88.96 - 1482.63 × 0.30 = 444.789; 444.789/5 = 88.9578 = £88.96 (to the nearest penny)

4. The correct answer is E. 4.6% =- 238.97/(238.97 +1482.63) = (238.97/1721.63) × 100 = 13.8805; 13.8805/3 = 4.6268 = 4.6%

5. The correct answer is C. 367g - To make 300g of pastry you need 110g of butter. 1 kg is 1000g. To make 1000g of pastry, you need 1000/300 x 110g of butter = 366.67g of butter

6. The correct answer is D. 750g - To make 300g of pastry you use 200g of flour. If you have 500g of flour, 500/200 x 300 = 750g of pastry could be made.

7. The correct answer is B. 275g - Each pie needs 250g of pastry. Therefore 3 pies require 750g of pastry. To make 750g pastry, you will need 750/300*110=275g

8. The correct answer is C. 5 - 4 pies per day for 7 days = 28 pies. 28 pies x 250g pastry = 7000g of pastry. 7000/300 x 200 = 4666.67g of flour = 4.67kg of flour. As flour is sold in 1kg bags, 5 would need to be bought.

9. The correct answer is D. 20 - First quarter = first three months; 5 + 6 + 9 = 20

10. The correct answer is A. February to March and September to October - The biggest monthly changes are from 6 to 9 (change of 3) in February to March and 8 to 5 (change of 3) in September to October

11. The correct answer is B. 28% - (9+7+6) = 22; (5+6+9+8+9+9+7+6+8+5+4+2) = 78; (22/78) × 100 = 28.205 = 28%

12. The correct answer is B. 6.5% - (5+6+9+8+9+9+7+6+8+5+4+2)/12 = 78/12 = 6.5

13. The correct answer is B. 26% - Total students = (3+24+38+17+4+6) = 92; (24/92)×100 = 26.087 = 26%

14. The correct answer is C. 93% - Total students = (3+24+38+17+4+6) = 92; 92 - 6 = 86; (86/92) × 100 = 93.478 = 93 %

15. The correct answer is B. 15% - 38 × 0.40 = 15.2 = 15

16. The correct answer is E. 41 - 17 × 0.16 = 2.72 = 3; 38 + 2.72 = 40.72 = 41

17. The correct answer is A. 45 - Total profit each week is £2,000. Dividing the total shelving by 2,000 and multiplying by the profit on pre-packed foods (602) is 45 (Option A)

18. The correct answer is D. 30 - There is now 70 metres to be proportioned over £1504 of profitability. 70/1504*645=30

19. The correct answer is B. 2442 - In the initial figures the other categories produced a weekly gross profit of £1,450. That is now reduced by 5% to £1,376. Add the profit on Fruit & Veg of £1,066 to show total profit earned of £2,442.

20. The correct answer is E. Cards, gifts and trinkets - £20,000 / 52 is £385. No other category displays closer to this figure as a weekly profit figure in either the initial or revised figures.

21. The correct answer is B. 151 - 182 × 0.83 = 151.06 = 151

22. The correct answer is A. 6.3g - 5% more salt than the RDA; The RDA = 6g; 6 × 1.05 = 6.3g

23. The correct answer is B. 0.89g - Weight per tub = 3100/7 = 442.85; Salt content is 0.2% = 442.857 × 0.002 = 0.8857 = 0.89 g

24. The correct answer is B. 114 - 48/6 = 8 = 8 times the RDA of salt: 6% of microwave meals contained more than 8 times the RDA of salt; 42/7 = 7 times the RDA of salt: 82% of microwave meals contain more than 7 times the RDA of salt. The study is looking at between 7 and 8 times the RDA of salt: 82% - 6% = 76%; 150 × 0.76 = 114 meals

25. The correct answer is B. 7 - Range = largest value - smallest value = 8 -1 = 7 months

26. The correct answer is D. 5 - Mean =average = (8+6+3+4+4+6+6+8+2+3+1)/11 = 51/11 = 4.6 months = 5 months

27. The correct answer is E. 6 - Mode = most occurring = 6

28. The correct answer is D. 4 - Median = central value of ordered values: 1,2,3,3,4,4,6,6,6,8,8: 4

29. The correct answer is: D. 39.12 cm - (23.47/3) × 5 = 39.1166 = 39.12 cm

30. The correct answer is: A. 2.77 kg - Weight(kg) is 6/13 of Volume (m^3). (6/13) × 6 = 2.769 = 2.77 kg

31. The correct answer is: B. 202.17g - Per tank: (310/4.6) × 1.5 = 101.08696; for both tanks = 101.08696 × 2 = 202.17 g

32. The correct answer is: D. 165:2 - Density: depth = 495:6 = 165:2

33. The correct answer is: C. £630.27 - GIC = 12% Gross so GIC = £949.44 × 0.12 or GIC = 113.9328
Net = Gross Salary - Student loan - GIC – Tax. Net = £949.44 - £22 - £113.93 - £183.24. Net = £630.26727 or £630.27

34. The correct answer is: E. £912.92 - Basic + 4% Basic = Gross. Gross = 104% Basic. Gross = 949.44/1.04 = 912.92

35. The correct answer is: D. £1.00 - Gross salary per hour = £949.44/184 = £5.16; Hourly tax = £5.16 × 19.3% = £5.16 x 0.193; Hourly tax = 0.99588 or £1.00 to the nearest penny

36. The correct answer is: E. £644.94 - New gross salary = £949.44 × 1.03 = £977.92; New GIC = £977.92 × 0.12 = £117.35; New Tax amount = £977.92 × (0.193 + 0.005) = £977.92 × 0.198 = £193.63; Student Loan contribution remains unchanged as it is charged per complete £600 of gross salary so New Net = Gross Salary - Student loan - GIC -Tax. New Net = £977.92 - £22 - £117.35 - £193.63 = £644.94.

Question Set 1 (questions 1 – 5)
Set A contains one black shape that is placed inside a white shape. Set B contains one white shape that is placed inside a black shape. All other shapes are irrelevant.

1. Set B
2. Set A
3. Set A
4. Neither
5. Neither

Question Set 2 (questions 6 – 10)
Set A always contains a 4-pointed star in the top right-hand corner. There is always at least one 4, 5 and 6-pointed star. Set B always contains a 4-pointed star in the centre. There is always at least one 4, 5 and 6-pointed star.

6. Set A
7. Set B
8. Neither
9. Neither
10. Set A

Question Set 3 (questions 11 – 15)
Set A always contains one object made up of two of the same shapes (one inside the other).
Set B always contains two objects, each made up of two shapes that are different to each other (one inside the other). The colours of the shapes are irrelevant.

11. Set A
12. Set B
13. Neither
14. Neither
15. Set B

Question Set 4 (questions 16 – 20)
Set A always contains three lines in contact with each other. There is also always at least one vertical and one horizontal line that are not in contact with any others. Set B always contains four lines in contact with each other. There is also always at least one vertical and one horizontal line that are not in contact with any others.

16. Set A
17. Neither
18. Set B
19. Neither
20. Neither

Question Set 5 (questions 21 – 25)
Set A contains one black square and at least one triangle of any colour. Set B contains one black circle and at least one white square.

21. Set A
22. Set B
23. Set A
24. Set B
25. Neither

Question Set 6 (questions 26 – 30)
Set A always contains a pair of identical and parallel straight lines. The squiggle shape is irrelevant
Set B always contains a pair of identical and parallel crescent shapes curved lines. The squiggle shape is irrelevant

26. Neither
27. Set B
28. Neither
29. Set A
30. Neither

31. The correct answer is: D
Explanation: The number of sides in the outer shape is equal to the sum of the number of sides in the inner shapes. There is always two small shapes inside a medium sized shape.

32. The correct answer is: D
Explanation: The number of sides in the outer shape is equal to the sum of the number of sides in the inner shapes. There is always two small shapes inside a medium sized shape.

33. The correct answer is: A
Explanation: The outer shape rotates 90 degrees clockwise. The inner shapes remain in place. The colours swap.

34. The correct answer is: B
Explanation: Shapes 1 and 3, and 2 and 4; swap effect. The small inserted shape remains in place. The stripe effect is perpendicular in the 2nd picture. The overlaps of shapes change so shape 2 is fully visible rather than shape 4.

35. The correct answer is C
The two shapes which are grey in the first picture rotate 180 degrees and change to white. The white shapes become black and the black shapes become grey.

Question Set 7 (questions 36 – 40)
In Set A there is always one shape enclosed within another. The inner shape has fewer edges than the outer shape. In Set B there is always a shape enclosed within another – the inner shape has more edges than the outer shape.

36. B
37. C
38. A
39. C
40. D

Question Set 8 (questions 41 – 45)
Set A always contains an oval inside another shape. Set B always contains a triangle inside another shape. The colours of the shapes are irrelevant.

41. Set B
42. Set A
43. Neither
44. Neither
45. Set A

Question Set 9 (questions 46 – 50)
Set A contains a set of exactly three identical circles. Set B always contains a set of exactly four identical circles.

46. Set A
47. Set B
48. Neither
49. Set A
50. Set A

Question Set 10 (questions 51-55)
Set A – there are two dots for each complete set of three triangles. Set B – there is one dot for each complete set of four triangles

51. Neither
52. Set B
53. Set B
54. Neither
55. Set A

1. The correct answer is C. Inappropriate but not awful – 2 marks (1 mark for B. Appropriate but not ideal or D. A very inappropriate thing to do) - Overriding the instruction of a senior is generally inappropriate but where there is a legitimate concern for patient safety then this would at least buy some time for the situation to be checked and changes made if necessary

2. The correct answer is C. Inappropriate but not awful – 2 marks (1 mark for B. Appropriate but not ideal or D. A very inappropriate thing to do) - As a medical student this is somewhat out of Sasha's remit however she may be able to get some useful information as she's specifically investigating one thing. This may be useful later when the situation is looked at.

3. The correct answer is A. A very appropriate thing to do – 2 marks (1 mark for B. Appropriate but not ideal) - The nurse is likely to be experienced within the ward and will also know the right channels to go through if an error has been made.

4. The correct answer is D. A very inappropriate thing to do – 2 marks (1 mark for C. Inappropriate but not awful) - Whilst this deals with the initial problem it is at the expense of the doctor patient relationship and trust. It is possible that the mistake is not a mistake but actually a factor Sasha isn't aware of. Questioning a senior is one thing, encouraging a patient to do likewise is worse.

5. The correct answer is A. A very appropriate thing to do – 2 marks (1 mark for B. Appropriate but not ideal) - This allows the patient to tell their story and, assuming nothing untoward has occurred, allows Dr Williams to explain the delay and defend the nurse. If there has been anything of concern to report then this will also come to light.

6. The correct answer is B. Appropriate but not ideal – 2 marks (1 mark for A. A very appropriate thing to do or C. Inappropriate but not awful) - Whilst this seems unfair on the nurse, who may not have done anything wrong, it may make for a better doctor / patient consultation.

7. The correct answer is C. Inappropriate but not awful – 2 marks (1 mark for B. Appropriate but not ideal or D. A very inappropriate thing to do) - This would make the patient feel like his concerns were being dismissed. Checking in with the nurse is wise but when done later the nurse may not report everything honestly if there has been anything poor about her conduct.

8. The correct answer is D. A very inappropriate thing to do – 2 marks (1 mark for C. Inappropriate but not awful) - This not only puts the nurse on the spot but also dismisses the patient's narrative as being less valuable that the nurses – in front of the patient.

9. The correct answer is C. Inappropriate but not awful – 2 marks (1 mark for B. Appropriate but not ideal or D. A very inappropriate thing to do) - Emily might find this doctor consistently criticises people, or otherwise. It might give her some peace of mind, but might make her feel worse if other students feel their marks are fair.

10. The correct answer is A. A very appropriate thing to do – 2 marks (1 mark for B. Appropriate but not ideal) - Hard as it is - it is a good discipline to always try and turn criticism into action to improve.

11. The correct answer is A. A very appropriate thing to do – 2 marks (1 mark for B. Appropriate but not ideal) - The doctor may be able to point to specific areas for Emily to work on. If he is being unfair then he won't be able to and Emily can move on.

12. The correct answer is D. A very inappropriate thing to do – 2 marks (1 mark for C. Inappropriate but not awful) - The surgery is described as urgent and simply asking for a postponement may compromise patient safety. It also seems to be a way for Kayla to avoid admitting to her error.

13. The correct answer is A. A very appropriate thing to do – 2 marks (1 mark for B. Appropriate but not ideal) - This is the most honest approach. It's possible that things can be sped up or that the test isn't as vital as Kayla thinks. Either way – this shows the most integrity and gets the whole team working on solving the problem.

14. The correct answer is D. A very inappropriate thing to do – 2 marks (1 mark for C. Inappropriate but not awful) - As the error was Kayla's it is not fair to ask a patient to make a clinical decision about an urgent surgery

15. The correct answer is A. A very appropriate thing to do – 2 marks (1 mark for B. Appropriate but not ideal) - This shows some initiative and could solve the problem but it still appears like Kayla is trying to avoid her mistake being found out.

16. The correct answer is C. Inappropriate but not awful – 2 marks (1 mark for B. Appropriate but not ideal or D. A very inappropriate thing to do) - Asking someone to apologise is unlikely to result in a genuine apology – or at least one which is taken as genuine. It might alert Leo to how his comments were taken though.

17. The correct answer is C. Inappropriate but not awful – 2 marks (1 mark for B. Appropriate but not ideal or D. A very inappropriate thing to do) - You can't really apologise on someone else's behalf. It does acknowledge the upset though which is good.

18. The correct answer is A. A very appropriate thing to do – 2 marks (1 mark for B. Appropriate but not ideal) - It's right to challenge rudeness in a discreet manner.

19. The correct answer is B. Appropriate but not ideal – 2 marks (1 mark for A. A very appropriate thing to do or C. Inappropriate but not awful) - This seems like real overkill as a formal complaint by Leo seems unwarranted. It would shut down the conversation though and maybe make Leo realise if he was being unreasonable.

20. The correct answer is C. Inappropriate but not awful – 2 marks (1 mark for B. Appropriate but not ideal or D. A very inappropriate thing to do) - This is quite a presumptuous course of action and Gabriella may well be justified if she feels she doesn't want to help.
21. The correct answer is B. Appropriate but not ideal – 2 marks (1 mark for A. A very appropriate thing to do or C. Inappropriate but not awful) - This is a respectful course of action to Gabriella but it is usually better to ask politely for what you need rather than hoping someone else will offer it.

22. The correct answer is A. A very appropriate thing to do – 2 marks (1 mark for B. Appropriate but not ideal) - This shows sensitivity to Gabriella's potential concerns about sharing her work. By laying it out on the table it enables a frank discussion and may make Gabriella's more inclined to help.

23. The correct answer is D. A very inappropriate thing to do – 2 marks (1 mark for C. Inappropriate but not awful) - There are rules governing treating your own friends and family for doctors. This would be frowned upon as an ear infection could not be described as a dire emergency.

24. The correct answer is A. A very appropriate thing to do – 2 marks (1 mark for B. Appropriate but not ideal) - This is likely to be the quickest way for his sister to get the medication she needs without breaking any rules.

25. The correct answer is B. Appropriate but not ideal – 2 marks (1 mark for A. A very appropriate thing to do or C.
Inappropriate but not awful) - Whilst not breaking any rules this course of action is unhelpful.

26. The correct answer is C. Inappropriate but not awful – 2 marks (1 mark for B. Appropriate but not ideal or D. A very inappropriate thing to do) - This is bending rather than breaking rules but it still inconveniences his colleague and also doesn't follow the proper channels to ensure safety.

27. The correct answer is D. A very inappropriate thing to do – 2 marks (1 mark for C. Inappropriate but not awful) - This sounds friendly but Bethany is disturbing the consultation. There is no mention of her explaining the situation or asking for permission to observe the consultation so nothing is achieved by this action at all.

28. The correct answer is A. A very appropriate thing to do – 2 marks (1 mark for B. Appropriate but not ideal) - Bethany may feel awkward about this but it is the best option. The GP may simply have forgotten or may know there is another system in place to ensure consent is given.

29. The correct answer is D. A very inappropriate thing to do – 2 marks (1 mark for C. Inappropriate but not awful) - As a medical student, it is important Bethany learns to ask difficult questions when required and takes responsibility for things - even things which aren't technically her responsibility.

30. The correct answer is B. Appropriate but not ideal – 2 marks (1 mark for A. A very appropriate thing to do or C. Inappropriate but not awful) - This is adding to the workload of the receptionists which Bethany doesn't really have any warrant to do. Far better to raise the issue with the practice manager or the GP himself.

31. The correct answer is C. Inappropriate but not awful – 2 marks (1 mark for B. Appropriate but not ideal or D. A very inappropriate thing to do) - Jamie really ought to see the correct Mr Smith if possible and follow the correct appointment order.

32. The correct answer is A. A very appropriate thing to do – 2 marks (1 mark for B. Appropriate but not ideal) - It is appropriate to apologise but also important to follow the appointment sheet where possible.

33. The correct answer is A. A very appropriate thing to do – 2 marks (1 mark for B. Appropriate but not ideal) - This may seem cumbersome but it's better than repeating this awkward situation.

34. The correct answer is C. Inappropriate but not awful – 2 marks (1 mark for B. Appropriate but not ideal or D. A very inappropriate thing to do) - An apology to the diabetic Mr Smith is appropriate but it is unnecessarily specific to apologise for a breach in confidentiality. This is likely to raise more questions and concerns than the apology can answer.

35. The correct answer is C. Inappropriate but not awful – 2 marks (1 mark for B. Appropriate but not ideal or D. A very inappropriate thing to do) - An apology is appropriate, and she probably should have gone to her GP, but Kristina doesn't know the details. Possibly this woman has not got a GP or is in a lot of pain and couldn't get an appointment for many days.

36. The correct answer is D. A very inappropriate thing to do – 2 marks (1 mark for C. Inappropriate but not awful) - It is not unreasonable for a patient to be angry after a six hour wait whilst in pain. There is no suggestion that the anger is aggressive or that there is any threat. This course of action is excessive and likely to cause more harm than it cures.

37. The correct answer is B. Appropriate but not ideal – 2 marks (1 mark for A. A very appropriate thing to do or C. Inappropriate but not awful) - This is factual but lacks any compassion

38. The correct answer is A. A very appropriate thing to do – 2 marks (1 mark for B. Appropriate but not ideal) - An apology is appropriate even though the reasons are justifiable. Kristina does not need to explain the situation but should provide the care she would usually provide.

39. The correct answer is A. A very appropriate thing to do – 2 marks (1 mark for B. Appropriate but not ideal) - This could be complex and problematic, or it might not be. Getting advice from people who know, or who know people who know, is a good choice.

40. The correct answer is C. Inappropriate but not awful – 2 marks (1 mark for B. Appropriate but not ideal or D. A very inappropriate thing to do) - This would be an option but if Melvin enjoys writing the blog and other people enjoy reading it then it would be premature to remove it without having to.

41. The correct answer is B. Appropriate but not ideal – 2 marks (1 mark for A. A very appropriate thing to do or C. Inappropriate but not awful) - In other circumstances this would be entirely appropriate but as Melvin is already nervous that his blog content may cause problems with the university it would be less than ideal to try and monetize his blog before sorting out this concern.

42. The correct answer is B. Appropriate but not ideal – 2 marks (1 mark for A. A very appropriate thing to do or C. Inappropriate but not awful) - Whilst wanting to show off your accomplishments in a personal statement, trying to make them sound 'more impressive' could class as exaggeration. On the other hand - good word choices and writing can emphasise good achievements.

43. The correct answer is C. Inappropriate but not awful – 2 marks (1 mark for B. Appropriate but not ideal or D. A very inappropriate thing to do) - This embellishment replies on the ambiguity of the word 'regularly' so isn't strictly dishonest. However - it is a slippery slope and other small embellishments may not be as easy to justify.

44. The correct answer is D. A very inappropriate thing to do – 2 marks (1 mark for C. Inappropriate but not awful) - This would be very unfair of George as Dean clearly would not have shown him his PS if he thought this would happen. This course of action has no benefits to anyone.

45. The correct answer is A. A very appropriate thing to do – 2 marks (1 mark for B. Appropriate but not ideal) - The best way to write a great personal statement is to get advice from the real experts.

46. The correct answer is D. A very inappropriate thing to do – 2 marks (1 mark for C. Inappropriate but not awful) - Although personal relationships should not interfere with someone's work, it is important to ensure that there is no conflict of interest between the patient and the people who are treating the patient. Hence, Adam should at least inform the consultant about the relationship who can then decide whether there would be a problem with Adam attending the consultation.

47. The correct answer is A. A very appropriate thing to do – 2 marks (1 mark for B. Appropriate but not ideal) - This is a very good course of action as it would ensure that the person-in-charge of the patient's treatment is notified of any potential conflict of interest between Adam and the patient.

48. The correct answer is C. Inappropriate but not awful – 2 marks (1 mark for B. Appropriate but not ideal or D. A very inappropriate thing to do) - This course of action would ensure that the patient is informed of Adam's relationship with him. However, the consultant should be notified before the patient of the relationship to avoid placing the patient in an awkward or stressful position.

49. The correct answer is D. Not important at all – 2 marks (1 mark for C. Of minor importance) - If plagiarism is suspected in someone's work, their ranking in the year is of no relevance. There should not be any special treatment given to anyone, regardless of their rank or social status, when it comes to academic or clinical malpractice.

50. The correct answer is A. Very important – 2 marks (1 mark for B. Important) - It is in Jack's best interest to ensure that the coursework is of good quality and it is an original work. The consequences of plagiarism can be quite severe and if Jack is affected as a result of Sarah's contribution, he can also suffer the penalty for not doing anything to stop the plagiarism even though he suspected it.

51. The correct answer is D. Not important at all – 2 marks (1 mark for C. Of minor importance) - The reputability of a journal is not essential as plagiarism is wrong regardless of the source. Moreover, all written work is cross-checked against a very large database comprising of every paper published and available online and against all other student submissions from most institutions

52. The correct answer is C. Of minor importance – 2 marks (1 mark for B. Important or D. Not important at all) - This might play on Jack's mind while dealing with this issue, but it is essential for him to keep in mind that the outcome of this coursework would affect both of them. And, therefore he should tackle this issue as quickly and prudently as possible.

53. The correct answer is B. Important – 2 marks (1 mark for A. Very important or C. Of minor importance) - This is an essential possible consequence to keep in mind. As the work has not been submitted yet, Jack should talk to Sarah and explain the situation to her. It could be that she unintentionally plagiarized her work so she should be given another chance to change it and make it original. All possible solutions should be explored before any 'official measure' needs to be taken.

54. The correct answer is A. Very important – 2 marks (1 mark for B. Important) - The patient's confidentiality is of utmost importance. It should not be violated unless another person's life is at risk because of the patient. Patients should not be discussed in public, especially on social media where anyone could potentially access the information.

55. The correct answer is C. Of minor importance – 2 marks (1 mark for B. Important or D. Not important at all) - Although the closed Facebook group might limit the number of people who will read about the patient, the information would still be seen by some people and there is no control over how it will be used. Sensitive information should not be shared, especially on public networks where it could be accessed by potentially anyone.

56. The correct answer is D. Not important at all – 2 marks (1 mark for C. Of minor importance) - Once patient confidentiality is breached, the manner in which the patient is discussed is not important as the patient information has been already been shared. Many improper disclosures are unintentional and not made in a negative manner but can still affect the patient significantly as details of their personal life are now available for other people to see and use.

57. The correct answer is B. Important – 2 marks (1 mark for A. Very important or C. Of minor importance) - If Jessica does report the post to the medical school, her flat mate could get into trouble and Jessica might feel awkward or guilty about it. However, Jessica can use this situation to her advantage by explaining to her flat mate the consequences of the post in a calm manner and suggesting to her to remove the post. This would resolve the problem easily and not affect Jessica's personal life.

58. The correct answer is D. Not important at all – 2 marks (1 mark for C. Of minor importance) - The patient's health is not an important factor when it comes to breach of patient confidentiality. Whether it is a healthy patient or a patient with severe mental health problems, a patient's confidentiality should never be breached in public and definitely not on social media.

59. The correct answer is A. Very important – 2 marks (1 mark for B. Important) - It is vital that Tamil has written consent for each child to take part in this activity. This is both a legal and moral consideration. Tamil really shouldn't take the two children without consent.

60. The correct answer is D. Not important at all – 2 marks (1 mark for C. Of minor importance) - The issue of consent is not to do with the danger levels of the activity.

61. The correct answer is D. Not important at all – 2 marks (1 mark for C. Of minor importance) - Consent is important
whether the children are going sky diving or to a museum

62. The correct answer is C. Of minor importance – 2 marks (1 mark for B. Important or D. Not important at all) - Knowing how disappointed children may be could spur Tamil on to ensure consent forms are returned.

63. The correct answer is A. Very important – 2 marks (1 mark for B. Important) - This is an accidental disclosure of several points of information. The key word is accident - something which can happen to anyone.

64. The correct answer is B. Important – 2 marks (1 mark for A. Very important or B. Of minor importance) - Vivien should take steps to let the teacher know their mistake and assure her than she will be discreet

65. The correct answer is A. Very important – 2 marks (1 mark for B. Important) - Professional behaviour is not always legislated for but is always appropriate

66. The correct answer is D. Not important at all – 2 marks (1 mark for C. Of minor importance) - Vivien should act as before – as if she has no knowledge of the situation

67. The correct answer is C. Of minor importance – 2 marks (1 mark for B. Important or D. Not important at all) - If the speaker has come on the stage declaring a medical emergency, it suggests the situation is urgent. Whether someone is qualified or not is of minor importance, Louisa should respond quickly and offer as much help as she can.

68. The correct answer is C. Of minor importance – 2 marks (1 mark for B. Important or D. Not important at all) - Although Louisa is not fully qualified and she may not be able to resolve the emergency fully, however she can still offer assistance and her training so far will mean that she can deal effectively with a medical emergency.

69. The correct answer is D. Not important at all – 2 marks (1 mark for C. Of minor importance) - If there is a circumstance where Louisa can offer critical help then there is a moral obligation to do so even if there is not social pressure.

Prepare and you WILL succeed!

Congratulations on completing the UCAT Success Toolkit – we hope it has been a useful part of your preparation. The whole Emedica team wishes you every success with your UCAT, your UCAS application and in your medical or dental career. Please do keep in touch and share your success with us!

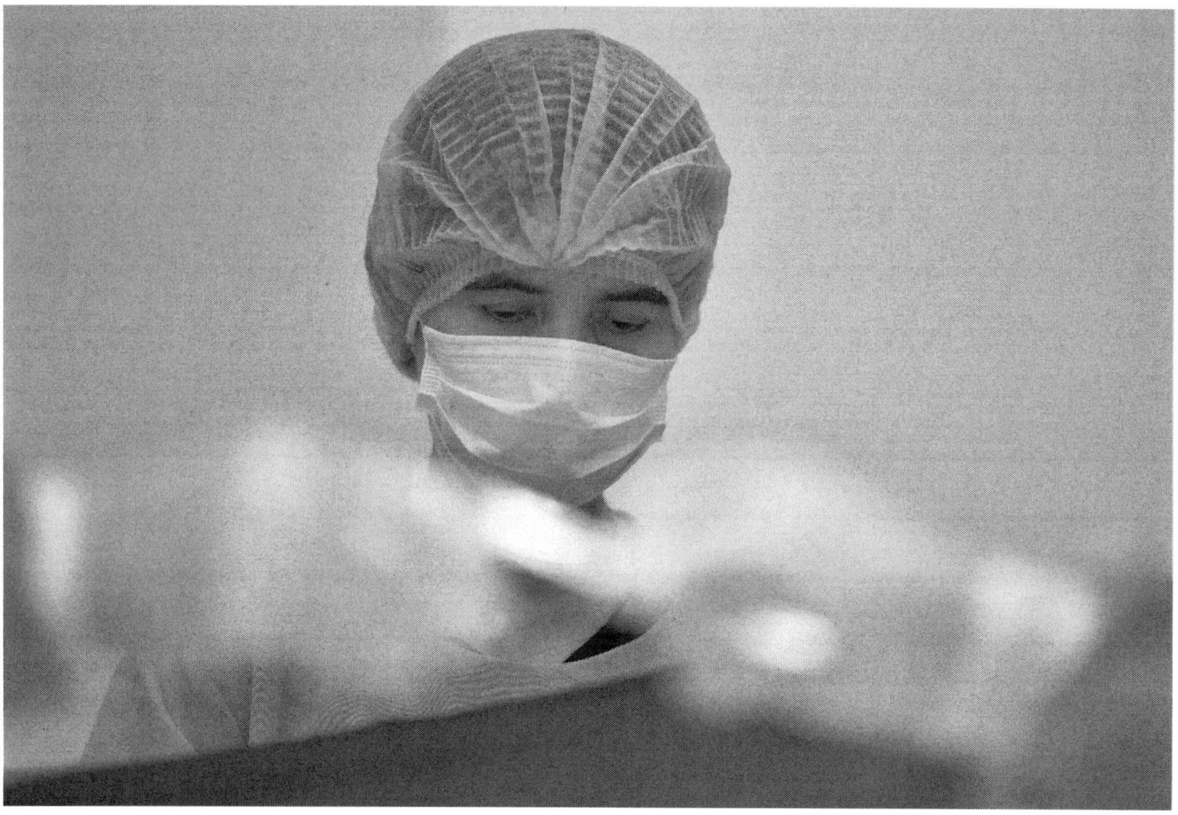